Diabetes
Its Medical and Cultural History

Outlines – Texts – Bibliography

Edited by Dietrich von Engelhardt

With 50 Figures

Springer-Verlag
Berlin Heidelberg New York
London Paris Tokyo Hong Kong

Prof. Dr. phil. Dietrich von Engelhardt
Institut für Medizin-
und Wissenschaftsgeschichte
Medizinische Universität zu Lübeck
Ratzeburger Allee 160
2400 Lübeck

Coverillustration: Ductus Pancreaticus, Engraving from a drawing by Johann Georg Wirsung (1600–1643), 17th century

ISBN-13: 978-3-642-48366-0 **e-ISBN-13: 978-3-642-48364-6**
DOI: 10.1007/978-3-642-48364-6

Softcover reprint of the hardcover 1st edition 1989

2127/3140/543210 – Printed on acid-free paper

Preface

"Diabetes is a puzzling disease. It is not very common and consists of a liquefaction of the flesh and limbs into urine." This is the first sentence of the classical treatise on diabetes by Aretaios in the first century A. D. While we may concur with the first part of this sentence, the second part of course no longer applies to the 1 1/2 to 2 million diabetics in the Federal Republic.

The strength and impotence of medical progress are impressively shown in diabetes. Reports of this disease and the search for therapeutic aid go back to antiquity; empirical knowledge increased extensively, the affliction was significantly reduced. Yet so far no medical advance had been able to overcome this disease.

It is profitable to direct one's gaze, again and again, back into the past. The decisive aspects of the historical development are the terminology and phenomenology of the disease, its etiology and treatment. But diabetes also always implies that the patient is a person, with speech, awareness and social relationships. Medicine is both science and art; disease fundamentally portrays a physical, psychical, social and intellectual phenomenon.

The present volume, after a brief sketch of the historical development of diabetes, contains, on the one hand, a series of important studies in the history of science as a guide to the aspects mentioned; on the other hand, it combines in a bibliography the important titles of the primary sources and the secondary literature. The references have not been revised and thus have been printed as they appeared in the original publication; the original illustrations have not been reproduced. Indexes of persons and subjects will facilitate orientation and aid further study. In general, it is to be hoped that this book may provide a clear overview as a stimulus to further individual research.

Many thanks are due to Bayer AG (Leverkusen), especially Drs. K.J. Preuß and U. Höhner, for supporting this publication. I am also grateful to the Springer company and Mrs. H. Hensler-Fritton for their competent and helpful assistance in publishing the book.

Lübeck, Autumn 1989

Contents

Antiquity

India and China

Renaissance – 19th Century

Historical Outlines

Outlines of Historical Development

a) Antiquity

As far back as Egyptian times there was mention of a disease with excessive urinary output and specific plans for treatment were advanced (Ebers papyrus, 1500 BC). The name 'diabetes' is attributable to Demetrios of Apamaia (2nd century BC) and is derived from the Greek word *diabeinein*, to go to excess, used as a substantive at that time as a circle and double siphon for the passage of fluid. Other terms of antiquity were urinary diarrhea, the thirst disease and dropsy of the chamber-pot *(hydrops ad matulam)*. The verbal distinction between diabetes inspidus and diabetes mellitus was first made in the 18th century (William Cullen and Johann Peter Frank) as well as numerous other terms for further varieties. In 1874, Adolf Kussmaul (1822–1902) used the expression *'coma diabeticum'* for the 'characteristic type of death in diabetics'. Etienne Lancereaux (1829–1910) distinguished a *diabète gras* and a *diabète maigre*, which called for different forms of treatment. The word 'insulin' was coined in 1909 by the Belgian, Jean de Meyer (1878–1934) for the hypothetical pancreatic hormone; later, Frederick Grant Banting (1891–1941) and Charles Herbert Best (1899–1978) adopted this term after having themselves initially proposed the word 'isletin'.

Aretaios (81–138 AD) gives the first exhaustive description of the symptoms, using the name diabetes: intolerable thirst, burning in the intestines, passage of large amounts of urine, and the two stages: chronic and acutely fatal. According to him, the causes of this disease were either an acute illness or a stomach disorder with poisoning of the kidneys and bladder. As treatment, Aretaios suggested purgation, a mild diet and steam baths. Of course, like all the other physicians of antiquity and the Middle Ages, Aretaios failed to observe the sweetness of diabetic urine. Galen (129–199 AD), the great authority of antiquity, considered that diabetes was not a disease of the stomach, but of the kidneys; like diarrhea, it consisted of an unaltered excretion of fluids. For Galen, treatment consisted of overcoming the acidity of the humors, slowing the movement of the blood and cooling the overheated kidneys.

b) Middle Ages

The Arab physicians of the Middle Ages continued in the old traditions and became engrossed in the theoretic and therapeutic knowledge handed down. They, too, were unaware of the sweet taste of diabetic urine. The cardinal symptoms were polyuria, polydipsia and subsequent physical wasting. Rhazes (850–930) warned against energetic physical exertion, also sexual intercourse *(concubitus mulierum)*. Avicenna (980–1037) adhered to the Galenic connection with the kidneys. Abs al-Laṭīf al-Baġdādī (1162–1231) published a specific treatise on diabetes (1225) which contains a wide range of treatment and an exhaustive discussion of the transmitted literature. The Byzantine physician, Actuarius (13th century) treated diabetes with rosewater. In the Latin Middle Ages little attention was paid to diabetes.

c) Modern Era

The modern era was marked by serious empiric research, theoretic interpretations and therapeutic proposals. An abundance of monographs and articles appeared in the 17th, 18th and 19th centuries dealing with diabetes, not just in recent times.

Paracelsus (1493–1541) discarded the traditional connection with the kidneys, as with the stomach, and brought biochemical principles to bear. For him, diabetes was a systemic disease, a corruption of the humors as the result of a disordered combination of sulfur and salts in the blood, overflowing into the kidneys, which became inflamed, and causing excessive urinary excretion: "Diabetes is nothing other than an excessive eagerness to pass urine, and the cause of this malady is excessive heat of the kidneys." Steam-baths should prevent this dangerous salt formation. Paracelsus certainly discusses sweetness of the urine in general terms, but not in connection with diabetes. Helmont, Sylvius and others followed the biochemical approach of Paracelsus.

It was in this chemiatric tradition that, in 1674, Thomas Willis (1621–1675) discovered the sweetness of the urine in diabetics – *"quasi melle aut saccharo inbuta"*; for the first time we have the decorative adjunct 'mellitus'. The identity with cane-sugar of the sweetish white mass obtained by evaporation was established in 1776 by Matthew Dobson (1745–1784). The chemically based confirmation of the identity of urinary and grape sugar was of course first made in 1838 by Apollinaire Bouchardat (1806–1886) and Eugène Melchior Peligot (1811–1890). Willis was able to report on intermittent diabetes, and also remarked on the increase in diabetes in his time; the relationship between diabetes and socio-economic conditions was to be repeatedly observed in the future, as noted by Bouchardat on the occasion of its decline during the Franco-Prussian War of 1870–71.

References to the sweetness of diabetic urine had already appeared in the Chinese and Indian medical writings of the 2nd to 6th centuries AD, but without exerting any influence on the development of Western European medicine, though the scientific value of these observations became a matter for controversial discussion in research.

The Age of the Enlightenment led to the distinction between diabetes insipidus and diabetes mellitus, as well as diabetes decipiens (sugar without polyuria), and to further subclassifications by Boissier de Sauvages (1707–1767), William Cullen (1710–1790) and Johann Peter Frank (1745–1821) in the style of the natural history classifications of Linnaeus (1707–1778). At this time, too, there were added pathologic approaches to the interpretation of diabetes, as by Giorgio Baglivi (1668–1707). On the other hand, a patho-physiologic interpretation – incomplete digestion of the chyle in the blood – was advanced by Thomas Sydenham (1624–1689).

As for treatment, this gained a new stimulus in the 18th century. In 1776, Dobson argued for an improvement in digestion and assimilation in view of the sugar excretion. However, in the received dietetic tradition, the diabetic treatises of the period now recommended patients to sexual abstinence and gaiety of mind *(sint animo hilariori aegri, a Venere plane se abstineant)*. Yet John Roll (d. 1809) exerted a decisive influence with his meat diet, advocated on the basis of his treatment of 48 diabetics in 1797. Rollo also goes into the problem of those patients who were unable to comply with this diet because of their aversion to meat and their vegetarian yearnings. His patient Meredith recovered on this diet. In the 18th century, evidence as to the hereditary nature of diabetes was reported as well.

The 19th century led to an insight into the significance of the islet cells of the pancreas in diabetes, based on the research of Paul Langerhans (1847–1888), Gustave-Édouard Laguesse (1861–1927), Oskar Minkowski (1858–1931), Josef von Mering (1849–1908), Bernhard Naunyn (1839–1925) and many other workers. In his thesis of 1869, Langerhans described the anatomy and histology of the pancreatic islet cells, as to whose function he was of course unable to express an opinion. With his famous *piqûre diabétique* (diabetic puncture) on the brain of dogs, Claude Bernard (1813–1878) showed the connection between the central nervous system and diabetes. The differential extirpation of the dog's pancreas by Minkowski and von Mering in 1889 produced an artificial diabetes. As far back as 1682, Johann Conrad Brunner (1653–1727) had observed polydipsia and polyuria in dogs after partial pancreatectomy, though without drawing the appropriate conclusions; the secretion of the pancreatic juice remained unknown to him and he declared the pancreas to be a superfluous organ. In 1893, Laguesse surmised the endocrine secretion of the islet cells and in 1898 Naunyn advanced a comprehensive theory of diabetes.

Further developments were concerned with the isolation of the active agent insulin in 1921 by Banting and Best, and its therapeutic application was crowned by its use, first in a dog, and in January 1922 in a man. In 1908, Georg Ludwig Zuelzer (1870–1949) had reported the first treatment of a diabetic consumptive with a pancreatic extract. The discovery of insulin itself is complicated and linked with a dispute over priority, still unresolved at the present time. The 1923 Nobel Prize was shared by Banting and MacLeod with Best and Collip.

These investigational endeavors of the past and their practical applications to diagnosis and treatment formed the basis for the advances of later decades, with numerous new insights into the causes and course of the disease and a profusion of new therapeutic techniques: oral antidiabetics, the transplantation of the pancreas and of insulin-producing tissue, the implantation of insulin pumps and gene therapy. There is also the differentiation of types of diabetes, e.g., types I and II, which called for a varied approach and relationship to the disease (Coping), and finally there are the epidemiologic studies, which deal with the complex interplay of heredity and environment in the development of diabetes.

d) Diabetes of the past

Diabetes is both a medical and a cultural topic; disease is never just an objective phenomenon, but always involves a suffering human being who possesses awareness and speech, lives in a social setting and adopts an attitude to his disease. Medicine is fundamentally both a science and an art; the doctor does not merely have to deal with objects, but also and always with the patients as subjects.

Noteworthy but less famous persons of the past, including doctors, suffered from diabetes. Diabetes made its mark in art and literature.

It is an ubiquitous disease, yet its relationship to times of prosperity and hardship is indisputable. That diabetics know themselves to be actively affected by economic conditions was emphasized by Friedrich von Müller in 1928: "My diabetics from prosperous circles (and diabetes is predominantly a disease of the rich) have been revealed by the bank as extraordinarily gifted hoarders". The variable distribution of diabetes is affected more by ethnic and religious differences, and hence differing dietary and life styles, than by genetics. Among the North American Indians there has been a lively increase in maturity-onset diabetes since the 40's of this century, whereas juvenile diabetes is rare here. The increase in diabetes among the second generation of insulin-dependent jews proves the importance of overweight as a causal factor. In 1907 J. P. Bose asserted: "What gout is to the nobility of England, diabetes is to the aristocracy of India".

History provides numerous examples of diabetics, though of course the diagnosis is not always confirmed. Thus whether, as has been asserted, Herod was actually afflicted with diabetes is extremely problematic. Geronimo Cardano (1501–1576) who, as a physician, handed down relevant case-histories, suffered from diabetes insipidus as he himself describes: "and then in the year 1536 . . . I developed urinary flux, and that in very marked fashion, about 40–100 ounces a day, and now I have had it for nearly 40 years and am still alive and suffer not at all from wasting – I still wear the same rings – or from thirst". The Saxon King, August the Great (1670–1733) was a diabetic, though the diagnosis was not established in his time; the first signs appeared in 1726 and an inflamed great toe had to be removed. Likewise, the Polish King, Michal Korybut Wisniowiecki (1640–1673) was affected by diabetes 50 years earlier.

Johann Georg Hamann (1730–1788) also suffered from diabetes. In a letter from the year 1786 the philosopher wrote: "Sedentary for 20 years, overfed through burning hunger and thirst, tense with passionate feelings". Hamann probably died in diabetic coma. In the French Revolution, Jean-Paul Marat (1744–1793), murdered on 13 July 1793 by Charlotte Corday in the bath he was taking to soothe his pruritus, was also assumed to be a diabetic though the symptoms we are told of rather contradict this.

The Brazilian Emperor Pedro II (1825–1891) suffered from diabetes from the 1870s, the first symptoms being increasing fatigue, intermittent fever and inflammation of the legs. The Emperor was treated by Adolf Kussmaul in August 1887 after having consulted Jean-Martin Charcot (1825–1893) in Paris; the winter of 1887–88 saw Pedro II in Italy and on the Riviera, where he met Nietzsche, and a pneumonia was successfully treated in Milan in May. The political overthrow occurred in 1889 and, from 1891, the Emperor lived in the modest Hôtel Bedford in Paris, associated with scientists and artists and was repeatedly subject to medical advice; he died of pneumonia on 5 December 1891.

The poet and musician, Peter Cornelius (1824–1874), Hippolyte Taine (1828–93), the Postmaster-General Heinrich von Stephan (1831–97) and the painter, Paul Cézanne (1839–1906) were other famous diabetics of the 19th century. Peter Cornelius began to complain of hunger and thirst in the sommer of 1874. His general practitioner diagnosed a severe sugar disease and advised a cure at Bad Neuenahr, but this led to only temporary improvement. Cornelius died on 26 October 1874, in the bosom of his family and under the friendly care of his doctor. Heinrich von Stephan had to undergo amputation of a foot because of his diabetes, and asked that on the casket in which his foot was placed there should be inscribed the phrase: "Here lies the foot which trod on no-one's neck". Cézanne betrays the social and psychologic effects of the disease in his behavior and letters.

The series continued in the 20th century. The Russian art critic and producer, S. P. Diaghilev (1872–1929), suffered from diabetes towards the end of his life. In June 1929, in Paris, he was informed of the diagnosis by Dr. Roger Dalimier, who treated him for discharging lesions of the entire body. Other physicians who treated Diaghilev included Dr. Talariko in London and Drs. Vittoli and Bidali in Venice. Diaghilev also had his problems with the prescribed diet. He died on 18 August 1929 at the Grand Hôtel des Bains in Venice, no longer able to make use of the insulin developed in 1921.

Other diabetics of the 20th century were the Berlin designer, Heinrich Zille (1858–1929), ironic even in the context of his own disease, and the composer, Giacomo Puccini (1858–1924), whose *Madame Butterfly*, composed during his period of illness, was termed the 'Diabetic's Opera'. The painter, Oskar Schlemmer (1888–1943) died of heart-failure after acute diabetes and jaundice, his weakened body no longer responsive to treatment. Schlemmer's artistic declaration from his inaugural address of 1932 may be attributed as much to his therapeutic regime as to his political position: "We need number, measure and precept if we are not to be overcome by chaos." It was actually during his illness that Schlemmer painted the hospital picture *The Night-watch and the Old Man*. His last diary entry of 1 April 1943 is a quotation from Rilke: "Art is not something we *select* from the world, but what is completely transformed into the glorious".

Many doctors have also suffered from diabetes and not uncommonly even died in diabetic coma: the gynecologist, Rudolf Chroback

(1843–1910), the ophthalmologist, Julius von Michel (1843–1911), the dermatologist, Albert Neisser (1855–1916), the anatomist, Max Fürbringer (1846–1920). George Sprague was attacked by the disease in 1921, but was saved by the insulin discovered in that year, went on to study medicine and devoted himself particularly to research and treatment of diabetes. George Richards Minot (1885–1950) was one of the first patients that Elliott Proctor Joslin (1869–1962) treated with insulin; for his discovery of a treatment for pernicious anemia, Minot was awarded the Nobel Prize in 1934. Another diabetic was Robert Daniel Lawrence (1892–1968), one of the founders of the British Diabetic Association.

But less important diabetics of the past and present also deserve mention: the "certain noble earl" of Thomas Willis in the 17th century and John Rollo's Captain Meredith of the 18th, who benefited from the meat diet. In the 19th century, there were the gardener, Wilhelm W., on whose diabetic retinopathy Eduard von Jäger (1818–1884) published a study in 1855, the first patient of Banting and Best, the children at the beginning of the insulin era whose fate was reported by W. Korp and E. Zweymüller in 1973. Numerous reports on patients of the present day have been published.

e) Literature and Art

For their part, literature and art have often taken diabetes as their subject, especially in modern times. Scientific films have been made on diabetes, diabetes has been publicized on postage stamps. Whether the Venus of Willendorf was a diabetic remains undecided. The 20th century is particularly rich in stories about diabetes, especially in the English-language literature: Angus Wilson *(A Sad Fall)*, Nancy Hall *(Love is not Love)*, Lamed Shapiro *(Journeying through the Milky Way)*, Pauline Clarke *(The Sharp One)*, Brian Lester Glanville *(The King of Hackney Marshes)*, Phyllis Reynolds Naylor *(Just One Small Part of Living)*, John Keefauver *(How Henry J. Littlefinger Licked the Hippies)*, Édouard Roditi *(Mademoiselle Blanche, or Diabetes Can Be Fun)*, Josef Kampos de Metro *(The Sluggard Heart)*, Stephen Dixon *(Cut)* are writers to be mentioned here with their stories.

Angus Wilson's *A Sad Fall* (1957) depicts the diabetic fate of old Miss Tanner, her diet regime, the social reaction, her own behavior, her appearance, the swelling flesh, her sensations, her assessment of the disease. She attributes the origin of her diabetes to agitation over the death of her husband; this derivation, to which the doctors sadly pay little attention, provides its own justification: "It helps me to know that the mind controls our miserable body."

In his *Buddenbrooks* of 1901, Thomas Mann has Senator James Möllendorpf fall ill with diabetes: "The instincts of self-preservation were so far absent in this old man that in the last years of his life he increasingly succumbed to a passion for cakes and pastry." As his family had barred access of their head to sweet confectionery, Möllendorpf rented a modest room where he could tuck into cakes and tarts undisturbed: "and there he was found lifeless, his mouth still full of half-chewed cake, the remains soiling his coat and scattered on the wretched table. A fatal stroke had forestalled his gradual decline."

Diabetes has also stimulated the poets, like the physician Angus McD. Morton in 1898 and later Cecil Striker in 1962, also Wilhelm Haenecke. The last ended his verses of 1969 with the cheering insight: "He who's stuck with insulin is helped the most by discipline, for many troubles on this earth can also show us virtue's worth." The poem *'Diabetes'* (1979) by the American writer James Dickey has particular poetic depth.

Diabetes is an impressive example of medical and cultural history, and progress in this field has been at the frontiers of medicine. Antiquity, the Middle Ages, the Modern Era and the present are the significant periods of historical development. The history of diabetes is always to be seen as of an anthropological nature; and this disease is also always manifest as a physical, mental, social and intellectual phenomenon.

Many problems still exist for the future: in the scientific, psychologic and social fields. The texts selected for this reader document the history and study of the disease. The bibliography of the primary sources and secondary literature will aid further private study. But at the center stands the sick man; it is to him that theory and practice apply, to him also must the future be consecrated.

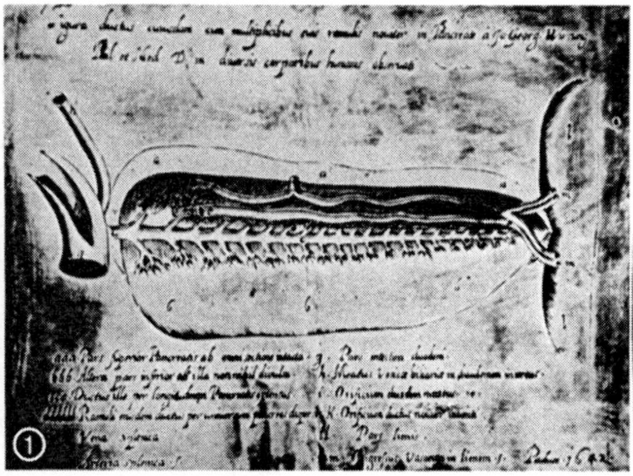

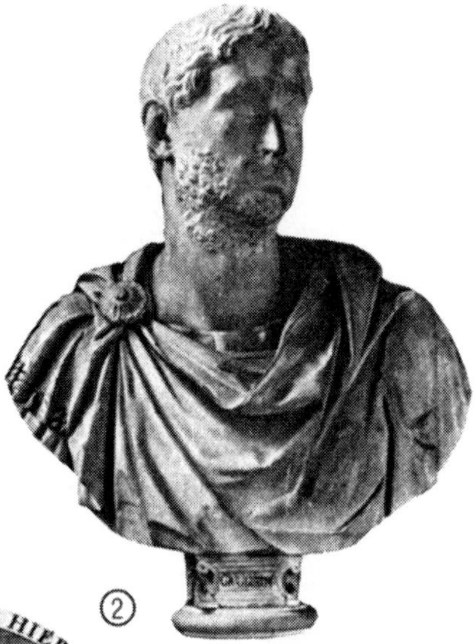

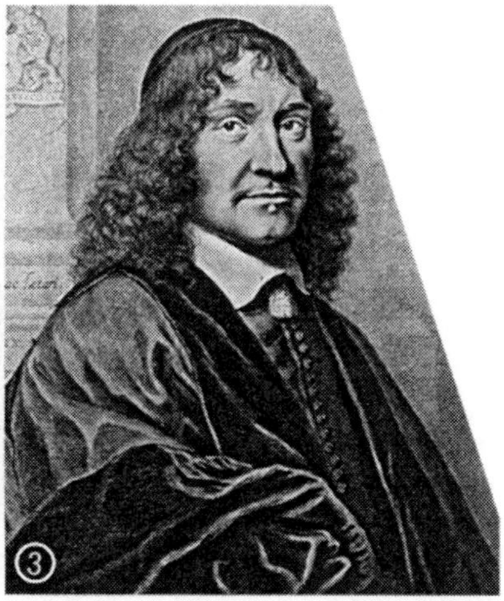

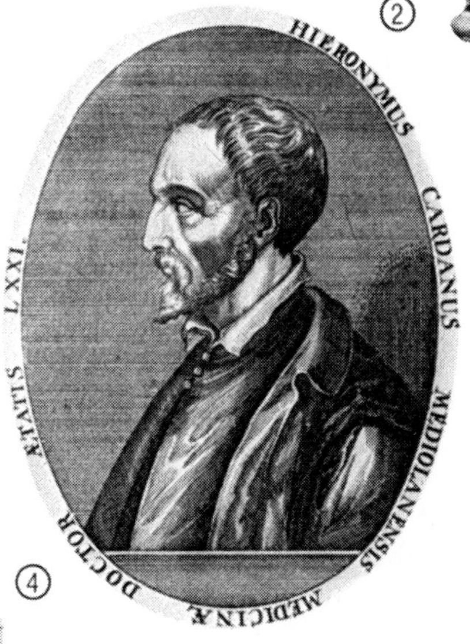

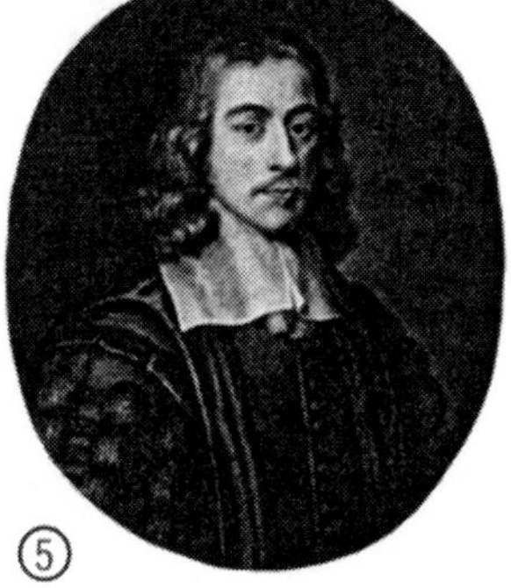

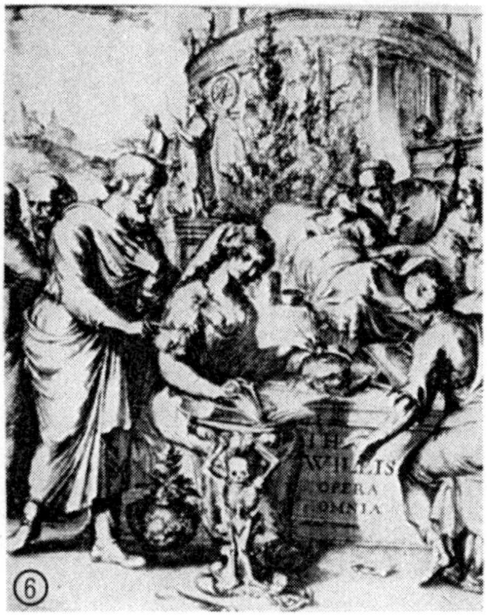

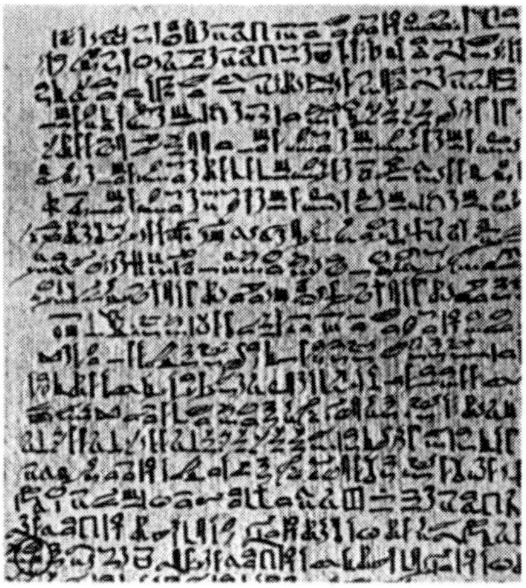

① Ductus pancreaticus, Engraving from a drawing by Johann Georg Wirsung (1600–1643), 17th century
② Claudius Galen (129–199) Marble, 2nd–3rd century

③ Franciscus dele Boë Sylvius (1614–1672), Engraving, C. van Dalen, 17th century. ④ Gerolamo Cardano (1501–1596), Engraving, about 1650. ⑤ Thomas Willis (1621–1675). Engraving, G. Vertue, 1742. ⑥ Title page: Thomas Willis: Opera Omnia, Amsterdam 1682. ⑦ Ebers Papyrus: Instructions for treating diabetes, 1550 BC

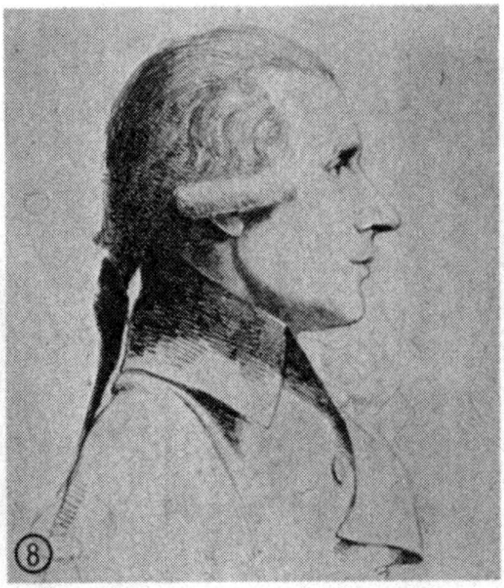

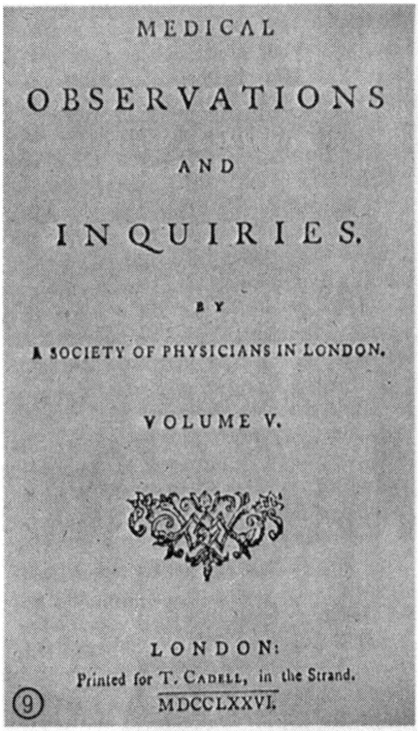

MEDICAL

OBSERVATIONS

AND

INQUIRIES.

BY

A SOCIETY OF PHYSICIANS IN LONDON.

VOLUME V.

LONDON:

Printed for T. CADELL, in the Strand.

MDCCLXXVI.

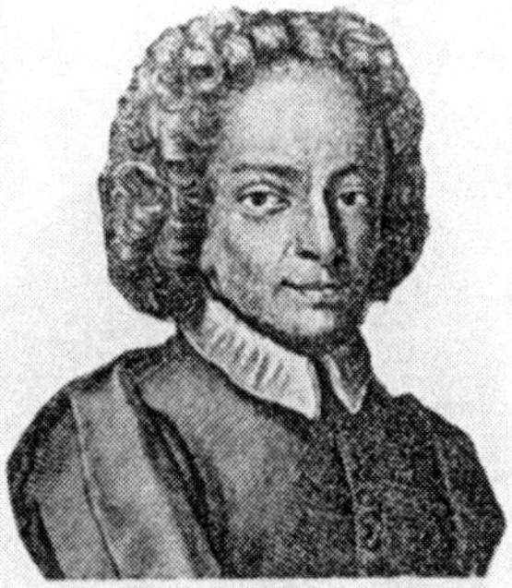

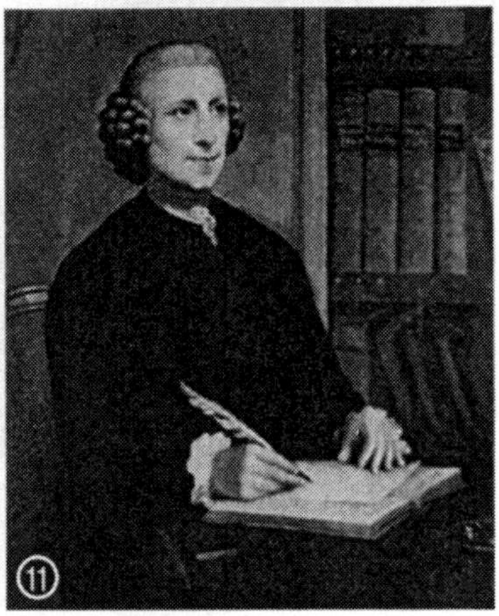

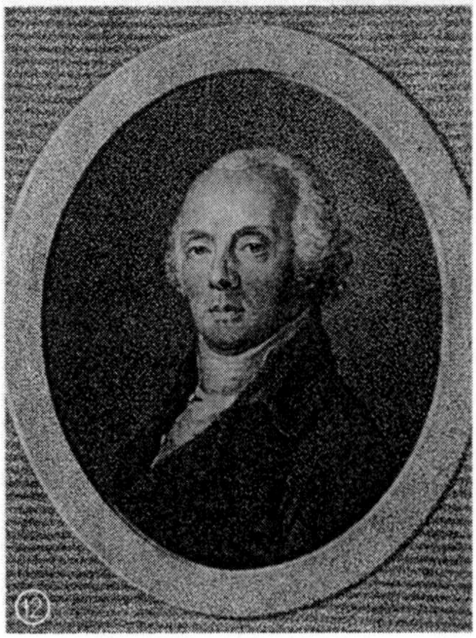

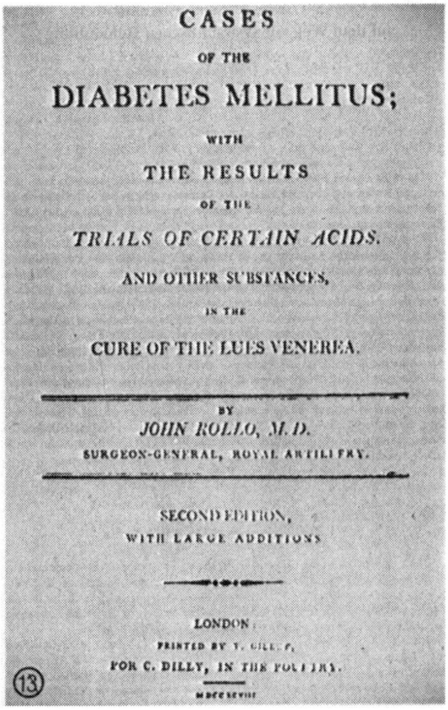

CASES

OF THE

DIABETES MELLITUS;

WITH

THE RESULTS

OF THE

TRIALS OF CERTAIN ACIDS,

AND OTHER SUBSTANCES,

IN THE

CURE OF THE LUES VENEREA.

BY

JOHN ROLLO, M.D.

SURGEON-GENERAL, ROYAL ARTILLERY.

SECOND EDITION,

WITH LARGE ADDITIONS.

LONDON:

PRINTED BY T. GILLET,

FOR C. DILLY, IN THE POULTRY.

MDCCXCVIII.

⑧ John Latham (1761–1843), Lithograph, W. Daniell, 1812

⑨ Title Page: Medical observations by a Society of Physicians in London, vol. 5, London 1776

⑩ Giorgio Baglivi (1668–1707), Engraving from a drawing by C. Maratta, about 1700

⑪ Francis Home (1719–1813), Oil, 18th century

⑫ Johann Peter Frank (1745–1821), Engraving, 19th century

⑬ Title page: John Rollo: An account of two cases of diabetes mellitus, vol. 5, London 1797

Literary texts

Only a few examples of the portrayal of diabetes in literature are supplied. The illustrations in this volume attest to the artistic connotations.

A Sad Fall

by Angus Wilson

Mrs Tanner stood in the porch watching the hired car disappear down the drive taking her son to the London train – first short lap of his long journey overseas. She waved once or twice; but it was not Jeremy's face that turned to smile at her, only Naomi's so she bent her heavy body ostentatiously to examine the loose paving in the front steps. Her sudden attention to the cracked paving would make clear her deliberate rejection of the smile, for her daughter-in-law knew well enough that the dilapidation of the house was one of the things that least concerned her. It was surely enough that she shared this war time rural isolation with Naomi, had allowed her to go alone with Jeremy for his embarkation; she had earned a right to a single act of rudeness to this stranger brought in by marriage. In any case Naomi was well aware of the mutual indifference upon which their friendly relationship rested.

From the drawing-room came the sound of a piano duet. Mozart or Beethoven – Mrs Tanner made no attempt to guess. Music was not one of the cultural horizons which her isolation and ill health had extended. Even her uninclined ear, however, noted Roger's stumbling treble in contrast to John Appleby's practised bass. She felt a now rare sense of pleasure in anticipating John's continued stay in her house. The weakening of once agonizing maternal love was not all that old age brought in compensation for its other more depressing physical weaknesses; for the first time for many years she had found real delight in the company of a stranger. He had become one of those few whom she could put trust in if she had a sudden seizure; in her new diabetic scheme of life such people were the elect. Of course, an attentive audience of any sort was relief to the imprisonment of solitude. Then too, John Appleby was not truly a stranger, but a wanderer returned from the happy lost days of Jeremy's youth. Nevertheless she knew that it was not just 'company' nor the past that had attracted her to the young man during his week's visit. Going into the hall lobby to leave the light tweed overcoat which the cold September afternoon had demanded, Mrs Tanner gave an unwonted glance to the dusty mirror and patted her white shingled hair into place on each side of her plump wrinkled checks. A look of almost coy merriment tempered the usual self-mourning gaze of her spaniel-brown eyes as she went upstairs to take her insulin dose before joining the others in the drawing-room.

In that room Roger crashed his square-topped fingers down on to the keys. 'It's no good,' he cried, 'I can't keep it up. You see I haven't kept my practising going this holiday,' and he broke into a long giggling laugh that seemed oddly hysterically-edged in so stolid and squareframed a boy.

'Yes,' said John Appleby, 'I do see.' His smile took from his deliberate tones their touch of rebuke. He got up from the piano stool and, crumpling his long thin body into an arm-chair, he began to fill his pipe.

The boy swung round on the other stool – a revolving one which he had brought to the piano from the desk in the dining-room. Legs apart, he drummed with his fingers on the stool's edge. He looked towards John, his lower lip pouting a little as though he feared his refusal to continue the duet had brought the conversation to an end. But John, as he sucked at his pipe, looked up at him over the bowl and between his suckings asked: 'Do you give up with most of your prep like that?'

His note was schoolmasterly, but this must have been long accepted between them, for Roger said, 'Yes, Professor,' and laughed. 'I get bored when things are difficult,' he added.

'Or you think you do,' John observed.

'I do,' Roger repeated, the touch of petulance underlining the cockney strain in his speech.

'So Tompkins is top of the form and not you. But you manage to get moved up each term, so why worry?' John's smile was quizzical. Roger's cheeks flushed, their high colour spreading up to the edge of his smoothly brilliantined fair hair. John's quizzical smile spread across his thin, monkey-like face. He shook his head, 'No, no, I mean it,' he said, 'it's the perfect recipe for sensible moderate success.'

If there was an undertone to the gay, friendly note of his voice, it was beyond the range of the boy's thirteen years. He swung round again on the stool, his plump bare knees catching the light as he moved. He began to play 'Chopsticks' then changed to 'The March of the Tin Soldiers'. 'I had a hen and she laid such eggs that I gave her trousers for her legs,' he sang. He bawled the words at the top of his voice.

Mrs Tanner, coming into the room, took in the boy's high spirits and smiled across at John. 'Heavens what a noise!' she cried. The boy stopped singing, but continued to play the tune. 'He's been lecturing me', he called over his shoulder.

'I made an observation,' John said, 'Roger took it as a rebuke.'

'It wasn't an observation,' the boy threw back, 'it was a jawing.'

'No doubt deserved,' Mrs Tanner concluded, 'however little you liked it.'

Roger refused the conclusion; 'Oh, but I did like it,' he said and swung round again, facing them rather primly, 'I don't mind a bit with him.'

'And I thought you were busy with your Mozart,' Mrs Tanner said.

'Beethoven,' John pretended to mutter, but cast a teasing look at her.

'Don't you make any of your observations to me, Mr Appleby,' she cried. Then, deflecting the conversation from herself, 'You mustn't take up all Mr Appleby's time, Roger, he's got his paper to write.'

'Oh my poor paper,' John said, 'you bring it in like a penance, Mrs Tanner. A hundred Hail Marys.'

'Well I don't like the idea of an old woman and a schoolboy coming between you and a certain vague number.' She brought out the technical phrase with a certain coquetry.

'Good Heavens. You've remembered it. I beg you not to clutter your head with such awful stuff.'

'It might displace some of the useless lumber,' Mrs Tanner said, 'there's precious little else there.'

'Oh, no, just the whole of Gibbon and *The Ring and the Book* and *Clarissa*.'

'I wish I'd never told you about my war time reading,' Mrs Tanner replied, 'it was simply a solitary old woman's chance of repairing a bit of her abysmal ignorance. In any case,' she went on, 'I thought scientists and mathematicians weren't interested in human beings of any sort let alone old women and schoolboys.'

'We live among them,' John smiled, 'we must learn to deal with them. Otherwise we should leave it all to humanists like Hitler.'

'Hitler was vilely inhuman.'

'It's the same thing upside down. Too much attachment.'

Mrs Tanner could not make anything of it, but if she intended to voice her perplexity she was prevented by Roger. 'I bet Hitler isn't dead really,' he cried, 'Is he? You know about it, don't you, Mr Appleby, that's your job, spying.'

'Now, Roger, I've told you you're not to question Mr Appleby about his job.'

'But I'm not questioning him, Mrs Tanner. I'm just telling him he's a spy. Anyway what's clever about spying? I'll spy on you today, Mr Appleby, and you won't know I'm doing it.'

John spoke in a heavy German accent, 'Good morning, General Hannay,' he said, 'I did not recognize you at first in those grey flannel knickers.' Roger gave way once more to his giggling laughter.

'General Hannay,' Mrs Tanner said firmly, 'must set the table for luncheon. You and I will have to share the chores, Roger, while Mrs Jeremy's in London. We usually have a roster of three,' she explained to John.

'Oh, there's plenty of time,' Roger said.

'No there is not. I've taken my insulin. I shall want my food sharp at one.'

The boy's face assumed a look of reverence. Mrs Tanner's diabetes involved holy rituals. 'I'll go straight away,' he said, 'is it fish?'

'Yes,' Mrs Tanner laughed, 'I'm afraid it *is* fish, Roger.'

As the boy opened the door to leave, he turned to John. If he seemed for a moment coy it was no more than the coquetry their visitor inspired in Mrs Tanner. 'If I promise to practise will you take me to the cinema tomorrow, Mr Appleby?' he asked.

'I'll take you to the cinema, but without any promises. We don't appease any more, you know, in our brave new world,' John said, and then, as though in fear that his moralizing had offended the boy, he added, 'Who knows we might see a Gumbleduck.'

Whatever the intimacy offered, Roger did not receive it well. 'How could we?' he asked, and went out of the room.

Mrs Tanner let herself down into a deep arm-chair, slowly filling its every crevice with her bulging flesh. She took up some sewing from the side-table. 'I hope you realize what you're letting yourself in for,' she said. 'There'll be only Roger and me to talk to in the whole place.' She waved her hand, incongruously small for her fat body, around the sitting-room to indicate the vast spaces in which he was, to be bored.

It was in fact, John Appleby reflected, only a moderate sized room in a smallish house with a smallish garden, less than half the size of the house the Tanners had occupied when he had visited them in his adolescence, yet she habitually spoke as though she was the unwilling mistress of a large estate. With his usual methodical approach to human behaviour, he sought an answer to the paradox and guessed that a house without servants seemed vast to her in the work it imposed.

He smiled with the teasing gallantry he had come to use with her. 'I like talking to *Roger* very much,' he said, 'He's both sensible and ordinary. An extremely pleasant combination in a small boy.'

Mrs Tanner, playing her part, pretended not to notice the teasing omission. 'I'm so glad you like him,' she said, 'you're certainly very good with him. Not that he's at all difficult. I can't tell you how pleased Naomi and I were that out of all the evacuees he should be the only one who hasn't drifted back to London. I oughtn't to say it, of course, because, poor child! its dreadful that his Mother shouldn't want him. But from the very start he gave me no trouble. I suppose, as you say, he is a very ordinary boy. He'll never set the world on fire, but then the others only set the *house* on fire or lied or wetted their beds. Not a very pleasing sort of extraordinariness and certainly not the sort that an old woman of seventy wants to cope with. All the same, Roger or no Roger, I warn you that the house will be no place for an intelligent man to spend his leave in, you've only seen it when Jeremy and Naomi were here, you don't know how dead it can be.'

'I can't remember,' he answered, 'that Jeremy showed any sign this week of wanting to talk to anyone but Naomi, or Naomi for that matter of noticing anyone but him. She put up the better show of pretending, of course, but then I'm not *her* old schoolfriend. But they were neither of them aching to be sociable. All the same as far as I remember I've had a great deal of very pleasant conversation and it hasn't all been with Roger.'

Mrs Tanner laughed but once again she disregarded the compliment, 'They're terribly in love,' she cried, 'you must forgive them, *I* try to even though he is my son. As a matter of fact,' she said, 'old age and infirmity free one from a lot of encumbrances and one of them is an excessive mother love.' She had bent over her sewing so that John speculated whether she was hiding a face that could belie her assured tone. 'I can honestly say that I was glad to let Naomi go alone to see him off in London,' she said emphatically, 'I've ached for him at times during these war years, of course; after all he is my only one and I worry too when he's been in London during air raids. But I live much more with a past Jeremy now than with the real one. That's one of the reasons I've been so pleased to get to know you. You're a link with his past. Of course, it's only *one* of the reasons,' she added with a smile.

It was John's turn gracefully to ignore the compliment, 'I hope you're not worried about his going to Calcutta,' he said, 'he'll be in less danger there, you know, than he was in London.'

'Oh heavens,' she cried, 'I'm not so blindly selfish that I'm unaware of the enormous luck we have had that he should be doing this intelligence work, whatever it is.' She threw him an amused glance; it was one of the customary jokes of their friendship that she should be a little arch about the secret work that he and Jeremy were engaged in. 'Oh no, he's safe enough. I feel quite guilty about it at times. One of the few compensations of my isolation down here is not having to face the other poor women whose wretched men are *not* safely in Intelligence. Naomi feels it at the hospital. So many of the nurses are married or engaged to pilots. Perhaps Jeremy's going to Calcutta will at least give her the peace of conformity with the others.'

John raised his eyebrows slightly, Mrs Tanner put down her sewing and, removing her amber-rimmed spectacles, she turned her large, anxious yellow-flecked brown eyes upon him. 'No, I don't mean it like that. Not even unconsciously, I'm sure of it. I really *don't* grudge her Jeremy's love.' She stroked the pale lemon silk of the cushion cover she was sewing as for a moment she pondered. 'Of course, I can't help remembering that *she* will have Jeremy again in a world of peace and decency. While as for me, a fat diabetic old woman – who can say how long this awful Japanese war will last? But it's not really him I'm thinking of. I've honestly and truly let him go. No, it's of myself. Oh, I know it's only a vegetable life I live down here and it'll never be much more. But to have got through this awful time, to have seen the horror fade away in Europe. For I'm sure it will. And then to face years more of it. I'm sorry I can't believe in this Far Eastern war or the necessity for it. I want so much to see a world of gentleness again. That's why,' she smiled, 'I've loved your courtesy in bothering with me and Roger. You're so gentle in a violent, hurrying world.'

'Oh,' John exclaimed, I'm civil enough, I suppose.' He ran his hand through his long black, hair, pulling his head down to the chairback so that his high-check-boned white face stared out at her against the dark red fabric. 'I shouldn't,' he added, 'put much trust in a world of gentleness again though. It'll take an age to teach manners again – if they *ever* come back.'

This time Mrs Tanner's brown eyes showed no gleam, they were all hurt spaniel, Charles I, reproach.

'Oh, it's more than manners that we need. It's love.'

John, pipe between his teeth, ventured no more than, 'Ah?'

'Oh, yes,' Mrs Tanner appealed, 'surely. I know something about it. You see,' now her eyes seemed old pools of wisdom, 'I used to love possessively, holding tight – husband, son, a London house I was proud of. Well, I lost them all. Or at least I lost Oliver, and then my health went, and the meaning of my life in London went from me. I think I learnt then that holding tight could only hurt me and others. That was why I was able to let Jeremy go. And as to personal possessions – well, you see the state of this house and the garden! I allow them to be no more than somewhere I live in, some place where I can take their air. Of course,' she laughed, 'I can't do much else anyway with only a charwoman and no gardener. But all the same,' she changed to the serious with a degree of ostentation, 'I have learned a little at last of how to love, I think, to love without holding.'

Again John grave only the slightest interrogative, 'Ah?'

'It's allowed me, for example, to be good friends with Naomi, simply because she's the woman my son loves.' Provided with no comment, Mrs Tanner drew to her conclusion quickly. 'Well, anyway that's the way the world has got to learn to love if we're ever to be done with all these horrors. And I think it will.'

The fitful, yet strong September sunshine had lit upon John's chalk-white furrowed forehead. Mrs Tanner took it as a way out of her one-sided conversation. 'Shall we seize the sunshine while it lasts?' she asked. 'If, that is, you don't mind walking at a fat old woman's slow pace.'

'We've talked so much about me and so little about you,' Mrs Tanner remarked, as they walked at indeed a very slow pace across the ill-kept lawn, 'women and especially old inquisitive women can be such a nuisance that I have purposely not asked questions. But that doesn't mean I'm not curious, of course I am.'

'A lecturer in Mathematics at Oxford,' John replied, 'Educated at Shrewsbury with Jeremy Tanner. The best of educations surely?'

'Oh, indeed,' Mrs Tanner laughed, 'my father was headmaster of the school, you know. I always felt it had gone down by the time Jeremy went there. But then I was bound to.'

'Well,' he went on, 'what else is there? Born in Brighton thirty-two years ago, father a stock-broker. Oh, and, of course, engaged twice but never married.'

If he supposed that the romantic note was what Mrs Tanner was waiting for, he seemed to be wrong, for she exclaimed impatiently, 'Oh, I know all that. But were you happy as a child? I'm sure you must have been, and yet no woman can quite believe it about other people's children. And sometimes you seem so silent.'

'I'm sorry,' John laughed, 'I'm usually listening.'

'Oh, you're a wonderful listener, who else would have allowed me to go on about my wretched diabetes as you have? Oh it's absurd of me, of course; you're bound to be abstracted with your brain, but you're so kind and put up such a show of interest that when for a moment you're not absolutely with one it seems strange.'

John reached over and began to free a tall head of Michaelmas daisy from the bindweed that entangled it.

'Oh, if you once begin,' Mrs Tanner said, 'there'll be no end to it. Look at it, what a wilderness.' And indeed the herbaceous border seemed a mass of weed – docks, polygonum, thistles and, over all, bindweed – only the Michaelmas daisies still fought a losing battle. 'I warned you,' she cried, 'I've just let it all go. I can manage a few roses but for the rest I've let it go – and it's released me. Old age must beware of property.' John too released the daisy and it swayed back to its weedy height.

'And they loved you, your parents?' Mrs Tanner asked.

'They were ideal,' John replied, 'We respected each other. They helped me to grow up and then, just when I had, they died.'

For a moment Mrs Tanner could make nothing of it, then she cried, 'There! I knew it. I'm never wrong. You *were* loved. Good, gentle, friendly people always have been. It's the one thing I'm proud to have given Jeremy – a loved childhood and ...' But once again her thoughts led on to silence. Then as the grass path passed between the rhododendrons of the shrubbery out on to a meadow, she said, 'Well, there it is. Our famous view. You said you liked it yesterday when it was clouded in mist, but now you can see what the mist hid. The vague red and grey to the left is Ludlow. And there you have Wenlock Edge. And beyond you're supposed to see The Long Mynd and on to the Welsh hills. And so you could I suppose if Wenlock Edge was not so high.' She had a number of such little jokes to express her love-hatred of her home of exile.

'As a matter of fact, I think I can,' John said.

'Oh, I don't believe it. And if you can, what do you see but a faint dark shape. And they call that *seeing* the Welsh hills.' Nevertheless she was pleased. She turned back to the shrubbery, striking at the struggling arms of rhododendrons with her ash-plant. 'Is this seat too wet?' she asked, but before he could answer, she had sat down. 'Don't ever get fat,' she said, 'or rather-don't get too fat, for you could do with some extra weight.'

Before John sat down next to her, he carefully folded the mackintosh he was carrying and made a cushion for himself. 'I was really interested about the diabetes, you know,' he said.

'Oh, my dear boy!' Mrs Tanner exclaimed, 'all the same I'm sure you're right, it began with the shock of Oliver's death.'

'It's only a hypothesis.'

Mrs Tanner, however, would have no modifications. 'And none of those wretched doctors have seen it.'

'It wouldn't have helped really, if they had, would it? It couldn't have brought your husband back.'

'It always helps to know that our wretched bodies are under the control of our minds,' Mrs Tanner declared, 'it's a great comfort.'

John smiled, 'The modern world should hold great comfort for you then,' he said.

'No,' she went on, 'your understanding of that has given me even more confidence in you. You see, every illness brings its fears and, although, of course, it's quite irrational, the only thing I fear is having one of those dreadful seizures when people are around whom I don't trust. It's quite absurd as I say, because it's only a question of regular meals, and if I go out I carry some sugar with me just in case. All the same there's some people I have confidence in. Roger, for instance, although he's only a small boy and now you, but not, I'm afraid, Naomi.'

John took out his pipe and knocked it on the wooden bench. 'You say these things about Naomi, and yet what I so admire is your friendly relationship with her. It can't be easy for two women together for all these years – and anxious years.'

'Oh, it's not so bad. Of course she's difficult at times, but then so am I. She comes back from the hospital tired and then she tells me everything she's going to do. "I'm just going to put on a kettle for the hot water bottles, Mother", or "I'm only going upstairs for some wool, Mother". As if I wanted to know. But there, as you say, two women living together.'

'That's interesting,' John observed, then he said by way of solution, 'she probably needs to protect her tiredness from comment, so she covers it up with trivialities.'

'There you are,' Mrs Tanner cried, 'you see you understand us all. Naomi and me and little Roger.'

'Oh, Roger!' John said, 'he's not difficult surely.'

'No, but you've won his confidence so quickly. What was all that about Gumbleducks?'

'Oh, it's an imaginary race of little men with whiskers and top hats that his father made up for him.'

'Ah!' Mrs Tanner put in, 'he doesn't tell us things like that. I thought he'd forgotten his home, poor boy."

'I was interested,' John remarked, 'because he's really such a sensible boy. He lives in the present. No ties or fears. I thought I'd found a chink. But I was wrong. He was resentful when I brought it up. He knows that this life is here and now. The Gumbleducks are over.'

Mrs Tanner sighed, 'I'm afraid so,' she said, 'with those dreadful parents.' She hoisted herself to her feet. 'Time for my meal,' she declared. 'All the same,' she said, 'I'm right about love. We all need it but not too much. I was so interested when I read about Dr Johnson. He needed love so much – too much, of course, that's why he behaved so badly when poor Mrs Thrale married her Piozzi.'

'You know your Johnson too?' John asked.

'Why shouldn't I?' Mrs Tanner asked laughing.

'No reason, I just haven't known many mothers. And those I have didn't read much. My mother never read.'

'She was probably far too busy. I used to be until all this illness and exile happened. But don't think I understand half of what I read. Only about people. Yes,' she declared, 'I can really judge people. After all, you know, I kept house for my father after mother died and headmasters of public schools entertain a wide range of people. And then Oliver was a very successful barrister. Oh, yes, I know the world. But not books. Do you know many lawyers?' she asked.

John took a moment to answer, 'I'm so sorry,' he said, 'I thought I saw something creeping by the corner of the roof.'

'The cat,' Mrs Tanner said, a little nettled.

'No,' John cried, 'it's Roger. Heavens: his idea of spying.'

Mrs Tanner looked towards the square two-storeyed Victorian house and there, spread flat against the purplish tiled roof, was Roger, shuffling this feet sideways along the guttering. He was dressed in an old coat of Jeremy's, its belt flying loose, and an old felt hat of Mrs Tanner's.

'Oh! he mustn't' she said, 'those tiles are so loose.'

'Well, don't call to him,' John said, but he spoke too late.

'Roger!' she cried, 'Roger! come down!'

The small head turned, displaying a large pair of dark glasses. 'I don't know what you mean,' he called, 'I'm mending Mrs Tanner's roof. I've come in from Ludlow special to do it.'

But Mrs Tanner was not playing. 'Come down, Roger,' she called sternly.

'Oh, all right! But I spied on you all the way to the meadow and you didn't see me.'

'No,' said John, 'you're a first rate spy. But you'd better come down now. Mrs Tanner wants her lunch.'

The boy began hastily to edge his way back to the corner of the roof above a derelict conservatory. Too hastily, for his foot wedged in the guttering and as he pulled at it to release himself, he threw his whole weight on to the rotting lead. It was the cracking of the guttering rather than Roger's scream that made Mrs Tanner retch. For a moment she saw him clinging batlike in the flapping black coat against the shining tiles, then something loosened and he fell down through the sunshine pool of glass beneath. For a second John stood trying in vain to distinguish the boy's screams from the crash of breaking glass, then he sprinted across the lawn.

When Mrs Tanner arrived panting, John seemed to be letting the small, stolid body roll back face down to the ground where it had fallen. 'He's alive,' he said and, not looking up, he turned the boy's face towards him and began to wipe the blood away. 'He's unconscious. Concussion probably. He must have caught his head in falling. I daren't move him. I think a rib may be broken.' He looked up at her, 'Telephone for a doctor and an ambulance at once,' he said. He seemed angry.

Mrs Tanner cursed her size as she tried to hurry to the house, but she welcomed relief from the nausea which the spattered blood in the greenhouse had brought upon her. When she returned from the house, John had slid his mackintosh and his coat under the boy, he had also torn a sleeve from his shirt and had tied it in a bandage below the boy's elbow.

'The ambulance is coming from Ludlow, but it may not be here for twenty minutes,' Mrs Tanner said. She produced a small bottle of brandy.

'No, no, no stimulants,' John said impatiently. She lowered herself to the ground with difficulty. 'I've asked the hospital people to phone to his mother,' she said wearily.

'Look,' John said, disregarding the information, 'you sit by him while I get a basin of water. Call me *if* he comes to.' She could see nothing to do but hold Roger's hand, but every now and then she stroked the fair hair from his forehead. In a minute John was back with a bowl of warm water and a napkin. He began methodically to wipe the wounds in the boy's legs and arms.

'I daren't touch the bits of glass. In any case these cuts are not serious. There was a haemorrhage of the arm but I've stopped that for the time being.'

Mrs Tanner said, 'Thank God you were here.' She stroked Roger's hand and gazed at his square little face, whiter now than John's. It was this whiteness that gradually made her panic. 'Why doesn't the ambulance come?' she said, and then again, 'they'll be too late, I know they will. Oh they can't let him die, poor little Roger,' she cried, 'I shall never forgive myself if he dies.'

John got up and stood over her, 'Look,' he said, 'he is feeling no pain, that's the important thing. It doesn't matter if he does die.'

For a moment she could find no words, then she said, 'How can you say that? He's a good, fine boy.' Anger added to hcr growing hysteria, she began to weep.

'Yes,' he said, 'a very good, decent, ordinary boy. And with luck he'll grow up into the same sort of man. But there are millions of good, decent, ordinary men. It just *doesn't* matter.'

Mrs Tanner fought to hold back her tears. A moment later, she said appealingly, 'You said that didn't you to help me? You thought it would help me.'

John turned round from his kneeling position beside the boy's legs, 'Good Heavens,' he cried, 'do you think this is a time to bother about helping *you*?' A minute later he turned round again, 'I'm sorry,' he said, 'if the remark upset you, please think I said it to help or anything else you like.'

It came to Mrs Tanner that she was alone with John Appleby; she got up slowly from the ground, 'I'm going into the house to pack a small bag,' she said urgently, 'I shall go with the ambulance. I must be at the hospital tonight.'

'Of course,' John said and turned back to this task.

She hurried along the gravel path to the house and almost ran to the kitchen. Her panic died as she swallowed her dose of sugar. Such fears, of course, were entirely irrational.

in: *A. Wilson: A bit of the map and other stories, Harmondsworth 1957, S. 141–156*

The Song of Diabetes

by Cecil Striker

This ingenious poem, in the manner of Longfellow's "Hiawatha," was read by its author, Dr. Cecil Striker, at the Banquet of the 12th Annual Meeting of the ADA in Chicago, June 7, 1952.

In the office of the doctor,
In the sanctum of the specialist,
Sat the diabetic patient.
Seven cardinal symptoms had he,
Seven means of recognition.
High blood sugar, malnutrition,
Nagging weakness, all these had he,
Polydypsia, polyuria,
Polyphagia, glycosuria,
And the doctor started speaking,
"I am here to guide and warn you,
Here to treat you and instruct you.
Two great friends have diabetes,
Singled out from all the others.
Basic therapy is diet,
Insulin when indicated.
Some there are, who need no insulin;
Diet only may control them.
Magic savior is insulin
For those others who require it.

Follow faithfully your orders,
Comrade make, of diabetes,
Working with it, not against it,
Thus avoiding psychic conflict.
Life expectancy is lengthened,
Yea, assured is normal living!

T' was not always so, my patient,
In the days before Minkowski,
In the days of poor prognosis,
In the days before von Noorden.
Long before the days of these men,
Claude Bernard, experimentor,
Studied enzymes of digestion,
Medullary sugar center,
Store of glycogen by liver,
Fathered modern physiology,
Paved the way for later research,
For all those who followed after.

Many men there were who labored
On the puzzle of the pancreas.
There was Max von Pettenkofer
Classical investigator,
Carl von Voit on dietetics,
Rubner of the calorimeter,
Heat and energy he measured,
Lusk and Benedict his followers;
Langerhans for islands noted.
Kussmaul recognized air-hunger,
Labeled now as Kussmaul breathing.
Naunyn, coiner of a new word,
Coined the new word, acidosis;
Magnus-Levy treated coma;
Emil Fischer, noted chemist,
Henry Sherman for nutrition.
These were men who laid the background,
Pioneers, these research giants;
Built the bridge between the patient
And the laboratory findings."

When the patient left his office,
Long the doctor sat and pondered
On the cause of glycosuria,
On the function of the liver.
Fate of glycogen he pondered,
On cholesterol reflected.
D:N ratio he thought of,

Ketone bodies, oxysteroids.
Factors chemical he mused on,
On this segment of the problem.
Thought then, of another segment,
Of the role of the adrenal,
Of hypophysis secretion.
Pancreas beta cells considered
And the alpha cell production;
Of the mystery of the granules.
Thyroid, ovaries and testes,
How essential their secretions.
All the endocrines considered
And the need for homeostasis.

As he mused thus, meditative,
Science spoke then, to the doctor;
Spoke to him of diabetes
And of all its complications,
Sending terror to its victims,
Sending grief and death among them.
Spoke to him of acidosis,
Painted him a vivid picture
Of the patient acidotic,
Of the patient sorely suffering;
Hard this breath came through his nostrils,
Through his teeth he buzzed and muttered.
Retinopathy depicted,
Dreaded macular involvement,
With its tragic blinded victims
Hearing voices call in darkness.
And arteriosclerosis
With its manifold involvements,
Such as striking early onset,
Of diseases coronary.

Then of legs and feet spoke science,
Spoke of crippling claudication,
Of restricted ambulation,
Painful, cramping, locomotion;
Of the failure to recover
From a superficial trauma;

Deeper, deeper, damage spreading.
Patient plagued by fear of gangrene;
With the sloughing wound enlarging,
Pain and apprehension mingled,
Who, by doubt and anguish tortured.
Then presented serious problems.
Spoke of worsened diabetes,
Spoke of worsened minor lesions,
Then of diabetic gangrene,
Gangrene with its poor prognosis.
Spoke of need for amputation
And the points of amputation;
Mentioned Lisfranc, subpatellar,
And the higher mid-thigh region.

Warned of kidney complications,
Of severe albuminuria,
Casts, edema, and uremia,
Kimmelstiel, their designation.
Warned of insulin reaction
With pre-prandial cephalgia;
With diplopia and confusion,
Cold and clammy perspiration,
Dizziness with wheeling, whirling,
Whirling, round and round, and downward.
Loss of consciousness may follow
Sometimes death, alas, ensuing.
Miscellaneous others mentioned,
Carbuncle, pruritus vulvae,
Painful osteoporosis,
And peripheral neuritis.

Sad, the doctor as he listened,
Sad, because of dismal warnings,
Still, he smiled when he remembered
All the tools at his disposal.
Thought of insulin, rejoicing,
Of the men who gave it to us;
Paused to cheer for Best and Banting,
Names to celebrate forever!
From the snares of previous failures,

From the case report of Barron,
Came the concept of extraction.
All alone worked Best and Banting,
Labored long and tedious hours.
From tenacity came triumph,
Came the joy of isolation,
Came the proof, the confirmation.
Thought then of the work of Joslin
With his passion for perfection,
Indefatigable worker
With unquenchable endurance;
With meticulous instruction
For strict control of patients, and
Statistical analysis
Of clinical material.
Thought of other great clinicians,
Thought of scientific methods,
Thought of work in laboratories,
Thought of all the dietitians.

And the doctor's grateful spirit
Set him in a mood for singing:
"Sing, oh song of diabetes
Of the happy days to follow,
In the land of glycosuria,
In the pleasant land and peaceful.
Sing the mysteries of the pancreas,
Sing the blessings of the insulins;
Buried is dread malnutrition,
Buried is starvation diet,
Buried hypoproteinemia,
Massive hepar is forgotten."
Hailed the use of all the insulins
And gave thanks for their inventors,
Thankful for their skill and wisdom,
Thankful too, for new improvements
Protamine and NPH with
Prolonged action in the body,
These discovered by the scholar
Hagedorn, the sage of Denmark.
Cheered the gratifying prospect

For the diabetic children,
For their rehabilitation,
Normal growth, and good nutrition;
Cheered the child who takes his hypo,
And his fine cooperation;
Doomed, before, to rapid wasting.
Cheered because that child is living.
And he hailed a great achievement:
Pregnancy of diabetics,
Long a sad and sorry story,
Now, a joyous, safe experience,
As the faithful diabetic
Bears a child unto her husband,
With the beauty of its mother,
And the vigor of its father.

Then the doctor, looking forward,
Looking, then, toward future progress,
Dreamed of greater knowledge, insight,
Into diabetic problems.
Dreamed a dream of insulin, of
Molecule complex and heavy,
Of its structural arrangement,
Of its chemical components.
Abel isolated sulphur;
Might more fractions be discovered,
Fractions which might be effective
In the treatment of the patient?
Might not synthesis be realized,
Oral insulin perfected,
Newer chemicals discovered
Finding cause for diabetes?
Dreamed of chemistry of glucose
And of energy production;
Of the metabolic process,
Tissue chemistry, and enzymes.
Dreamed of new and complex factors,
Of the role of hexose phosphate
In obscure phosphorylation;
Mystery of deamination;
Of sulphydryl radical with

Its importance undetermined,
Future place of isotopes, of
Glutathione and alloxan.

All these ideas, all these problems
Thoughtful doctors have in common;
All the members of this conclave,
Making A.D.A. their symbol.
Bound together, dedicated,
Organized to help the patient,
Organized to teach the doctor,
A.D.A. their torch resplendent!

in: *Diabetes 1 (1952), 492–493*

The Clever Diabetic (1969)

by Wilhelm Jaenecke

Cleverer than Archimedes
Is the man who with good sense
Puts a halt to diabetes;
For good sense alone can shield you
From misfortune, sickness, danger.

If you're lacking insulin
You must act accordingly,
For, alas, it is Man's fate
That his innards often fail.

Truly, though it's not too late,
Diet is the magic word
To embellish all your days
You must kick the sugar ways.

I will state the truth quite harshly,
No more cakes or pies or tartlets,
And all other sweets at table
Shun as much as you are able.

In your future life you'll strive
Always moderate and measured,
You'll achieve 'most any goal
If your guide is self-control.

You will stay both trim and slim,
Avoid sickness, thank the Lord,
Watch the fatties' jealous looks
At your meagre calories.

Where there's a lack of insulin
The best help is self-discipline,
And often need on earth can be
A virtue from necessity.

in: *der diabetiker 7 (1969) 277*

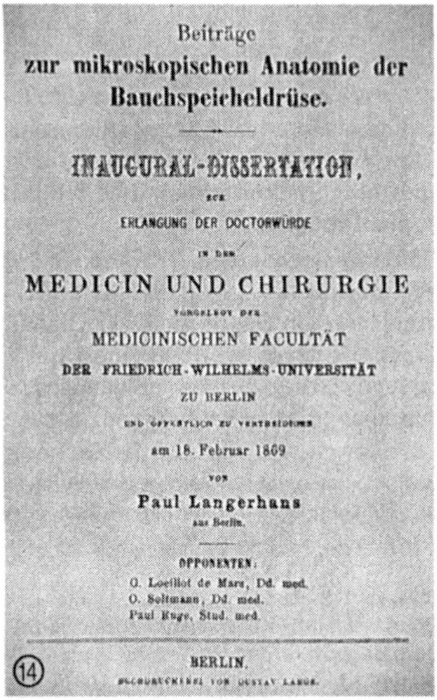

Beiträge
zur mikroskopischen Anatomie der
Bauchspeicheldrüse.

INAUGURAL-DISSERTATION,
ZUR
ERLANGUNG DER DOCTORWÜRDE
IN DER
MEDICIN UND CHIRURGIE
VORGELEGT DER
MEDICINISCHEN FACULTÄT
DER FRIEDRICH-WILHELMS-UNIVERSITÄT
ZU BERLIN
UND ÖFFENTLICH ZU VERTHEIDIGEN
am 18. Februar 1869
VON
Paul Langerhans
aus Berlin.

OPPONENTEN:
O. Loeillot de Mars, Dd. med.
O. Soltmann, Dd. med.
Paul Ruge, Stud. med.

BERLIN.
BUCHDRUCKEREI VON GUSTAV LANGE.

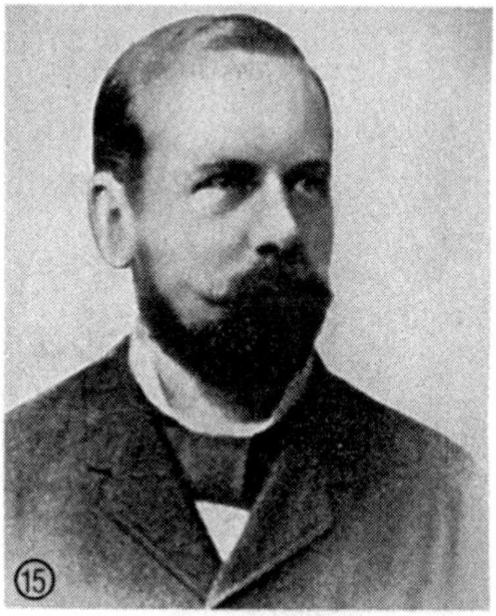

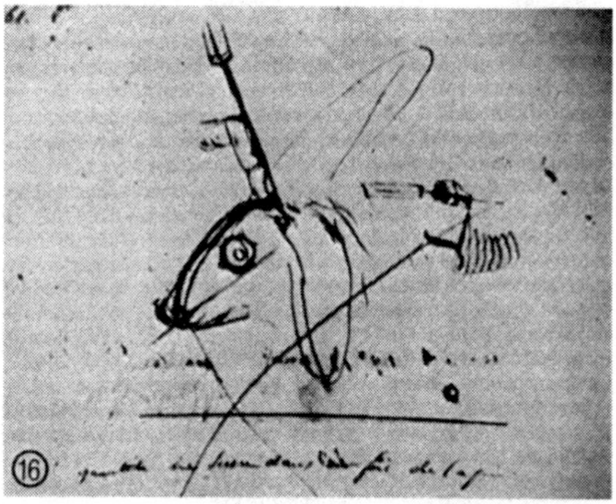

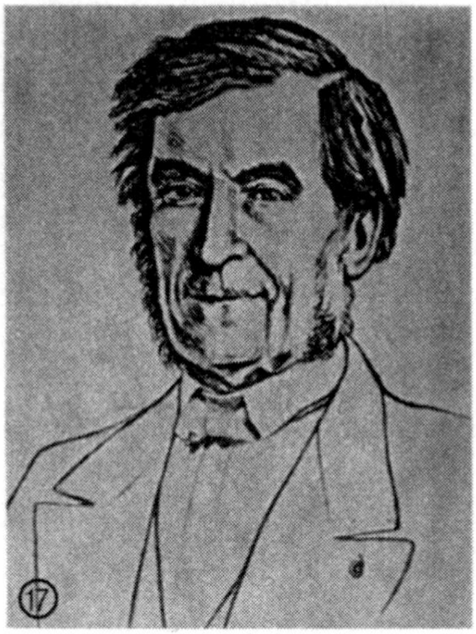

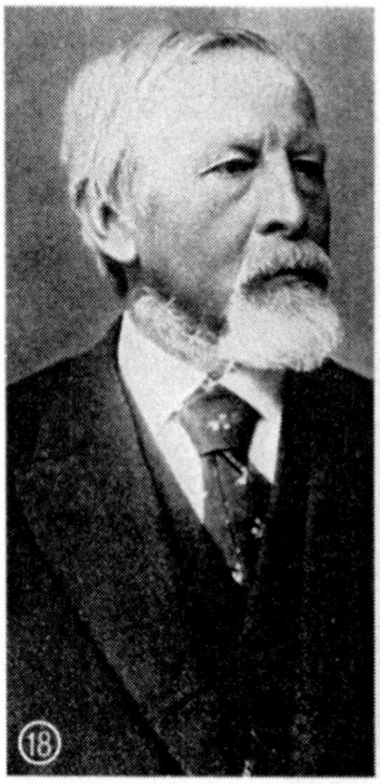

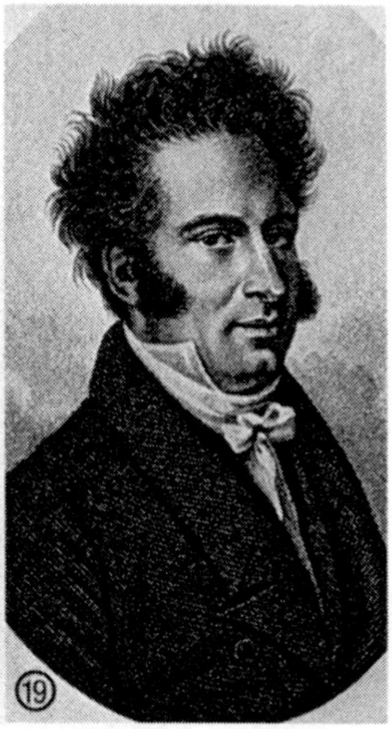

⑭ Title page: Paul Langerhans: Contibutions on the microscopic anatomy of the pancreas, Thesis, Berlin 1869
⑮ Paul Langerhans (1847–1888), Photograph, about 1880
⑯ Claude Bernard: Bernard's (diabetic) puncture, 1850
⑰ Appollinaire Bouchardat (1806–1886), Drawing, 19th century
⑱ Adolf Kußmaul (1822–1902), Photograph, about 1900
⑲ Michel Eugène Chevreuil (1786–1889), Engraving, A. Tardieu, 1825

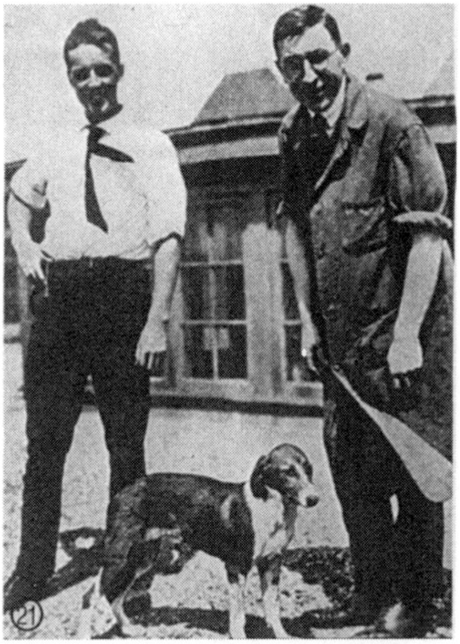

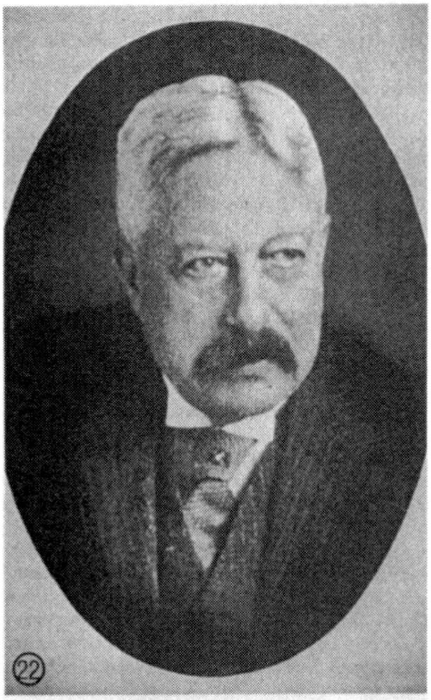

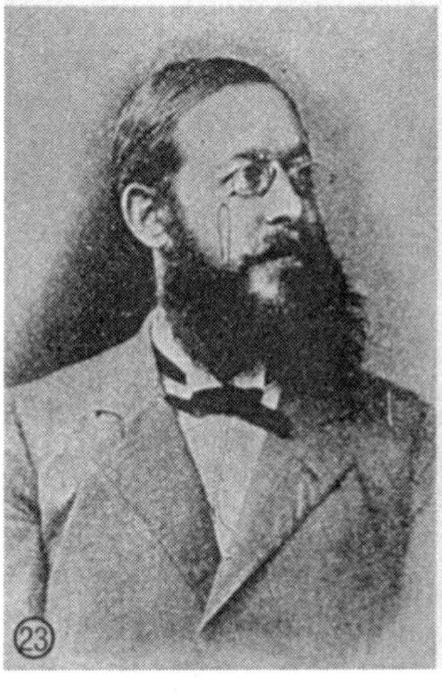

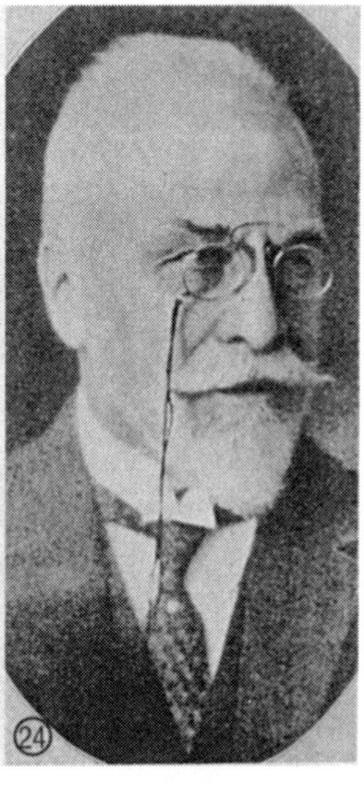

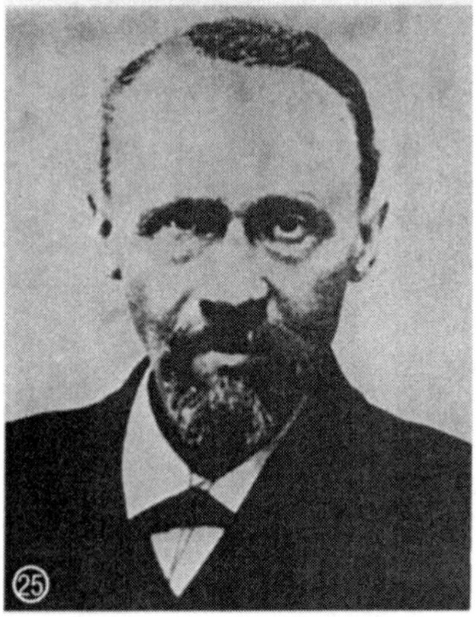

⑳ Georg Ludwig Zuelzer (1870–1949), Photograph
㉑ Frederick Grant Banting (1891–1941) (*right*) together with Herbert Charles Best (left) and the dog Marjorie, Photograph, about 1920
㉒ Carl Harko von Noorden (1858–1944), Photograph
㉓ Joseph von Mering (1849–1908), Photograph, about 1900
㉔ Oscar Minkowski (1858–1931), Photograph
㉕ Gustave-Euduard Laguesse (1861–1927), Photograph

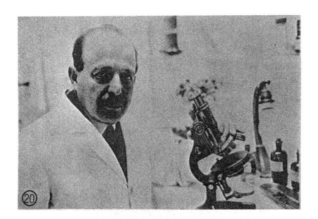

Texts Relating to the History of Scientific Study

Some exemplary texts have been selected from the literature of scientific history dealing with overall development, and others covering limited epoches and specific aspects. The spelling and punctuation have not been modernized, nor have the remarks and references been altered.

General Development

The History of Diabetes mellitus
Hans Schadewaldt (1975)

Diabetes, Sugar Consumption and Luxury Through the Ages. A Question Posed by History
Erich Ebstein (1928)

Antiquity

Diabetes
Karl Kalbfleisch (1958)

Synonyms for Diabetes in Antiquity and Their Etymology
Hermann Orth (1964)

News, Notes and Queries. On the Term Diabetes in the Works of Aretaeus and Galen
Folke Henschen (1969)

Aretaeus the Cappadocian. His Contribution to Diabetes Mellitus
Eugene J. Leopold (1930)

India and China

Epistemological Fashions in Interpreting Disease. The Deleterious Effects of Western Terminology on the Application of the Scientific Tradition of Chinese Medicine (illustrated by the Case of diabetes mellitus vs. sitis diffundens (hsiao-k'o))
Manfred Porkert (1977)

The Urinary Flux of the Ancient Indians, Prameha (with Special Reference to the Carakasamhita)
Reinhold F. G. Müller (1932)

Renaissance – 19th Century

Paracelsus and the Sugar Disease
Hans Schadewaldt (1977)

The First Description of the Symptoms of Experimental Pancreatic Diabetes by the Swiss Johann Conrad Brunner (1653–1727)
Ole Christian Zimmermann

John Rollo
Alexander Marble

Matthew Dobson (1735–1784).
Clinical Investigator of Diabetes mellitus
anonymous (1967)

Then and Now: 100 Years of Diabetes mellitus
Horst and Joseph Schumacher (1956)

On the Development of Anatomical Research on the Pancreas from Vesalius to Bichat. Part I: from Vesalius to Kerckring
Hans-Michael Dittrich and Herwig Hahn von Dorsche (1975)

On the Development of Anatomical Research on the Pancreas from Vesalius to Bichat. Part II: from Borelli to Bichat
Hans-Michael Dittrich and Herwig Hahn von Dorsche (1978)

From the History of Diabetes with Particular Reference to the Pancreas
Erich Ebstein (1924)

First Steps in Claude Bernard's Discovery of the Glycogenic Function of the Liver
Mirko Dražen Grmek (1968)

The Priority Dispute between Claude Bernard and Victor Hensen about the Discovery of Glycogen
Rüdiger Porep (1971)

Paul Langerhans – Of Islets and Islands
Günther Wolff (1978)

The Discovery of Pancreatic Diabetes. The Role of Oscar Minkowski
Bernardo Alberto Houssay (1952)

Apollinaire Bouchardat 1806–1886
Elliot P. Joslin (1952)

The First Case of Diabetic Retinopathy (Eduard von Jaeger, Vienna 1853)
Franz Fischer (1957)

The History of Traumatic Diabetes
Viggo Thomsen (1938)

Insulin Precursors – a Historical Sketch. The First Attempts at Treating Diabetes with Pancreatic Extracts
Karl Heinz Leickert (1975)

Karl Petrén. A Leader in Pre-Insulin Dietary Therapy of Diabetes
Russell M. Wilder (1955)

Discovery of Insulin

On the History of the Discovery of Insulin
Joseph H. Pratt (1954)

Problems of Priority in the Discovery of Insulin
Eric Martin (1971)

Right and Wrong Avenues of Exploration in German Insulin Research
Paula Drügemöller and Leo Norpoth (1953)

50 Years of Insulin Treatment at the Vienna Hospital for Children the Fate of Diabetic Children from the First Insulin Era
W. Korp and Ernst Zweymüller (1973)

The Beginning of the Diabetic Association in England
Robert Daniel Lawrence (1952)

The Early History of the American Diabetes Association
Cecil Striker (1956)

General Development

The History of Diabetes mellitus

by Hans Schadewaldt

Introduction

"Diabetes is a mysterious illness." This statement made in antiquity by the physician Aretaeus of Cappadocia (ca. 81–138 A. D.) is still valid today. For almost two millennia the real cause of this strange ailment remained obscure. Finally, when pancreatic diabetes was discovered in 1889, and when insulin became part of the pharmaceutical armoury in 1922, it was thought that the cause and the etiological therapy of diabetes had been found. At that point, the new discoveries led to a new set of problems which presented research with further challenges. There was resistance to insulin, the action of the pancreas hormone on the metabolism of carbohydrates and fats, and new insights into pathology and electron microscopy, to cite but a few. The fact that in the first century A. D. Aretaeus could say that *". . . (Diabetes) is not at all frequent in humans"*, while in 1964, at the 5th Congress of the International Diabetes Federation in Toronto, Paul S. Entmacher and Herbert H. Marks stated that 1 in 900 healthy 25-year olds is diabetic and that this rate becomes 1 in 200 between the ages of 25 and 44, and 1 in 50 among 45 to 65-year olds, rising to 1 in 20 after the age of 65, has given much food for thought on various levels; even so, to this day the exceptional increase in cases of diabetes throughout the world cannot be explained fully.

In recent decades diabetes research has produced a deluge of literature, far too much to be mastered by any one person. The last attempt at coping with it was made by my Freiburg teacher Joseph Schumacher (1902–1966) who compiled the "Index to *Diabetes mellitus*" in 1961 on the basis of decades of study. The section on *"Literatur zur Geschichte"* ("Data on the History") consisted simply of four closely printed pages of titles, which we mention here as a guide to secondary texts (Schumacher, 1961, pp 61–64). The Index is also preceded by an equally detailed introduction (Schumacher, 1961, p. 1–34). However, we should like to single out two works that are mentioned in this index since these are monographs.

In 1952, the director of the Athens Diabetic Center, NIKOS S. PAPASPYROS, brought out a relatively modest book, "The History of Diabetes mellitus" in 1952 which is a usefulgood survey of the subject. In 1964 and enlarged and revised edition was published. Also, as valuable as ever is the work of MAX SALOMON (1837–1912), who, in 1871, compiled a *"Geschichte der Glycosurie von HIPPOKRATES bis zum Anfange des 19. Jahrhunderts"* ("History of Diabetes from Hippocrates to the Beginning of the 19th Century"). Of the voluminous writings published since the appearance of the 1961 "Index Diabeticus", we would mention only the monographs by GÜNTHER WOLFF (b. 1922), *"Zucker, Zuckerkrankheit und Insulin"* ("Sugar, Diabetes, and Insulin") (1955) and ERWIN LAUSCH'S *"Diabetes, Siege, Hoffnung und immer neue Rätsel"* ("Diabetes, Victories, Hopes, and still more Problems") (1971).

The older historians – as indeed most authors even today – chose to treat the history of diabetes purely chronologically. However, a few authors have attempted to group at least the main periods and keep them apart from one another. For instance, MEINDL has divided the history of diabetes according to its manifestation among non-European people and among those of the Occident, and also in the various periods of antiquity, the Eastern Roman Empire, the Arab world, the Middle Ages and the time of Paracelsus, followed by the so-called age of *"Diabetes anglicus"*, a therapeutic era, and an era of research into the relationship between the pathologic, physiologic and chemical metabolic processe involved. In 1919, FREDERICK MADISON ALLEN (1879–1964) proposed four phases, calling the earliest, from antiquity until the 17th century, the *period of clinical description of cases*; the second the *diagnostic period,* which he considers to have begun with THOMAS WILLIS' (1621–1675) discovery of sweetness in the urine (1674), and to have reached its climax in 1776, when MATTHEW DOBSON (1745–1784) identified the sweet substance as sugar; he called the third period that of *empirical treatment* culminating in his view in the introduction of a meat diet by JOHN ROLLO (d. 1809); the last, *experimental period,* began in 1847 with the work of CLAUDE BERNARD (1813–1878) on the problems of sugar metabolism (PAPASPYROS, p. 1).

A fourfold division, although a very different one, was suggested also by J. POULET, GERFIELD GEORGES DUNCAN (b. 1901) named the individual periods in 1951 after their most outstanding representatives: thus he called the period 1898–1914 the *Naunyn* era, 1914–1922, the *Allen* era, 1922–1936, the *Banting* era, 1936–1943, the *Hagedorn* era, and 1943–1951, the *Best* era (DUNCAN, 1951, p. 9 ff. J. P. H. HOFFMANN, p. 2).

From such studies it became clear by the time of the preliminary work on the script for the first historical film on diabetes by

Farbwerke Hoechst, which was first shown in 1966, that a purely chronological treatment of the history of diabetes was not feasible, but that it should be viewed as a kind of "hour-glass". There seemed to have been three mutually independent trends of research which did not converge until the last decades of the 19th century and which culminated in the discovery of insulin in 1921, forming, so to speak, the waist of the hour-glass. These were, first, the study of *clinical symptoms,* and, secondly *pathologic and anatomic research,* following the discovery of the functions of the pancreas, and the development of *biochemistry,* which led gradually to an understanding of the metabolic processes in the organism. Clinical work, pathology, and biochemistry are the three branches from which modern diabetes research has evolved (SCHADEWALDT, 1968). We therefore propose in the historical account that follows to examine in turn *clinical symptoms, anatomic and pathologic conditions of the pancreas,* and the *evolution of biochemical knowledge*, and then, starting with the discovery of insulin, to deal with modern methods of fighting diabetes.

Terminology

If we assume that the physician ARETAEUS (ca. A. D. 81–138) preceded GALEN (129–199), then it was he who first used the term *"diabetes"*. It stands as such at the beginning of his impressive description of the illness, although it has been impossible to decide to this day whether we are dealing with *diabetes mellitus,* as many features suggest, or with *diabetes insipidus,* ARETAEUS said:

> "And that is the reason, I believe, why the sickness has been called *diabetes,* as if it were a wine siphon, because liquid is not retained in the body but uses the human being like a tube through which it can drain itself off" (ARETAEUS, p. 133, SCHADEWALDT, 1968).

ARETAEUS' contemporary, GALEN, used the same term, and he too seems to have felt that the name *"diabetes"* could by no means be assumed to be familiar to all the physicians of his time. For he adds to his account that the sickness might be called not only *diabetes* but *Diárrhoia eís oúra,* i. e., *polyuria,* or *Hýderos eís amída (chamber-pot craving),* which soon entered the whole of medical writing in the Latin form of *hydrops ad matulam* (GALEN, vol. 7, p. 394; SALOMON, p. 493). GALEN finally knew of a third name, *Dipsakos,* the *thirst sickness,* which aptly described one of the most important symptoms of diabetes (GALEN, vol. 7, p. 394). Nearly all the other ancient authors who dealt with this odd sickness, which must have been relatively rare in Greece at the time, felt that it was necessary to elucidate further when speaking of diabetes. Thus RUFUS OF EPHESUS (ca. A. D. 98–117), that is, a contemporary of ARETAEUS and GALEN, stressed the similarities between the clinical picture of diabetes and that of Leienteria, dysentery, and suggested a second name, Leiouria *(polyuria)* (RUFUS, p. 35; SCHUMACHER, 1961, p. 2). GALEN and RUFUS thus used two practically synonymous words for what they saw as the rapid flow of liquid through the body, besides the clearly older term *"diabetes"*. CASSIUS FELIX (5th century A. D.) still thought, when writing his work on medicine, that it was necessary to expand on the term diabetes. He wrote:

"The sickness was called diabetes by the Greeks because the porousness of the internal organs caused any liquid to be eliminated through the urinary tract as soon as it was drunk, as if gushing though empty space."

It was not until we come to a – fortunately surviving – work about acute and chronic illness written in the 5th century A. D. by the Byzantine physician Caelius AURELIANUS that we learn, in a chapter about pathologic thirst, of the man who presumably coined the word. For it says:

"Apollonius of Memphis declared that a form of pathologic thirst is caused by liquid retention and another form through an incapacity to retain water, for whatever the patient drinks is immediately eliminated as if it has passed through a tube; and, in agreement with most physicians, he asserts that that type of thirst that leads to retention appears in three different kinds. But DEMETRIUS OF APAMEA has made a clear distinction between pathologic thirst and the illness in which everything that is drunk immediately is passed as urine, which he called diabetes."

As DEMETRIUS OF APAMEA was a 3rd century B. C. successor of the Alexandrian physician ERASISTRATUS, we may assume that this idea originated in that period: there was already a clear differentiation between the two basically different types of *"hydrops"*, the one in which the body retains water, and the other, in which water is eliminated immediately, a *"hydrops cum et sine retentione."*

Finally, in the 5th century A. D., a new term appeared – besides those we have mentioned – in the *"Compositiones medicamentorum"* a work produced in 17 A. D. by the Roman physician SCRIBONIUS LARGUS, who listed the word *"enkausis"*, meaning "burning" under stomach illnesses, and this Greek form was also used in the same context in the Latin version of the treatise. As this refers to an illness in which all the stomach fluids are dried out so that the patient is forced to drink jugfuls of water but can never quench his thirst, it almost certainly must be diabetes, or *"dipsakos"*, the pathologic thirst described by Greek physicians (ORTH). However, the term *"dipsakos"*, pathological thirst, survived and, besides GALEN, AETIUS, ALEXANDER OF TRALLES and PAULUS OF AEGINA are known to have used it. ARETAEUS himself considered that the word was derived from the name of a snake called *"dipsas"* whose bite produced unbearable thirst in the victim (ARETAEUS, p. 134). But the name *diabetes,* dating from the 2nd century B. C., quickly prevailed and is now used throughout the world.

German is the only language in which other names gained currency, besides the universally accepted term *diabetes*, i.e., *Zuckerharnruhr* or *Zuckerkrankheit* ("polyurie" or "sugar sickness"), which naturally could not appear until the decisive symptom, sugar in the urine, was ascertained.

Study of Clinical Symptoms

It is surprising that there is not a single reference to diabetes in the Corpus Hippocraticum. Nor does the technical term, which was clearly introduced not earlier than the 2nd century B. C. by DEMETRIUS OF APAMEA, occur in the Corpus Hippocraticum, nor do we find an account of the course of diabetes in any of the numerous highly sophisticated descriptions of illnesses. This has astonished historians of medicine to this day. However, we must remember that diabetes was relatively rarely diagnosed in antiquity. Even GALEN tells us that he only saw two cases in his life, and ARETAEUS, too, mentioned that this illness was rare among humans.

Not only in the Corpus Hippocraticum, but in the Egyptian papyri on medicine, which were edited and annotated so admirably a few years ago by HERMANN GRAPOW (1895–1967), there is no mention of any illness that resembles diabetes. Of course, these medical writings, especially the Ebers Papyrus, which seems to date from 1550 B. C., gives a number of remedies against a socalled "excess of urine" (DEINES, GRAPOW, and WESTENDORF, vol. 4,1, p. 134 seq.). The view of several authors that these are prescriptions for diabetes are not supported by any specific clinical evidence in the papyri themselves (PAPASPYROS, p. 4; WOLFF, 1955; HOLSCHER and KENDE, p. 23; OTTEN, p. 10).

This problem is posed differently in ancient Indian Sanskrit medicine, as for instance in the textbooks of the *Susruta, Charaka* and *Vagbhata*. These famous medical writings, which seem to have been produced between 300 B. C. and 600 A. D., but whose precise chronology remains uncertain, contain many references to illnesses in which *Iksumeha* (urinary sugar flux) or *Madhumeha* (honey urine) occur, and further evidence that we are dealing with real cases of diabetes is found in the additional mention of *Hastimeha*, i.e., a *"polyuria as found in a randy elephant"* or the remark that ants or insects would be attracted to such urine (SCHUMACHER, 1961, p. 4; L. L. FRANK).

The question whether ancient Indian physicians already knew of the sugar content in diabetic urine is still controversial (CHRISTIE; MEINDL, p. 5 seq.; SALOMON, p. 520; SECKENDORF; R. F. G. MÜLLER, 1942; L. L. FRANK). Urinary disorders were often thought to be related to craving for fat. Incidentally, many of the complications commonly found in diabetes today are already mentioned in ancient Indian writings. Thus all three works connected abcesses and carbuncles with urinary abnormalities, together with increasing fatigue and lethargy: this, as well as accounts of shortness of breath, somnolence and vomiting in later stages of the illness, suggests ketosis and diabetic coma (PAPASPYROS, p. 4 f.). There are therefore many indications that diabetes may have been known to ancient Indian medicine. But it is strange that this knowledge was not passed on from Indian medicine to the Greeks.

It remains uncertain whether BARACH was right in asserting that as long as 1700 years ago the Chinese and Japanese recognized that the urine of diabetics was sweet, so much so that it attracted dogs, a statement made without reference to any source and subsequently repeated uncritically by PAPASPYROS (p. 5).

The theory that sugar in the urine was recognized is contradicted by the neglect by the Chinese of urine as a basis for diagnosis (MEINDL, p. 19). On the other hand, in 1973 *GARRY* J. TEE pointed out that the relevant literature contains a treatise on diabetes written by LI HSÜAN as early as 750. The author, in his turn, had used an earlier source by CHEN CHHÜAN (d. 643). In 1970, JOSEPH NEEDHAM (b. 1900) and LU GWEI-DJEN asserted, after studying that work, that it really does contain reference to the sweetness in diabetic urine, which the authors find comparable with the observations made by WILLIS in 1674.

Whereas the term "diabetes" is used – or also used – by all post-Hippocratic medical authors when describing the relevant clinical picture, the name is missing from the first classic description by AULUS CORNELIUS CELSUS (25 B. C. to 50 A. D.) in which he stated that in cases where the urine exceeded the amount of liquid drunk and was passed painlessly, there was danger and wasting. In such cases it was necessary to take exercise and have massage, preferably in the sun or by a fire. The urine was apt to be thin, but if it became thicker physical exercise and massage had to be increased. It was also important to avoid all remedies that normally acted as diuretics. CELSUS (25 B. C.–50 A. D.) attached great importance to reducing food intake and to drinking acid wine, although in general drinking should be discouraged. Individual symptoms listed were *polyuria without spasmus, marasmus* in the advanced stages of the illness and life-threatening coma. CELSUS correctly pinpointed two of the main requisites in the modern treatment of diabetes, namely physical exercise and a correct diet. All the above symptoms can be safely assumed to refer to diabetes mellitus.

We have already mentioned that GALEN, who codified and annotated the whole of ancient medical knowledge and whose work correspondingly influenced medicine in the next 1500 years, had by his own admission seen only two cases of diabetes. At first GALEN suspected that this odd illness was caused by a kidney complaint. That organ, he thought, showed a weakness similar to that of the stomach and intestine in cases of "leienteria" which GALEN compared with diabetes: just as stomach and intestinal complaints often led to raging hunger, because the stomach craved to be filled, so the kidney craved fluid, on the ancient principle of *"horror vacui"*, but could only eliminate unmetabolized liquids (GALEN, vol. 8, p. 394 seq.). Thus GALEN was the first to connect diabetes with the organ that eliminates urine, i.e., the kidney, and for centuries this theory was reverted to again and again, linking the cause of diabetes with kidney trouble.

The best description of the clinical symptoms of diabetes came from ARETAEUS of Cappadocia (d. ca. 138 A. D.), who stated clearly that the seat and cause of the raging thirst was to be found in the stomach, and that the changes in the kidney and bladder, which he did not deny, should be regarded as side-effects. In another, earlier part of his work we find the classic description of diabetes, which was subsequently elucidated in detail in numerous works (GEMMILI; HENSCHEN; LEOPOLD; LESKY; REED; SALOMON, p. 491 seq., MANN; MEINDL, Appendix p. 10; OTTEN, 1966, p. 20; SCHADEWALDT, 1968).

ARETAEUS thought that the main cause of the illness lay in the stomach, its main symptom being a tormenting thirst, which the physician had to do his utmost to alleviate. To this end the stomach had to be cleansed with the aid of a time-honored laxative which ARETAEUS called *"hiera"* and poultices with sweet-smelling herbs were to be applied to the stomach region. Great importance was attached to diet.

All Byzantine medical writers followed GALEN in looking again and again to the kidney for the cause of diabetes, and like GALEN recommended siccative remedies to eliminate body moisture (ORIBASIUS, RUFUS, AETIUS OF AMIDA, ALEXANDER OF TRALLES, PAULUS OF AEGINA).

However, the Eastern Roman physician JOHANNES ACTUARIUS (d. 1283), who lived in the 13th century but already heralded the Middle Ages, rejected two ancient theories that had become dogma, although he accepted the rest of Galen's teaching. He did not share the view that the diabetic eliminated an amount of urine greater than the amount of liquid ingested and that the marasmus, *"macies"* was due to a dissolution of "flesh and fat", but believed that intake of fluid and elimination of urine were in equilibrium; he no longer shared the view that diabetic urine was the unaltered liquid taken, basing his explanation on the altered color of the urine. It is surprising that none of the physicians we have mentioned so far, not even ACTUARIUS, who wrote one of the first monographs on uroscopy and suggested differentiated diagnoses on the basis of urine examination, recognized the sweet flavor in the urine of diabetics.

The so-called Islamic physicians who took the relay from antiquity, did not really contribute anything significantly new. All of them – be it RHAZES (ca. 850–923), AVICENNA (980–1037) or AVENZOAR (ca. 1092–1162), eagerly embraced the tradition of GALEN, AVICENNA alone contributed something new to the discussion by introducing an Arab description for diabetes, namely *"Aldulab"*, which means water wheel, and also by distinguishing between *"lubricitas remum"*, the diabetes of the Greeks and simple harmless *"multidudo urinae"*, thus perhaps being the first to differentiate between a diagnosis of *diabetes mellitus* and one of *diabetes insipidus* (SCHADEWALDT, 1968; MEINDL, p. 35; HEINZEMANN, p. 5). AVICENNA has been credited with two additional discoveries, frist, the mention of further symptoms – besides the triad (polydipsia, polyuria and marasmus) known to antiquity – namely, physical, mental, and sexual weakness and the occurrence of carbuncles and gangrene, and secondly the alleged discovery of the sweetness of diabetic urine (SCHNEIDER).

This raises the problem of the rediscovery of the leading symptom, which, like the question whether the ancient Indians knew of the sugar content of diabetic urine, has led to lively controversy in recent years (BARACH; METTLER, p. 358; PAPASPYROS, p. 11; ACKERKNECHT, p. 144; POULET; SCHNEIDER; LEVINE; NOTELOVITZ). In 1971 HANS JÜRGEN THIES showed in a brilliant study, that the view according to which AVICENNA was aware of the sweetness of diabetic urine was based on a mistranslation made by a Tunisian colleague in 1913 which appeared in a French newspaper (RODIN; THIES, p. 27 seq.). When THIES compared the Latin translation of AVICENNA's diabetes chapters with his own German version – which, incidentally, he checked against the original Arabic – and the French translation by DINGUIZLI, he was able to show that DINGUIZLI arbitrarily changed the passage which speaks of a sweetish tendency in the odor of the urine that showed an excess of blood in the urine and that *hydromel* should be differentiated from *urine*, to mean that the dried urine had a sweet-flavored residue reminiscent of honey.

A. RESHEF showed that the famous Jewish physician and philosopher MAIMONIDES (1135–1204) in his "Aphrodisms", could cite 23 cases of diabetes, 20 in men and 3 in women as opposed to GALEN's sparse two. MAIMONIDES was surprised at the astonishing increase in cases, but ascribed this to the hot climate in Egypt, where he spent most of his life, and to the "soapy" water of the Nile (LEIBOWITZ, 1966, 1972).

From then on almost every encyclopedia of medicine and many monographs treated diabetes in the manner of GALEN. For the period 1500 to 1670, SECKENDORF has cited no fewer than 100 authors who dealt with diabetes.

It was not until PARACELSUS (1493–1541) that a significant new element was brought into the debate. He had already distanced himself considerably from the old Galenic system in his writings and was the first to take a fresh etiologic view by suggesting that diabetes had its cause in the presence of a so-called "dry salt", which could attach itself to the kidneys and affect them as tartar did a cask of wine. In fact, he was the first to have the concept of diabetes as a general illness and sought its origin in some change in the composition of the blood (PARACELSUS, vol. 5, p. 103 f. and 145; vol. 11, p. 15 f.). This "salt" generated in the blood caused, PARACELSUS thought, the thirst in diabetics: its precipitation in the kidney and finally in the urine, where PARACELSUS had already observed octahedral crystals (MEINDL, p. 39; SALOMON, p. 304) he ascribed to a failure of a regulating force, the so-called *"archeus"*. In this connection PARACELSUS also spoke of a *"dulcedo"* of the urine (SECKENDORF), but by this he did not mean a sweetish sugary taste (PARACELSUS, vol. 5, p. 103). It seems highly likely that, during his experiments to obtain that "salt" by distilling urine, he may have found a residue of grape-sugar (PAPASPYROS, p. 12). Even if we cannot ascribe the detection of urinary sugar to PARACELSUS, it is undeniable that his theory on the origins of diabetes greatly influenced further research and directed attention away from the kidney as the local seat of the illness to an examination of the blood and the general metabolism.

However, many of PARACELSUS' contemporaries and successors, e.g., JEAN FERNEL (1497–1558), MARCELLO DONATI (1538–1602), ANDREA CESALPINO (1519–1603), clung to GALEN's view that diabetes had its seat in the kidney and that it originated in a kidney complaint and in an excessive production of urine, which was in itself identical to the fluid consumed. On the other hand, the view first propounded by PARACELSUS that the causes of diabetes are to be found in other factors, especially the blood, gradually began to make its way (HELMONT; DE LE BOË SYLVIUS; SALOMON, p. 510; MEINDL, p. 44).

WILLIS was clearly the first to investigate the sweetness of the urine and in 1674 he reported on the detection of a honey-like flavor. He pointed out that diabetes had previously been a rare disease which had become more common in his day; he also considered the polyuria to be a blood disorder, but added the strange sweet taste to the symptoms that were already known: *". . . quasi melle aut saccharo imbutam, mire dulcescere."* According to WILLIS, the honey-like taste of urine was due to a precipitate of "salt" and "sulphur" in the blood, which underwent a kind of putrefaction process as a result of an increased influx of liquefied body substances. In this way WILLIS combined the ancient views of corruption of the blood with iatrochemical concepts which culminated in the attempt to make certain localized chemical substances responsible for all illnesses. Thirst and the craving to consume ever larger quantities of liquid were explained by the rapid loss of fluid entering the blood-stream and the salts deposited in the blood. This also served to account for the weight-loss and growing weakness through a wastage of body tissue. Therapy consequently consisted of preventing the deposition of "salt" and "sulphur" which he though would be accomplished by means of fattening foods like rice and certain gum preparations, as well as a milk diet and above all alkaline chalky fluids.

The detection of the sugary taste of diabetic urine was to have direct consequences although it was another century before an English chemist, MATTHEW DOBSON (1745–1784), succeeded in retrieving a residue from diabetic urine which resembled brown sugar. For it was now noticed that not all cases of *"polyuria"* exhibited the symptom described by WILLIS, and MICHAEL ETTMUELLER (1644–1683), in his posthumous *"Opera"* which appeared in 1685, was the first to distinguish between *"diabetes notha"* and *"diabetes vera"*. *"Diabetes notha"* exhibited the symptoms typical of sweet polyuria, whereas these were absent in *"diabtes vera"* (ZANDER, p. 44 seq.). The differentiation between true and false diabetes was also made in 1711 by MICHAEL BERNHARD VALENTINI (1657–1729) (VEITH).

Another factor that undoubtedly led to further differentiation, apart from the detection of a sweet honey-like flavor in the case of some diabetics, was the classification of illnesses compiled in 1783 by FRANÇOIS BOISSIER DE SAUVAGES (1706–1767) – on the lines of CARL VON LINNE'S (1707–1778) classification of plants – in which he listed 7 kinds of diabetes.

In 1794, stimulated by SAUVAGES' classification, JOHANN PETER FRANK (1745–1821) undertook the differentiation of 3 separate types of diabetes, which he called *"diabetes insipidus seu spurius"*, *"diabetes mellitus seu verus"* and *"diabetes decipiens"* (deceptive polyuria) (MAIWALD).

The adjective "insipidus" was used earlier, in 1769, by WILLIAM CULLEN (1709–1790), who grouped diabetes under neuroses, and applied the term "diabetes mellitus" to the type in which a sweet substance is found in the urine and to the other, in which this substance appeared to be lacking, "insipidus" (tasteless). CULLEN, incidentally, mentioned the liver as well as the kidney as seat and source of the illness.

FRANK'S clear classification finally led to the differentiation of these two forms of polyuria. Most other authors who dealt with the subject at that time contributed little that was new. With the differentiation between diabetes mellitus and diabetes insipidus and DOBSON'S identification, a few decades earlier, of the sweet residue in diabetic urine as sugar, the basic clinical symptoms that are still valid to this day were defined. Glycosuria was added to the symptoms known in antiquity.

Two further significant discoveries concerning the clinical symptoms of diabetes should be mentioned. In 1880 ETIENNE LANCEREAUX (1829–1910), who had been making an intensive study of diabetes since 1877 and was the first to suspect a link with the pancreas, created a subdivision of two different kinds of diabetes: *"diabète maigre"* and *"diabète gras"*. LACEREAUX had noticed that *"diabète gras"* responded relatively easily to an appropriate diet whereas *"diabète maigre"*, resisting all therapeutic efforts, continued to develop and was incurable (POULET).

In 1874 ADOLF KUSSMAUL reported on the "strange manner of death in diabetics". He had been able from 1872 closely to follow three cases of acute diabetes, all of which ended fatally, in which he observed a strange kind of "dyspnoea" – today named *"Kussmaul's hard breathing"* after him – increased cardiac activity, notable agitation with groaning and screaming with jactitation, and in the final stage a loss of awareness such as he had previously seen only in a uraemic coma. In view of the similarities of the clinical picture to uraemia, although differing from it considerably in the hard breathing, he called it *"diabetic coma"* and thereby introduced yet another important clinical symptom into the study of diabetes; in his day, it was an indication of the approaching end, although fortunately today it can often be controlled. In almost every case the patients concerned exuded a smell like apples or violets: in 1857 WILHELM PETTERS (1820–1875) was the first to attribute this to acetone shown to be in diabetic urine. In 1860 JOSEPH KAULICH (1830–1886) was able to confirm this and produced the first clinical picture of *acidosis*.

However, we should mention that, as early as 1711, VALENTINI described a case in which the patient's body gave off a pungent smell, which was also given off by the urine. Clinical pictures resembling comas had also been observed before KUSSMAUL in 1842 by WILLIAM PROUT (1785–1850); in 1854 by HENRY MARSH (1790–1860); and in the same year, by THEODOR VON DUSCH (1824–1890).

Anatomic and Pathologic Findings

Whereas in antiquity ARETAEUS ascribed diabetes to a basic stomach disorder and his contemporary and adversary GALEN saw the kidney as the seat of the illness – a theory that dominated medicine for centuries – THOMAS SYDENHAM (1624–1689) initiated the theory that the digestive tract was a more likely source of diabetic complaints, and RICHARD MEAD (1673–1754) saw the liver as the culprit, while CULLEN considered diabetes a neurosis stemming from the whole nervous system. But the organ that held the true solution to the problem, the pancreas, remained practically unnoticed until the 19th century, at least in connection with diabetes (SCHADEWALDT, 1964; SCHIRMER; E. EBSTEIN, 1924; M. FRANK, 1916).

Undoubtedly the pancreas was known to HEROPHILUS (325–280 B. C.) and ERASISTRATUS (310–250 B. C.), two Greek physicians working in Alexandria, whose writings, however, have been passed down only through GALEN. The famous Pergamon physician also reported that RUFUS, and before him even EUDEMUS around 300 B. C., knew of that odd organ but there was no agreement on its function. There were three theories on its functions. The Alexandrian doctors seemed to think – and this must be treated with great caution – that certain fluids, similar to saliva, were secreted from this gland into the intestines, although GALEN thought that unlikely (GALEN, vol. 4, p. 646). He himself held the view that the gland was simply one of the organs intended to fill certain hollow spaces – as did, it was believed, the parotid gland – or, possibly, to protect the blood-vessels on the spinal column from the pressure they might sustain when the stomach was full (GALEN, vol. 3, p. 344).

The followers of Hippocrates, on the other hand, regarded this glandular body as a kind of sponge that soaked up fluid from the intestine and eventually passed it on into the mesentery (GALEN, vol. 8, p. 561). In view of the high esteem in which the Greek physician was held in the West, it is not surprising that his theory that the pancreas had a merely mechanical protective function ran like a thread through medical works throughout the Middle Ages and to the beginning of modern times. The organ was often considered analogous to the thymus, which, however, becomes atrophied in adults and turns into an insignificant fatty body.

In German popular parlance the pancreas was called *Bauchdrüse, große Magendrüse, Wampenbries, Gekrösedrüse, Magenrücklein* (stomach gland, intestinal gland, stomach backing, etc.) (E. EBSTEIN, 1924; HÖFLER), and its function regarded even by anatomists as that of a support *(fulcimentum)* or cushion *(polvinarum)* (M. FRANK; SCHADEWALDT, 1964; SCHIRMER, p. 10; CLAESSEN).

Then two new anatomic discoveries threw a fresh light on the debate: in 1641 MORITZ HOFMAN (1622–1698) was the first to discover the *"doctus pancreaticus"* in the turkey. Soon afterwards, JOHANN GEORG WIRSUNG (1600–1643) succeeded in finding a similar duct in a human body, but he did not really know what to do with it and wrote to his Paris teacher, JEAN RIOLAN (1577–1657) to ask him about its function. As WIRSUNG was killed shortly afterwards in a duel, we have only the letter referred to and a copperplate engraving ordered by him on which his discovery is recorded (SCHIRMER, p. 14; MORGENSTERN).

This disposed of the old thesis that the pancreas was a support or filler, but now a long quarrel ensued as to whether the duct served to absorb the fluid from the liver and spleen – as RIOLAN conjectured in his reply – so that the pancreas was a kind of filter through which the chyle could be cleaned, or whether a fluid was secreted from the gland through the duct, as THOMAS BARTHOLIN (1641–1673) surmised. Soon afterwards DE LE BOË assumed correctly that lymph was produced by the blood in the gland itself and then transmitted to the intestine where it was mixed with food (GRAAF, p. 34). Now interest became concentrated on the lymph itself, and in 1664 REIGNIER DE GRAAF (1641–1673), a student of DE LE BOË, set up the first experiment to clarify its function (GRAAF, p. 65 f.; METTLER, p. 126; SCHADEWALDT, 1964).

A second author, BERNHARD SWALWE (d. ca. 1680) wrote a book on these questions without, however, recording any significant new experiments. Thus, in the last decades of the 17th century it was clear that the pancreas must be a gland secreting a gastric juice, but the significance of both the organ and its secretion was clearly understood. In 1798 the anatomist SAMUEL THOMAS SOEMMERRING (1755–1830) coined the German name *"Bauchspeicheldrüse"* (abdominal salivary gland) which has survived to this day.

From 1682, JOHANN CONRAD BRUNNER (1653–1727), born in Schaffhausen and later personal physician in Düsseldorf and professor in Heidelberg, pursued the question of pancreatic function in the animal organism: he hoped to find an answer by means of experimental ligature and extirpation. Undoubtedly these experiments led to the appearance of temporary diabetes symptoms, but BRUNNER did not recognize them and missed the discovery of pancreatic diabetes by a hair's breadth. It was not until 1889, some 200 years later, that proof thereof was produced by MERING's and MINKOWSKI's experiments.

BRUNNER has left an impressive illustration of his procedures. He obviously recognized and described the most important symptoms of diabetes, polydipsia, polyphagia, and polyuria, and clearly described the atrophy of the endocrine parts through dissection.

BRUNNER believed that his experiments proved the pancreas to be a dispensable organ, and this explains why research turned away from the pancreas to other apparently more interesting subjects. Thus BRUNNER's impressive animal experiments inhibited research into diabetes and the pancreas for almost 200 years (ZIMMERMANN, MAJOR).

In 1775, 100 years after BRUNNER, THEOPHILE DE BORDEU, a French physician (1722–1776) was the first to express the view that every organ could put certain substances not only into the organs of evacuation but directly into the blood where they would affect the whole organism. This theory, put forward with great caution, was supported in a dissertation by JULIEN JEAN CESAR LEGALLOIS (1770–1814), who stated that certain substances were obviously mixed into the blood from the body and would produce specific effects on sites other than those where they originated. Of course, it was not until 1878, when the anatomist RUDOLF HEIDENHAIN (1834–1897) observed the effect of certain nerve stimuli on glandular secretion that the older, purely mechanical theory of saliva production was laid to rest. It was not until 1904, first, when WILLIAM MADDACK BAYLISS (1860–1924) and ERNEST HENRY STARLING (1866–1927) established their theory of the so-called "chemical regulation" of the secretionary processes and then, a year later, when, on W. B. HARDY's suggestion, STARLING in his famous Croonian Lecture adopted the term hormones – from *hormáo* = I send – for these "chemical messengers"and inscribed it in medical terminology that the circle was closed that began with BRUNNER's experiments with extirpation of the pancreas and led to the explanation of the causes of pancreatic diabetes.

Meanwhile other initiatives came, not from anatomy but from pathology. In 1789 THOMAS CAWLEY was able to describe unambiguous diabetic symptoms, like polyphagia, polydipsia, polyuria, glycosuria, marasmus and convulsions – which today would be considered as comatose – and in this connection drew attention to the fact that on dissection of the dead patient, the pancreatic duct was blocked by calculi, but he did not dare to incorporate his pathologic findings into the clinical picture of the illness (E. EBSTEIN, 1924; SCHIRMER, p. 42. f.; SCHADEWALDT, 1964; SPIEGELHOFF, p. 53 seq.).

It seems that in 1864 JOSEPH ALEXANDER FLES(?) (1819–1905) was the first to link the atrophy which he found in the pancreas on dissection – although in this case the liver was equally affected – with diabetes mellitus in the patient when he was alive. FLES had already reported treatment of cases through oral administration of calf's pancreas which was supposed to have a beneficial effect on the digestive shortcomings. However, the fatal outcome could not be prevented (SCHADEWALDT, 1964).

We have already mentioned that MORGAGNI paid little attention to the pancreas and does not seem to have carried out a single dissection on a diabetic. In 1854, almost 100 years later, RUDOLF VIRCHOW (1821–1902) triggered off a renewed interest in the gland among anatomists and pathologists. He asserted broadly:

". . . so it is reasonable to assume that the pancreas prepares certain substances for the liver and that this gland secretes not only outwardly but also inwardly into the blood . . ."

Meanwhile, in the second decade of the 19th century, a kind of reaction to the romantic movement in medicine set in the shape of a new era of exact scientific research in Germany and also in France. Particular attention was paid to physiologic processes and soon detailed knowledge of the function of pancreatic juices could be gathered. This development originated in France from 1817 on with FRANCOIS MAGENDIE (1783–1853), and in Germany with FRIEDRICH

TIEDEMANN (1781–1861) and LEOPOLD GMELIN (1788–1853) as well as JUSTUS VON LIEBIG (1803–1873) and his school, who founded the new discipline of "animal chemistry" in 1840 (MANI, p. 249 seq.). The capacity of pancreatic juices to break down carbohydrates as well as fats and proteins was first mentioned by JOHANN NEPOMUK EBERLE (1789–1834) in the monograph he published in the year of his death. In 1867, WILLI KÜHNE (1837–1900) succeeded in isolating the pancreatic enzyme that breaks down protein, which he named "trypsin" in 1877, after ALEXANDER DANILEWSKI (1839–1923) in 1862 had succeeded in obtaining the active digestive principle by grinding down pancreatic substance with sand.

In 1867 KÜHNE was working in RUDOLF VIRCHOV's Institute of Pathology so that it was hardly accidental that a young research student, PAUL LANGERHANS (1847–1888), began to study the microscopic anatomy of the pancreas in that institute. In 1869 he published his 32-page thesis for the doctorate which now is considered one of the classics of medicine (V. BECKER; HELLMANN and KÄLJEDAL; KLOPPE; GIACOMETTI and BARSS; MORRISON; VOSS; CAMPBELL). In the first instance it deals with the differentiation of the different groups of cells in the pancreas, which BERNARD had already noticed before LANGERHANS, LANGERHANS managed to differentiate nine separate groups of pancreatic cells. Without going into their physiologic function, LANGERHANS described the ninth group, the "island cells" later named after him:

"Their content ist homogeneous, glossy and free from any kind of grain, their nucleus light, round, and of medium-size. Their diameter is 0.0096 to 0.012 mm, that of the nucleus 0.0075 to 0.008 mm.

These cells mostly lie close together in large numbers, peculiarly distributed in the parenchyma of the gland . . . They are thus distributed in the parenchyma (in the old sense of the word) of the gland crowded together in somewhat rounded heaps at regular intervals . . ."

LANGERHANS's modest thesis did not have a single illustration, which explains why it did not make a greater impact and why neither he nor VIRCHOW subsequently returned to this line of research. Nevertheless the cells described by LANGERHANS are mentioned again and again in the literature of the years that followed (KÜHNE and LEA; SAVIOTTI; HEIDENHAIN; PODWYSSOTZKY; GIBBES; LEWASCHEW). In 1893 it was EDOUARD LAGUESSE (1861–1927) who called these cell groups *"îlots de Langerhans"* after their original reporter and noted that they existed already in the fetus, in fact were found more frequently there than in the adult subjects, which later led BANTING and BEST to turn to calf embryos in their experiments to obtain insulin.

Of course, the quest to solve the puzzle of the function fulfilled by these strange island cells did not end there. LANGERHANS had to admit that he *"saw no possible explanation"*. Some authors assumed that they were dealing with lymphoid cells (KÜHNE and LEA; SOKOLOFF; MOURET, 1894; MacLEOD, 1927, p. 1), a view which LANGERHANS had already rejected (HARRIS and GOW; DIAMARE, 1895; SCHÄFER, 1895) and which lost all credibility in 1902 when GENTES was able to observe that in cases of leukemia Langerhans islets did not share in the hypertrophy that affected the whole lymphatic system.

Some thought that a co-enzyme for the exocrine functions was produced in these cells, perhaps in conjunction with the spleen (HARRIS and GOW; SAJOUS), but this theory was contradicted by the absence of evacuatory ducts, the persistence of the islets of Langerhans after the destruction of the secretory pancreatic tissue and other similar objections. Nor was there any evidence for the view that these cells represented a reversion of spent acinar glands (LEWASCHEW TSCHASSONIKOW). This was chiefly contradicted by the rich blood-supply to that system.

We can say that the internal secretion of the pancreas, which VIRCHOW had already suspected, was first traced to the so-called islets of Langerhans by LAGUESSE in 1893.

Here we must mention briefly that as early as 1899 VINCENZO DIAMARE (1872–1960) had postulated two types of cells in the islets of Langerhans (TSCHASSOWNIKOW; SCHULZE; SSOBOLEW; DEWITT; BENSLEY; FERNER).

In 1907 SIR WILLIAM ARBUTHNOT LANE (1856–1943), who has hitherto been wrongly regarded as the discoverer of these two cell systems in the islets of Langerhans, called the two cell types A- and B-cells and differentiated them according to the solubility of the granules.

Until the middle of the 19th century the kidneys, the stomach and finally the liver were thought to be the site of diabetes. It is therefore not surprising that pathologists were more apt to investigate diabetics' liver and kidneys, taking little notice of the pancreas. In particular, the research done in 1847 by CLAUDE BERNARD (1813–1878), which led to the discovery of glycogens in the liver, diverted interest to that important organ, which obviously had a special part to play in the formation of sugar. Then, in 1849, the publication of information on BERNARD's "piqûre", a procedure whereby a transitory glycosuria could be induced, drew attention to the vasomotor nervous system, a term introduced in 1840 by BENEDICT STILLING (1810–1879) (SCHUMACHER, 1961, p. 17). This was the basis for the theory of so-called *"angioneurotic diabetes"* (UHLE; SCHRADER; P. J. BECKER; KÜHNE; SCHIFF).

Medical scientists were fascinated by the possibility that the destruction or stimulation of certain nerve tracts or the effect of certain poisons, like curare, chloroform, ether, etc., or even simply the shackling of animals used in experiments could induce artificial glycosuria (PAVY; ECKARD; KLEBS; MUNK; HENSEN; NAUNYN); and in 1897, long after MERING's and MINKOWSKI's epoch-making experiments of 1889 and KUSSMAUL's clear-cut description in 1874, it was even possible for ADOLF VON STRÜMPELL (1853–1925) to describe the diabetic coma as "the most important symptom due to the nervous system". In 1892 JULES THIROLOIX (1861–1932) could still speak of *"diabète nerveuse"* and EDUARD PFLÜGER (1829–1910), the German physiologist, became a passionate champion of this concept and a bitter and personal opponent of the supporters of *"pancreatic diabetes"*.

Probably the first to postulate, in 1852, the close link between diabetes mellitus and pancreatic disorders was the French pharmacist, hygienist and chemist APOLLINAIRE BOUCHARDAT (1806–1882). Then, in 1875, NIKOLAUS FRIEDREICH (1825–1882) also concluded, after thorough discussion of a case he had himself observed, that the combination of the two illnesses was not a coincidence, though he still explained it as due to the sympathetic nerve ganglia, especially the celiac ganglion and the celiac plexus (SPIEGELHOFF, p. 54). LANCEREAUX was more positive about the direct etiological connection between pancreatic illness and diabetes, and in 1877 was the first to regard this special – as he thought – form of diabetes, which often seemed to be identical with *"diabète gras"*, as *"diabète pancréatique"*.

Admittedly, the experiments, carried out from the time of BERNARD onwards, in which the pancreatic duct was blocked by means of fat or paraffin in order to obtain precise indications of pancreatic function led to atrophy of most of the gland but never to diabetes. Whereas BERNARD, in his experiments carried out from 1855 onwards, was mainly concerned with the effect of pancreatic lymph on the digestion, in 1884 CHARLES LOUIS XAVIER ARNOZAN and LOUIS VAILLARD (1850–1935) drew attention for the first time to this strange discrepancy between the atrophy of the whole gland following the blocking of the pancreatic duct and the absence of diabetic symptoms.

Two years later, in 1886, JOSEPH VON MERING (1845–1908) succeeded, with the aid of phlorizin in inducing a so-called *"experimental transitory diabetes"*, which – as soon became apparent – was due to the poisoning of certain pancreatic areas which particularly affected the islets of Langerhans. Even so, the anatomic and pathologic evidence remained inconclusive. During an edifying historical survey of pancreatic diabetes, which he gave in Strasbourg in 1929,NAUNYN, OSKAR MINKOWSKI's (1858–1931) famous teacher, said (or so his students report):

"There is nothing more tedious than the dissection of a diabetic, except the dissection of two diabetics."

Thus, in 1889, MERING's and MINKOWSKI's short (barely one page in length) report on *"diabetes mellitus after extirpation of the pancreas"* had the effect of a thunderbolt. In earlier years the pancreas of animals had already been removed in daring experiments. BERNARD, who had attempted the extirpation of the gland on several occasions, thought it was not feasible because of its close connection with the duodenum and went on – as we have said – to destroy the gland by injecting fat into Wirsung's duct. Nor did other authors succed in removing the gland entirely (BERNARD and COLIN; MARTINOTTI; KLEBS).

MERING and MINKOWSKI undertook their experiment in connection with a completely different problem and, as MINKOWSKI himself admitted, owed its success to chance (NOTHMAN). MERING had been concentrating in Strasbourg mainly on reabsorption of fats. But even ligature of the excretory ducts of the pancreas was insufficient to keep pancreatic lymph from the intestine because there were a number of pancreatic channels of which the authors could not yet know. MINKOWSKI suggested to MERING that he should extirpate the pancreas. He had acquired particular dexterity from similar experiments, and so, on the very day of their conversation, the first dog was operated on with MERING's assistance. Neither of the two physicians imagined that the dog would experience any further problems since it had safely recovered from the operation and the wound had healed. MERING himself had to go away for a week because of illness in his family, and the dog, which had been fully housetrained before, urinated several times indoors and made life hell for the laboratory servant. Acting on a sudden hunch, MINKOWSKI examined the urine and found a high proportion of sugar. He quickly operated on a few more dogs, which he tested to make sure they were free of sugar before the operation, and all of them developed severe diabetes.

MERING's and MINKOWSKI's highly economical but scientifically precise and incisive report is a shining example of how such findings should be presented.

The first short report mentioned not only the fact of glycosuria but the typical clinical symptoms of a rapidly fatal case of diabetes. The authors had also determined the sugar content in the blood and found hyperglycemia, had shown that there was acetone in the urine, had disproved the angioneurotic thesis claiming that diabetes could be caused by an injury to the celiac plexus, and finally, through experimental transfusion, had proved that the diabetogenic substance could not be in the bloodstream: therefore the hypothetical diabetic poison did not exist and the pancreas itself had to be the source of the illness, since a dog with its pancreas intact did not develop diabetes in spite of a transfusion of blood from a diabetic dog.

This, one would think, fulfilled all the criteria for proving that the pancreas was the site of diabetes, yet MINKOWSKI met with bitter opposition from EDUARD PFLÜGER (1829–1910), who continued until 1908 to attack these experiments involving extirpation of the pancreas and claimed that the results were due to an injury to the celiac plexus in the abdomen during the operation.

The most decisive confirmation of all, was the fact that ligature of the excretory ducts led to atrophy of the gland, but not to diabetes, whereas their total removal resulted in the appearance of diabetic symptoms leading to death. This showed that the pancreas must contain an anatomical substratum whose absence was responsible for the development of diabetes. MERING and MINKOWSKI did not yet mention the islets of Langerhans. Their significance did not become clear until subsequent experiments succeeded in destroying the exocrine parts of the pancreas through ligatures while leaving the islets of Langerhans intact.

NICOLAS DE DOMINCIS, who was undertaking similar extirpation experiments in Italy at the same time, reported on them in 1889, DE DOMINICIS thought that diabetes was not – as MERING and MINKOWSKI believed – caused by direct action, but by an indirect effect on the inhibiting exocrine function. This led to abnormal breakdown of foodstuffs and the production of diabetes toxins, whose secondary effect was the development of glycosuria. Shortly afterwards, ENRICO RENZI (1839–1921) and ENRICO REALE in Italy and THIROLOIX, GLEY, HEDON and MOURET in France also succeeded in inducing diabetes symptoms in animals through the removal of the pancreas.

MINKOWSKI soon found that feeding pancreas to dogs whose own pancreas had been removed did not lead to any improvement in their diabetes. But when he implanted pancreas subcutaneously, the symptoms disappeared relatively soon. Starting in 1892, HEDON, too, successfully undertook such transplants and was able, in 1898, to conclude on the basis of his experiments that the pancreas secreted an internal substance that was essential for the metabolism of sugar.

From 1909 to 1913, HEDON, like MINKOWSKI, carried out parabiotic experiments in which he linked a healthy dog with one without a pancreas and he noticed a decrease in the sugar elimination of the dog without a pancreas. When the parabiotic experiment was stopped, the diabetic animal immediately exhibited typical diabetic symptoms again (LOUBATIERES, 1953, DULIEU).

A further step in the elucidation of the seat of diabetes came from the observation that diabetic patients frequently exhibited changes in the pancreas, especially in the islets of Langerhans (HANSEMANN; SPIEGELHOFF, p. 54). In 1895 CHRISTIAN DIECKHOFF, for instance, identified 49 different kinds of pancreatic disease in 53 cases of such disease.

From 1893 onwards, LAGUESSE's work made it increasingly clear that the islet cells actually had to be regarded in terms of an intervally secretory organ. In 1899 DIAMARE was able to detect such a cell system in every type of animal he examined. Then, between 1900 and 1906, WALTER SCHULZE, EUGENE LINDSAY OPIE and LYDIA DEWITT(b. 1859), and SSOBOLEW (1846–1919), independently confirmed the results of ligature experiments that DITTMAR FINKLER (1852–1912) had reported in 1880 as incidental findings during his investigation of the necrosis of fatty tissue.

SSOBOLEW, EUGENE LINDSAY OPIE(1873–1962) in 1900 ANTON WEICHSELBAUM (1845–1920), in 1901 E. STANGL, in 1901 JAMES HOMER WRIGHT (1871–1928) and ELLIOT PROCTOR JOSLIN (1869–1962) as well as HERZOG in 1902 had found in several cases of diabetes that islets of Langerhans were missing or that there was hydropic degeneration with formation of vacuoles, calcification and sclerosis. In 1906, WILHELM HEIBERG (1853–1920) of Copenhagen developed a special method for counting the islets exactly and found that the count was consistently low in diabetics (MACCALLUM; LUSK; MINKOWSKI, 1929; SCHUMACHER, 1961, p. 21).

These experiments and findings gradually allowed the theory of *"pancreatic diabetes"* to supplant that of *"angioneurotic diabetes"* (BERNARD, PFLÜGER). As long ago as 1909 JEAN DE MEYER (b. 1878), a Belgian, coined the word *"insulin"*, long before the precipitate itself was discovered. The word was also used by SIR ALBERT SHARPEY-SCHÄFER (1850–1935) in 1916.

Biochemical Findings

It was not until 1674 that WILLIS rediscovered one of the most important indisputable symptoms of diabetes, the sweet flavour of the urine, but it still took some time before *"honey sweetness"* of diabetic urine was identified as sugar, and finally as glucose, WILLIS himself still believed that the sweetness in the urine was due to a compound of salts and sulphur. It was not until 1776, a century later, that the Liverpool physician DOBSON was the first successfully to obtain a residue from the urine of several diabetic patients which was the equivalent of sugar in flavor and appearance (SCHADEWALDT, 1968; SALOMON p. 551 seq.; EBSTEIN 1915, p. 17; LIPPMANN).

It was also capable of fermentation and when blood serum was left to stand it too acquired the sweet flavor. However, DOBSON did not succeed in isolating a sugar-like substance from the blood serum. When the patient was better, it was impossible to obtain that white residue. This led DOBSON to the conclusion that diabetes could not originate in the kidney, since the blood evinced a flavor similar to that of the urine. The sweet flavor in the blood he was also able to detect in healthy people. The sugary substance must be an interim produkt of digestion and was still as capable of fermentation as barley containing a large amount of sugar. Thus diabetes had to be a general metabolic disorder accompanied by inadequate digestion, and seemed to resemble fermentation. Thus DOBSON was the first to identify the similarity to sugar in the residue found in diabetic urine, as he was the first to observe hyperglycemia in diabetics and the presence of sugar in healthy blood; he was also the first to point to fermentation of diabetic urine as a diagnostic method.

DOBSON'S observations were taken up immediately by his Edinburgh compatriot FRANCIS HOME (1719–1813), who, in 1780, developed the *fermentation test,* the first clinical method of testing diabetic urine. From one pound of urine, i.e., about 360 g, he was able to extract one ounce of the sugary substance. In 1788–1789 CAWLEY had diagnosed diabetes on the basis of the presence of sugar in the urine, JOHANN PETER FRANK, too, distinguished between neutral and sugary-sweet urine, and thickened diabetic urine over fire to extract a honey-like, brown sugary substance. He noticed the spontaneous fermentation of tartaric or acetic acid and he was able to obtain crystals allegedly of saccharic acid, ethyl alcohol and vinegar. When he wrote that during evaporation pleasant scents could be noticed, he must have been referring to acetone or acetoacetic acid (MAIWALD).

A third, English physician, JOHN ROLLO (d. 1809) who deserves special mention for his contribution to the treatment of diabetes through diet – he introduced the so-called meat diet – carried out a series of tests on the blood of two diabetic patients whom he was able to follow closely. He noticed that diabetic blood did not decompose after being left for days, whereas healthy blood showed traces of deterioration after as little as four days. Although ROLLO was unable to produce direct proof of the sugar content in the blood, he was able to halt the process of degeneration in healthy blood by adding a little sugar, which showed indirectly that there was a strong probability that sugar was present in diabetics (SALOMON, p. 378).

But it was still unclear what kind of sugar it was. In 1806 and 1815, DUPUYTREN, THENARD and MICHEL EUGENE CHEVREUL (1786–1889) surmised that it must be grape-sugar. Although in 1811 WILLIAM HYDE WOLLASTON (1766–1828), to whom we owe the first examination employing some kind of paper chromatography, was unable to prove the presence of sugar in diabetic blood by the relatively crude method of the period, whereas as early as 1802 PIERRE FRANÇOIS NICOLAS and C. V. GEUDEVILLE claimed to have established the presence of sugar in diabetic blood by means of a qualitative method, finally, in 1835, FELICI AMBROSIANI was able to obtain small colorless sugar crystals from both the urine and blood of diabetics (SCHUMACHER, 1961, p. 14; HOFFMANN, p. 10). Finally, in 1838, EUGENE BOUCHARDAT and EUGENE MELCHIOR PELIGOT (1811–1890) succeeded in confirming CHEVREUL's surmise that the sugar found in diabetic urine was glucose. At around the same time the fact that normal blood contains sugar became known, especially through the work of FRANCOIS MAGENDIE (1783–1855) in 1846 and BERNARD in 1855, but it was not until 1862 that FREDERICK WILLIAM PAVEY (1829–1911) expounded the direct link between hyperglycemia and glycosuria and demonstrated their mutual dependence (HOFFMANN, p. 14).

The fact that the isolated sugar was glucose soon led to the development of simple urine tests. The oldest, after HOME's above-mentioned "fermentation test", was KARL AUGUSTUS TROMMER's (1806–1879) which he announced in 1841. He used a copper sulfate solution and caustic potash as reagent. In 1848, the Stuttgart chemist HERMANN VON FEILING (1812–1885) published the formula named after him which was already capable of giving a quantitative value for the sugar content in the urine (WOLFF, 1955). These and other methods developed at the time (MOORE, 1844; HELLER, 1844) were based either on the reduction of certain copper solutions through glucose or on the fermentation of sugarcontaining urine, a notable example being the test devised in 1850 by KARL GOTTHELF LEHMANN (1812–1863) (SCHUMACHER, 1961, p. 14) with which BERNARD carried out his first diagnoses of blood sugar. The principle of reduction was also the basis of subsequent tests, as for instance those made in 1883 by the Swedish chemist EMIL NYLANDER (1835–1907), for which bismuth subnitrate was used, and those favoured in America in 1907 by the physiological chemist STANLEY ROSSITER BENEDICT (1844–1936) which again were based on the reduction of copper sulfate. First published in 1874, the test devised by the American chemist WALTER STANLEY HAINES (1850–1923) represented a further step towards a rough quantitative estimate, and was considerably improved in 1920 (HAINES int. al.).

Evidence for sugar in the blood was far more problematic. For his first examinations of blood sugar, BOUCHARDAT needed vast quantities of blood to test about 300 ml. Until 1908, when IVAR CHRISTIAN BANG (1869–1918) first introduced microanalysis with 10 ml, attempts at routine examinations to determine blood sugar met with three major difficulties. It was extremely difficult to separate the protein from the sugar in the blood. Each analysis took a long time: 2 days in the 19th century, and a whole took 3 hours as late as 1908 (BANG, 1908). It was not until 1910 that the test could be carried out in under 30 minutes. Finally, a relatively large quantity of blood was needed. Following the microanalytic methods of BANG and his collaborators, greater importance attached to the methods used by of ROBERT CURTIS LEWIS (b. 1888) and BENEDICT in 1915, which needed only 0.5 ml of blood, those used by VICTOR CARYL MYERS (1876–1951) and C. V. BAILEY (1887–1953) in 1916, which, incidentally, were used in 1921 by the medical student, BEST, and those used by KNUT OLOF FOLIN'S (1867–1934) and HSIEN WU'S (1863–1955) in 1919, as well as HANS CHRISTIAN HAGEDORN'S (b. 1888) and NORMAN B. JENSEN'S well known procedure, dated from 1923.

Thus, by the middle of the 19th century, it was clear that diabetes was a disorder of sugar metabolism, but it was not until BERNARD'S brilliant research that the process of sugar formation was explained. This were preceded by BERNARD'S experiments to induce a *"diabète artificiel"*, on which he first reported on 23 February 1849 to the prestigious "Société de Biologie" in Paris (GRMEK, 1966; YOUNG; PFLÜGER, 1905; SELMI).

After a lengthy research, which began in 1853, BERNARD was finally able to prove – with the aid of the "cathétérisme cardiaque" which was first demonstrated at a lecture on 9 January 1855 (SCHUMACHER, 1961, p. 16) – that sugar was always present in the blood stream between the liver and the lung, whereas there was very little or none at all in the blood in the portal veins. This confirmed him in his view that the liver must be the organ producing the sugar. In 1855 he called the parent substance of the sugar first *"fécule animale"*, but he soon changed it to *"matière glycogène"*. In 1857 he succeeded in isolating glycogen.

In the same year, two German research workers described this parent substance of sugar in the human organism; these were

MORITZ SCHIFF (1823–1896), who ungrudgingly acknowledged BERNARD's prior claim, and VICTOR HENSEN (1835–1924), thought by some as having discovered glycogen independently of BERNHARD, who did not fully acknowledge HENSENS achievement (POREP, 1970, 1971; HARMSEN, 1932, 1934; WOLFF, 1960; ROSEMANN, 1932; MANI 1964 and 1967, p. 539).

BERNARD's discovery that the liver was the site in which sugar was produced from glycogen and that there must be – BERNARD used the term first in 1855 – a *"sécrétion interne"*, together with the observation of a certain amount of sugar in normal human blood – BERNARD thereby showed the existence of an unequivocal *"normal glycemia"* and differentiated it clearly from *"hyperglycemia"* – and finally the fact that hyperglycemia following kidney failure led to the retention of sugar in the blood and consequently to glycosuria – all these findings failed to reveal the identity of the substance that finally led to diabetic coma. Sugar was a physiologic substance indispensable to the organism, whereas diabetic coma showed symptoms that could not be accounted for solely through an excess of sugar in the organism. Since the end of the 18th century it had been known that in the final stage of their illness diabetics exuded a smell like *apples, violets, or chloroform.* This was described by FRANK as early as 1794 and ROLLO in 1797.

Finally in 1850, ERNST BRAND (1827–1897), again noticed a strange applelike smell in the breath of diabetics, and this came to be recognized as an indisputable symptom of severe diabetes. In 1857 WILHELM PETTERS (1820–1875) demonstrated that a substance with a similar smell that was found in diabetic urine was acetone. In 1860 this was confirmed by JOSEPH KAULICH (1830–1886). Many symptoms of diabetes, particularly those accompanied by psychological troubles or effects on the nervous system were thereafter explained as acetone poisoning, until 1874 when KUSSMAUL, while studying diabetic coma and the hard breathing in the final phase, experimented with pure acetone on human subjects and animals and showed that only very large quantities could have a narcotic effect. But he could never find symptoms like those he had found in diabetic coma. FRANZ VON TAPPEINER (1816–1902) (SCHUMACHER, 1961, p. 11) also observed only a transitory confusion, but with no harmful effects, in spite of considerable doses. In 1882, a Breslau physician, EMMO LEGAL (1859–1922) published the test procedure using sodium nitroprusside solution that has been named after him (BERG 1962b). This facilitated further research.

As early as 1865, CARL GERHARDT (1833–1902) had found ethyldiacetic acid, which he regarded as the parent substance of acetone, in diabetic urine. In 1885 RUDOLF VON JAKSCH (1855–1947) confirmed the theory proposed in 1881 by BERNARD TOLLENS (1841–1918) that acetic acid was in fact the parent substance of acetone (SCHUMACHER, 1961, p. 11; STADELMANN). Finally, in 1884, MINKOWSKI and, at the same time, RUDOLF EDUARD KÜLZ (1845–1895) were able to identify β-oxybutyric acid in the blood; the explained NAUNYN's observation of the excessive acidity of the blood, to which he had given the name *acidosis* in 1898 (NAUNYN, p. 175 seq.) and which was now thought to be responsible for the coma.

The origin of this substance was controversial. While at first it was ascribed to abnormal fermentation processes (PETTERS, KAULICH), and thought to originate in food sugar, in 1897 GEORG ROSENFELD (1861–1934), FELIX HIRSCHFELD and HANS CHRISTIAN GEELMUYDEN (1861–1945) were able to prove that acetonuria and acidosis were due chiefly to lack of carbohydrates and, paradoxical as it might seem, it vanished when food rich in sugar or starch was given. Then it was debated whether the acetone matter was produced from protein or from fat in particular (EMDEN, SALOMON, SCHMIDT); on the other hand, fat was viewed in terms of ROSENFELD's classic dictum – which he ascribed to NAUNYN himself – that normally "fats are burnt up in the fire of carbohydrates". It was not until 1905 that FRANZ KNOOP (1875–1946) succeeded in showing, by proving the betaoxidation of fatty acids, that acetone matter was the product of the faulty breakdown of fats (BERG, 1962b). It became clear that acidosis was not the cause but the effect of the diabetic condition, and that acetone and acetoacetic acid were not diabetic toxins but side-effects of severe diabetes.

The Discovery of Insulin

In 1971 the 50th anniversary of the discovery of insulin by FREDERIC GRANT BANTING (1891–1941) and CHARLES BEST (b. 1899) was celebrated throughout the world. However, it is certain that before BANTING and BEST other researchers were using effective pancreatic extracts without – with a single exception – having tested these on human beings (DEROT; LEBENSOHN; SCHMIDT; BIBERGEIL; STÖCKER; KENEZ; ELAUT; KLEEBERG; PESTEL; GROEN; MELLINGHOFF; ALLAN; BEST; COLLIP; FLETCHER; CAMPBELL; MACLEOD; SELYE; FEASBY; PRATT; BRÜGEMÖLLER and NORPOTH; RICHARDS; MURLIN and KRAMER; RIOS; STEIGERWALDT; KLOPPE; SCHNEIDER; LEVINE; PAVEL; MURRAY; MARTIN; GOLDNER; STEIN; LEIBOWITZ; LEICKERT; DRURY; WALDBERG; WRENSHALL et al., MURLIN, 1972; CHEYMOL; STRIKER; HORNOR).

After the successful experiments in removing the pancreas, which led in every case to the development of diabetes mellitus in the dogs that had been operated on, MINKOWSKI already attempted to replace the missing pancreas, whose removal had obviously caused the condition, by administering of pancreas orally since, at the time, the administration of thyroid gland tissue had produced very good results in cases of hypothyroidism. But as early as 1890 MINKOWSKI had to acknowledge that the method of enteral administration was not promising. What he called "pancreatine", dried fresh pancreas, had no effect on diabetes.

Equally disappointing results were experienced in 1894 by JOHANN KARL GOLDSCHEIDER (1858–1935), in 1895 by WILHELM SANDMEYER (b. 1863), in 1897 by HUGOUNENQ and DOYON, and by HESS (1902) and PFLÜGER (1905), GOLDSCHEIDER also combined eremas with pancreatic tissue and tried pancreatic glycerine extracts and pancreas pills. It is surprising that KARL LOENING (b. 1877) as late as 1922 and ERNST VAHLEN (b. 1865) in 1924 advocated two oral medicines called *"metabolin"* and *„irrebolin"* with which they had allegedly been successful. However, there was no confirmation of this claim from anyone else.

MINKOWSKI now changed his technique and began to inject pancreas extracts which he had prepared with a saline solution and administered subcutaneously. But his remedies were ineffective, Reporting on a trial in 1893, he was already forced to admit his failure, especially as an abcess developed at the site of the injection, making further experiments inadvisable.

In the same year, 1893, the Italian physician FERNANDO BATTISTINI (1867–1929) published a report on two cases of diabetes in which he had observed a diminution of glycosuria after injecting a pancreas extract. In his published report, written in German, BATTISTINI mentioned a number of predecessors, e.g., the English physicians MACKENZIE, WOOD, WHITE and SIBLEY, but of those only WHITE had injected pancreatic fluid in minute quantities subcutaneously. The others administered pancreas extract orally. In most cases there was no appreciable lasting improvement. BATTISTINI forgot to mention his countryman ANDREA CAPARELLI. In 1894 GOLDSCHEIDER attempted to treat 6 diabetic patients with injections of glycerinized extract of pancreas, but without success. In 1894, PAUL FÜRBRINGER (1849–1930) was equally unsuccessful with two patients, who showed no objective improvement, nor did ERNST VON LEYDEN (1832–1910) and FERDINAND BLUMENTHAL (b. 1870) fare any better (OSER, LISSER, VANNI, LEICKERT).

Whereas all these experiments were based on MINKOWSKI'S conviction that the active principle for the prevention of diabetes must reside in the pancreas itself, OTTO COHNHEIM (b. 1873) started from a different thesis. For RAPHAEL LEPINE (1840–1919) had assumed that in diabetes, pancreatic deficiency was due to a disorder of glycolysis, and in 1903–1906 COHNHEIM attempted to treat dogs and cats with expressed muscle fluid which he mixed with pancreatic extract. He claimed that this compound considerably reduced the elimination of sugar in the urine. However, his optimistic notion could not be confirmed. It was not until the news of the discovery of *"isletin"* that EUGEN GLEY (1857–1930) agreed to a document which he had deposited at the "Société de Biologie" in Paris on 20 February 1905, being opened and read there on 23 December 1922.

In 1891 and 1892, following the Mering-Minkowski extirpation experiments, GLEY had made similar experiments. After hardening the exogenous part of the pancreas, he produced an extract from the remaining part of the gland which, according to LAGUESSE would contain the lymph of the islets of Langerhans as carrier of the active substance. With this he was able to achieve a considerable reduction of sugar in the urine of his experimental animals. He used intravenous injections. Though these experiments were supposed to have been started as early as 1891, they were not taken up again until 1902, probably because their author was busy with other tasks.

In the annex to his report of 1922, GLEY referred to an observation made in 1911 by HEDON, according to whom the injection of a serum from pancreatic venous blood considerably reduced glycosuria in diabetic dogs, and who thereby proved the thesis of a secretion within the pancreas. By implanting sections of pancreas subcutaneously, MINKOWSKI had succeeded in curing glycosuria in animals whose pancreas had been removed, and HEDON confirmed this observation. It is a pity that GLEY did not carry his experiments through at that time for he was on the right track. But as he did not publish his findings until 1922, he cannot be considered to have any prior claim as discoverer.

ALEXANDER RENNIE (1859–1940) and THOMAS RICHARD FRASER (1841–1919) started from a completely different premise; they were the first to make us of the fact that in certain kinds of bony fish the islet mechanism is separate from the excretory organ of the pancreas – something HERMANN STANIUS (1808–1883) had already observed in 1848.

However, in 1904 DIAMARE and A. KULIABKO were able to show that this strange structure was practically identical to the islets of Langerhans in the pancreatic tissue of higher animals.

In 1907 RENNIE and FRASER were thus able to open up fresh prospects for obtaining the substance of the islets and this was to be of great importance in the subsequent production of insulin. Admittedly, they themselves had given the mechanically crushed mash made from the islet substance orally to only five diabetic patients for two months and carried out only one experiment with subcutaneous injections, an experiment that was moreover unsuccessful. If they were able to report a considerable improvement, especially a lessening of glycosuria, this was most likely due – as MELLINGHOFF (p. 14) rightly suspected – to the strict diabetic diet administered at the same time.

Finally, in 1910, ERICH LESCHKE (1877–1933) published a comprehensive thesis in which he described all his experiments (for the most part completely discouraging) with pancreatic extracts. He came to the conclusion that *"the existence of this hypothetical anti-diabetic substance seems highly questionable . . ."*

The important work done by GEORG LUDWIG ZUELZER (1870–1949), which MELLINGHOFF discussed in detail, belongs also to this period. In 1901, FERDINAND BLUM (1865–1959) had discovered the so-called *"adrenal gland diabetes"*. He was able to show that adrenalin injections were followed by a rise in the blood sugar content with consequent glycosuria. ZUELZER pursued this train of thought and postulated a mutual adrenalin-insulin intolerance that is now widely discredited. For twelve years, from 1902 to 1914, he strove to obtain an antidiabetic hormone from the pancreas as a supposed antidote to adrenalin. In 1903 ZUELZER made his first animal experiments with pancreatic extracts and found that rabbits in which he had previously induced hyperglycemia with adrenalin injection were free of glycosuria and had a reduced elimination of urine after being injected with his preparation. As he needed a fair amount of pancreatic material for his experiments, and he was unable to procure it on his own, he approached the Schering Company in Berlin, where MAX DOHRN (1874–1943) and ANTON MARXER helped him.

MELLINGHOFF has rightly pointed out that the criticisms made in 1954 by JOSEPH HERSEY PRATT (b. 1892) of ZUELZER's experiments, as well as of BANTING's and BEST's, were not justified; for he claimed that the extraction of insulin started from a false premise, since the pre-enzyme found *in vivo* in the pancreas was really only activated through enterokinase in the intestine. Experiments have shown that as a rule, shortly after an animals is slaughtered there is a spontaneous activation of trypsinogens in the pancreas. ZUELZER already realized that. But is was not until he – like BANTING and BEST – used alcohol instead of saline solution, as was common, to extract the substance, that he was on the right track. ZUELZER had already preferred fractionated protein and thus had removed a large proportion of the neutralizing or damaging protein substances from his preparations. These obviously contained the active precipitate, for animal experiments, begun in 1905, and above all the first test on humans, described initially in 1909, showed distinct, if ephemeral, results.

The first patient was already in a coma and moribund, and the lower leg had had to be amputated because of diabetic gangrene. After the injection there was a five-day improvement but then the patient died as no more extract was available. Tests on the urine for sugar, acetone, or acetoacetic acid were made as rarely as checks on blood sugar. However, in a second case the decrease in sugar and acetone elimination was spectacular and could be incontrovertibly demonstrated by the author. In a third case there were some unpleasant side-effects at first: a rise in temperature to 38,4° Celsius with the young diabetic patient vomiting repeatedly; the second injection led to shivering fits which MACLEOD later explained as *symptoms of hyperglycemia* (1927, p. 59). But MELLINGHOFF believes that these phenomena should rather be attributed to impurities in the preparations injected.

ZUELZER was able to claim definite success for his preparation – which he soon called *"acomatol"* – in 8 cases, although there were some serious side effects. Subsequently, JOSEPH FORSCHBACH, MINKOWSKI's collaborator at Breslau University Hospital, treated two gravely sick diabetics with ZUELZER's extract. There was a notable reduction in the elimination of urine and sugar for 48 hours, but the preparation had strong side effects, with a rise in temperature and increased vomiting, and the experiments had to be discontinued. But FORSCHBACH concluded categorically:

> ". . . that ZUELZER was the first who has successfully produced a preparation from pancreas that, when applied intravenously and when there is no change in the ingestion of food, reduces the elimination of sugar for a shorter or longer period."

Unfortunately, neither FORSCHBACH nor his mentor, MINKOWSKI, enquired any further into the peculiar side-effects: as far as they were concerned the experiments, which would almost certainly have led to the production of pure insulin, were finished.

When, in February 1914, 114 g of pancreas were successfully processed in the Hoffmann-La Roche laboratories, ZUELZER was actually in possession of a highly effective extract prepared by CAMILLE REUTER, but, when applied to experimental animals, it induced painful convulsions of a kind not previously observed. MELLINGHOFF thought this was undoubtedly due to a genuine hypoglycemic effect produced by a very potent extract. ZUELZER, however, believed there was a harmful toxin releasing a specific convulsions trigger and stopped all further work in this direction. After 1909 he remained silent on the subject of his "acomatol".

To summarize: ZUELZER's new method of alcohol extraction, distilled protein precipitation, and evaporation of the alcoholic extract in a lowtemperature vaccum seems to have produced a very effective preparation containing insulin. Although his first batches, which he started to use in 1903, caused side-effects, which must be attributed to impurities, the extracts subsequently produced in collaboration with Hoffmann-La Roche were indisputably very effective but clearly caused convulsions due to hypoglycemia which ZUELZER did not identify because he did not employ any procedure for measuring blood sugar. Thus ZUELZER was the first to use an effective preparation not only in animal experiments but in treating human patients: nevertheless, he cannot be regarded as the first to introduce insulin as a generally effective anti-diabetic remedy.

While some researchers set out on the principle that the exocrine section of the pancreas must be destroyed in order – as they believed – to eliminate the fermentation of that section which broke up the active substance of the islets of Langerhans, other attempted to get rid of undesirable impurities through a process of precipitation. This group included W. M. A. CROFTON who, in 1909, prepared an extract from expressed pig pancreas which he fed to diabetic patients (MURLIN and KRAMER, 1956).

In 1910, JOSEPH H. PRATT, who in 1954 was to air some highly critical opinions on the history of the discovery of insulin – many of which were disproved by WILLIAM RICHARD FEASBY (b. 1912) – came to the conclusion that the transplantation of pancreatic tissues prevented the development of diabetes in animals whose pancreas had been removed and that the pancreas had an internal secretion that influenced sugar metabolism (MURLIN and KRAMER, 1956).

It is against this background that we must view further experiments to obtain an effective pancreatic extract for the treatment of diabetes. In the first place, ERNEST LYMAN SCOTT, an American, must be mentioned in this connection (RICHARDS). He was familiar with ZUELZER's works which be quoted, as he did those of HEDON. First he tried to achieve the atrophy of the excretory parts through ligature of Wirsung's duct, but did not fully succeed. So he decided to treat fresh pancreas with sand and warm alcohol. There was no visible effect on the elimination of sugar, but when he began to use acidulated water instead of 95% alcohol he observed an appreciable reduction in the sugar content of the urine of three or four dogs. His thesis concluded as follows:

1. There is an internal secretion from the pancreas controlling the sugar metabolism.
2. By proper methods this secretion may be extracted and still retain its activity.
3. This secretion is easily destroyed by oxidation or by the action of the digestive enzymes of the pancreas.
4. The secretion is insoluble, or nearly so, in strong alcohol but is readily soluble in acidulated water.
5. The failure of previous workers to procure satisfactory results was due to their not preventing oxidation or the action of the digestive enzymes.

In a shorter article, published in a periodical in 1912, SCOTT again emphasized the importance of obtaining the extract with the aid of 85% alcohol because in fact the active element – as became clear later from the works of BANTING, BEST and COLLIP – is soluble in water and 80–85% alcohol, whereas in 95% alcohol it is precipitated (RICHARDS).

Between 1913 and 1916, JOHN RAYMOND MURLIN (1874–1960) and BENJAMIN KRAMER (b. 1887) also sought to isolate the anti-diabetic hormone (MURLIN and KRAMER, 1956). In 1915 when their investigations were still in progress, ISRAEL SIMON KLEINER (b. 1885) and SAMUEL JAMES MELTZER (1851–1920) published the successful results of their experiments in which they obtained a greatly thinned pancreatic suspension by means of a physiological saline solution; when this was injected intravenously into dogs whose pancreas had been removed there was a notable drop in blood sugar. Neither MURLIN and KRAMER nor KLEINER and MELTZER experienced the severe side-effects in their experiments that had led ZUELZER – especially after FORSCHBACH's negative results – to abandon this line of research.

In the post-war period, ROBERT AMMON (b. 1902) pointed out that just before the outbreak of the First World War his teacher, ERNST JOSEPH LESSER (1879–1928), had also achieved a drop in the blood sugar in frogs through treatment with pancreatic extracts and had interpreted the side-effects he observed as a hypoglycemic reaction. In his circle of friends the substance that lowered blood sugar was called "glucopausin". LESSER had published none of his findings, but his obituary in 1928 by his Polish pupil JACOB KARL PARNAS (b. 1884) indicates that he had witnessed LESSER's experiments.

Finally, before dealing with the discovery of insulin by BANTING and BEST, we must mention the work of the Rumanian scientist PAULESCO, who, during the 50th anniversary celebration of the discovery of insulin in 1971/2, was claimed by his contemporary ION PAVEL (b. 1897) to have been its real discoverer. In several works and numerous letters to well-known diabetes experts throughout the world and to the Nobel Prize Committee in Stockholm, PAVEL showed that, 5 months earlier than his Canadian colleagues, on 31 August 1921, PAULESCO had published a report in the well-known "Archives Internationales de Physiologie", preceded by four short notifications to the "Société de Biologie" in Paris between April and June 1921. The longer article in the "Archives Internationales de Physiologie" was accepted by the editors on 22 June 1921, the first lecture by

BANTING and BEST to the "Physiological Journal Club" in Toronto was given on 14 November 1921, the second to the "American Physiological Society" in New Haven on 29 December 1921 (CHEYMOL, PAVEL).

In 1916 PAULESCO, who had lived in Paris between 1888 and 1900 for purposes of study and research, began research on the pancreas which was apparently interrupted by the German occupation of Rumania during the First World War. Immediately after the war he resumed his work, which led in spring 1921 to the discovery of the active substance in he called "pancréine".

PAULESCO did indeed report his extremely interesting experiments in four communications in April, May, and June 1921, which he then summarized in the article in the "Archives Internationales de Physiologie". He obtained pancreatic material in highly sterile conditions and diluted it with distilled water. Then he placed the suspension on ice for 24 hours, finally filtered it and treated it with salt. When the substance was injected intravenously a dramatic drop in blood sugar, from 140 mg-% to 25 mg-%, occurred right from the first experiments, and a depancreatized dog died from hypoglycemia.

PAULESCO also found that these results lasted for about 12 hours, that there was a noticeable decrease in acetonemia and acetonuria, that the strongest effect would be felt some 2 hours after treatment and that normal, non-diabetic dogs showed a similar drop in blood sugar. But when the injections were given subcutaneously there were inflammatory side-effects and, no doubt, for this reason, PAULESCO did not dare to use the preaparation on humans.

PAVEL's claim to be the first to discover insulin was defended as early as 1969 by JAN MURRAY, and in 1971, after PAVEL's efforts became known, was given prominence in a further work (DEROT; MARTIN; HAZARD); others, however, pointed out that PAULESCO had already been mentioned in most accounts of the discovery of insulin, but, as he did not take the vital step of progressing from animal experiments to human patients, he could not claim any priority in the introduction of insulin, which was first injected successfully into a diabetic child, LEONARD THOMPSON, on 11 January 1922 (STÖCKER; MACLEOD, p. 69 seq.; YOUNG; LEIBOWITZ; GOLDNER; STEIN; ALLAN; WRENSHALL; HETENYI and FEASBY p. 45; WOLFF, 1971 and 1974).

Whereas BANTING and BEST chose a two-part procedure in their first experiments, first ligating the excretory part of the pancreas and then processing the atrophied organ after a waiting period of some 7 to 10 weeks, PAULESCO obtained his extract from the fresh organ. But BANTING and BEST soon changed to using glands from calf fetuses which, according to JUSSUF IBRAHIM's (1877–1953) findings in 1909, do not yet contain any protolytic enzymes. The production process was very similar, and both products clearly had the same properties so that a committee of the "International Diabetes Foundation", set up in 1970 specifically to examine this question under the chairmanship of FRANK GEORGE YOUNG (b. 1908) from Cambridge, came to this conclusion after carefully considering all relevant works published between 1893 and 1921 by 20 authors:

"There can be little doubt that PAULESCO as well as BANTING and BEST obtained a pancreatic extract which contained insulin and that the pancréine and the insulin present in the crude extracts in which the hormone was first obtained, are the same substance."

But whereas PAULESCO's attempts to develop the purification of the extracts further seem – for unexplained reasons – to have failed, BAINTING and BEST were able to overcome this hurdle, mainly thanks to the collaboration of JAMES BERTRAND COLLIP (1892–1965), the chemist, and arrived at a relatively well-tolerated preparation suitable for subcutaneous or intramuscular injection, which alone permitted its wide use on human beings.

It is a pity, as PAVEL rightly pointed out, that an error slipped into the translation of the first work by BANTING and BEST in the discussion of PAULESCO's treatise in the "Comptes Rendues des Séances de la Société de Biologie" in Paris.

Their second work, dated March 1922, no longer contains this mistranslation, which says – and is scientifically perfectly exact:

"More recently, MURLIN, KLEINER and PAULESCO have tried the effect of aqueous extracts of the pancreas intravenously, on depancreatized animals and have found transitory reduction in percentage of blood sugar and in the sugar excreted in the urine."

PAULESCO's more extensive work of 31 August 1922 appeared after the start of BANTING's and BEST's work in Toronto. The authors obviously did not know of it even later, but it must be said that BANTING and BEST, who had set out on their experiments to obtain insulin quite independently of PAULESCO, did not stop when problems started to arise, but sought ways and means of overcoming them.

PAULESCO's work, bearing in mind all we have said about his predecessors, was undeniably the most exact, although for instance the blood sugar estimation still needed – on PAULESCO's own evidence – 25 ml of blood for each single analysis. However, there is no doubt that the 1923 Nobel Committee was perfectly right to award the Toronto researchers the Nobel Prize for the discovery and production of insulin in Toronto as well as the first experiments with it on human patients. There was, however, a personal injustice in the attribution, for the prize was awarded onyl to BANTING and MACLEOD, while the student, BEST, and the chemist, COLLIP, went empty-handed. As is well known, BANTING immediately shared his prize with BEST, and MACLEOD arranged for half of his prize to be made available to COLLIP.

Now let us turn to the dramatic weeks and months that led, in Toronto, to the isolation of the active substance and its use on human beings. In July 1920, BANTING, who was just 29 years old at the time, after working as an army medical officer for four years, opened a practice as an orthopedic specialist in London, Ontario (Canada), where it seems that he was not over-busy in the first few months. On the evening of 30 October 1920 when he was preparing his next lecture, since he was also Professor of Physiology at the university, he picked up a recent issue of the "Journal of Surgery, Gynecology and Obstetrics" (November, number 5) containing an article by MOSES BARRON (b. 1883) that particularly interested him. This discussed the possibility, on the basis of earlier accounts of atrophy of the pancreas as a result of blocking Wirsung's duct following gallstones, of producing such atrophy through ligature of the duct. BARRON pointed out that, in 1884, CHARLES LOUIS XAVIER ARNOZAN and LOUIS VAILLARD had already demonstrated this and referred to the work of SSOBOLEW in 1902, of ALEXANDRE MANKOWSKI (b. 1868) and E. SAUERBECK in the years 1902–1904, and of KAMINURA in 1917.

BANTING had not previously worked on this problem, but he was so fascinated by the possibility of isolating the hypothetical internal secretory substance of the pancreas that he at once approached MACLEOD, the Director of the Toronto Institute of Physiology and the foremost expert in carbohydrate metabolism, asking him to let him have a laboratory and experimental animals for research in this field. It seems that BANTING, who was not really familiar with the accumulated literature on pancreatic diabetes, did not make a lasting impression on MACLEOD, but he nevertheless put a laboratory (a very primitive attic room) at his disposal during the vacation, together with ten experimental dogs, and seconded two students, who were working at the institute, BEST and E. CLARK NOBLE, to help with the experiments which were not to last more than eight weeks.

They were supposed to act as assistants in alternate months, and, as HANS SELYE (b. 1907) tells us, they tossed a coin to decide who should be the first. The lot fell on BEST, who stayed on after the end of the month as NOBLE was unable to take over at that point. This was the start of a uniquely harmonious collaboration between the 29-years old orthopedic surgeon and the medical student who had just turned 21.

BANTING started with the idea of achieving atrophy of the exocrine region by ligature of the pancreatic ducts and then, after 7–10 weeks, obtaining the extract containing the hypothetical hormone from the remaining islets of Langerhans; this was again to be tested on depancreatized dogs. And so, on 16 May 1921, the young researchers went to work, while MACLEOD was spending his summer vacation in Scotland. On 27 July 1921, after numerous setbacks, they were finally able to remove a dog's degenerated pancreas.

They simply crushed the extirpated material in a cool mortar and froze it in salt water. The mass was ground down and added to 100 ml of physiological salt. 5 ml of this extract was administered intravenously to a dog whose pancreas had previously been removed, and within 2 hours its blood sugar had dropped considerably. The analysis of the blood sugar, for which BEST used a method modified by MYERS and BAILEY from a 1915 procedure by LEWIS and BENEDICT, published in 1916, contributed greatly to the success of the work. Unlike PAULESCO, who needed 25 ml of blood for each analysis. BEST was able to manage with only 0.2 ml and thus to reexamine the dog frequently, sometimes as often as every half-hour.

Then BANTING had the idea of isolating the pancreas from the supposedly hormone-inhibiting trypsinogen by stimulating the gland with secretin and at the same time stimulating the vagus nerves. An extract thus obtained saved the moribund experimental dog and this showed that the substance initially called *"isletin"* by the Toronto researchers, could be obtained in the manner indicated, without impairment by pepsins. The method was, however, lengthy and difficult.

Then BANTING procured the pancreas of some four-month old calf fetuses from a slaughterhouse. In the course of the experiments, which continued to be successful, it turned out that the active substance could be extracted from the fetal pancreas more easily with acetone and acidulated alcohol than with a saline solution. This was originally BEST's suggestion. It was probably due to this that the legendary experimental dog, Marjorie, who is continually mentioned in works on the subject (STÖCKER, WRENSHALL, HETENYI and FEASBY, p. 61) was kept alive for 70 days after removal of the pancreas.

The decisive tests – there were altogether 75 experiments on the 10 dogs available – were made between 7 and 14 August.

The result was then communicated by both researchers on 14 November 1921 in a lecture, unedifyingly entitled *"Pancreatic diabetes"*, given to the Physiological Journal Club of Toronto University. This lecture formed the basis for the first publication of the findings in February 1922.

By a coincidence, it was at the end of 1921 that the young – also just 29 years old – chemist COLLIP came to Toronto to carry out some research of his own at MACLEOD's Physiological Institute. At BANTING's request, and encouraged by MACLEOD, he joined the "isletin" team and in a few months – he left Toronto again early in the summer of 1922 – he made a considerable contribution to the production of insulin in large quantities and to the standardization of the new preparation.

Thus, on 11 January 1922, it was finally possible to undertake the first experiment on patient, namely a 14 year-old diabetic boy called LEONARD THOMPSON, after BANTING and BEST had tested the tolerance of the new batch on themselves. The boy had been diagnosed as diabetic two years earlier, and in view of the high mortality rate among young diabetics there was little hope of saving him. He had been subjected to the fasting treatment advocated by FREDERICK MADISON ALLEN. He was in a critical state, utterly emaciated, when he arrived on 2 December 1921 at the Toronto General Hospital, where he was treated by WALTER R. CAMPBELL (b. 1890) and ANDREW ALMOS FLETCHER (b. 1889), who had been co-signatories in March 1922 of the second publication by BANTING, BEST and COLLIP. Their treatment led to an immediate improvement of the pathologic symptoms. Admittedly, the subcutaneous injections caused a sterile abcess, which drove COLLIP to further attempts to purify the preparation even more thoroughly. Meanwhile MACLEOD suggested to BANTING and BEST that they should change the English term *"isletin"* to *"insulin"*, a name proposed as early as 1909 by DE MAYER and in 1916 by SHARPEY-SCHÄFER; it was not used any more frequently in the first two publications than the name *"isletin"*, but then it quickly gained international currency.

The Toronto research team now had the first and unambiguous proof that they really had isolated the pancreatic hormone that could prevent diabetes, and a new era in diabetes therapy began.

BANTING, BEST and COLLIP wasted on time in taking out a patent on the process of insulin production in 1922, but (after paying a symbolic dollar for it) they made it over without delay to the Board of Governors of Toronto University, with the sole proviso that they should appoint an insulin committee and that the production of insulin by commercial firms should be subject to rigorous testing by that committee. All income from the sale of the patent has to this day been used for scientific research, particularly at the institute in Totento named after BANTING and BEST.

As early as 1922, BANTING, BEST, COLLIP, MACLEOD, and BEST's student colleague NOBLE were able to prove that insulin lowers the blood sugar even in normal rats. This made it possible to test the effectiveness of insulin on nondiabetic experimental animals.

This was particularly important when it was found that a blood sugar content of less than 45 mg-% caused convulsions resembling the symptoms of hypoglycemia. So it is not surprising that the insulin unit was originally considered as corresponding to the dose needed to induce such convulsions in a normal rabbit. The Toronto research team also worked with mice and calculated the mouse unit as a six hundredth of the rabbit unit.

COLLIP must be given the chief credit for the fact that as early as 1923 the insulin unit was defined by the Toronto Insulin Committee, in collaboration with the Health Organisation of the League of Nations, as *one third of the amount that reduces the blood sugar of a rabbit weighing 2 kilograms, which has fasted for 24 hours, from the normal value of 118 mg-%* to the convulsion-inducing value of 45 mg-% in 5 hours (BARR and ROSSITER; LACEY). Later, in order to conform to an international standard the insulin unit was no longer based on the reaction of an experimental animal but on a specific weight.

The award of the Nobel prize to MACLEOD has been criticised on the ground that he seemed to have hindered rather than helped BANTING's and BEST's research work, and many considered the award to be an error of judgment (e.g., CHEYMOL). But in a work published in 1972, JANOS KENES rightly pointed out that, despite certain tensions between BANTING and MACLEOD, the latter deserves considerable credit for the relatively rapid discovery of insulin and its mass production. MACLEOD put at the disposal of BANTING, a young man he did not know at all, not only a temporary laboratory and ten experimental dogs but a congenial assistant, BEST; and if he was relatively sceptical at the start of the work, this was undoubtedly because he was familiar with all the literature on the subject and all that had been done in 30 years to isolate the active substance, so far with no decisive result. As soon as MACLEOD learnt of the success of BANTING's and BEST's research work on returning from his European vacation, he immediately stopped all other research at the institute, and put his whole team to work on the isolation, purification and testing of insulin. It was he who persuaded COLLIP, the chemist – albeit at BANTING's request – to collaborate with the team, and it was due to his prestige that insulin became known, not only in Canada and the U.S.A., but in Europe as the most effective remedy against diabetes.

As soon, as the discovery of insulin was published, a number of authors naturally questioned the prior claim of BANTING and BEST as its discoverers, just as PAVEL did a few years ago.

Here we must mention especially the contribution of a certain DR. FRANGOON ROBERTS to the British Medical Journal of 16 December 1922, in which he refers to the precursors, and in particular to the experiments of E. L. SCOTT. His rather unpleasant polemic refused to give the Canadian research team any credit for any original work. It is interesting that SIR HENRY HALLETT DALE (1875–1968), later a Nobel prize winner, at once published a sharply-worded reply in which he emphasized the extraordinary significance of the discovery. DALE's remarks on the work of SCOTT also applies to all the other precursors:

"The important point is that SCOTT did stop, and that Dr. Roberts would not be writing about his work now if BANTING and BEST and the other Toronto workers had not gone much further" (FEASBY).

The rapid spread of the news of insulin immediately raised the demand for it: BANTING decided to treat diabetics in his own practice, and appointed BEST as director of the institute, which now strove to produce insulin on a large scale. The small laboratory at the Physiological Institute of Toronto University was not adequate for this purpose and production, which had developed a dangerous bottleneck between February and May 1922 was taken over by Connaught Laboratories, built during the First World War (WRENSHALL, HETENYI and FEASBY, p. 67).

It was fortunate that the leading managers of the American pharmaceutical firm Eli Lilly in Indianapolis were prepared to produce insulin under licence and under the supervision of the Insulin Committee. Finally, in August 1922, when ELLIOTT PROCTOR JOSLIN, a noteworthy Boston diabetes specialist received the first insulin samples, the drug was launched on its triumphant progress. In October of the same year 3000 ml of the insulin solution were prepared. In the following year insulin production was taken over by indigenous firms in German-speaking countries. In Germany it was produced by Hoechst, a company that had already been in touch with ZUELZER as early as 1910, although this did not yield any successful collaboration, and also by Bayer Dye Works, Kahlbaum, Schehring and Merck, and in Switzerland by the great Basel companies, Hoffmann-La Roche (Hoglandol), which had also tried to collaborate with ZUELZER in obtaining the active extracts, as well as Geigy and Sandoz (Insulin-Sandoz). Denmark, too, began its own production, and was soon able to announce some considerable improvements in insulin. In order to avoid delays in checking insulin batches, as was mandatory according to the patent agreement, the Toronto Insulin Committee created additional reginal bodies.

Following a suggestion made on 6 April 1923 by MACLEOD, MINKOWSKI founded such a body in Germany (DÖRZBACH and MÜLLER, LAUSCH, p. 115). KARL VON NOORDEN (1858–1944) immediately supported the introduction of insulin into therapeutic procedure and also assumed clinical testing in Germany (DÖRZBACH and MÜLLER). But until production was in full swing, it was occasionally necessary here and there to produce insulin on the spot, according to BANTING's and BEST's instructions.

This was done in June 1923 by LEO POLLAK (b. 1878), an internist, together with SUSY GLAUBACH at the Pharmaceutical Institute of the University of Vienna (KORP and ZWEYMÜLLER; LESKY; WAGNER; KLEEBERG), FERDINAND SCHMIDT has pointed out that from May 1924 onwards, independently of the development of insulin by Hoechst Dye Works, which was continuously available from the end of 1923, WILHELM SAILER (1882–1942), a Mecklenburg country pharmacist began to work in his own laboratory on a preparation of beef and pig pancreases obtained from the main Hamburg abattoir, and this was soon mass produced by a DR CHRISTIAN BRUNNENGRÄBER company in Rostock and marketed as "Germano-Insulin".

The quest for a method that would produce a greater yield of insulin continued. The first step in this direction was made by JOHN JACOB ABEL (1857–1938) who succeeded in 1926 in crystallizing insulin (MURNAGHAN and TALALAY). This caused a dispute with BEST, MURLIN and ALLEN, who were striving for a biuret-free insulin distillation, whereas ABEL's experiments had convinced him that crystallized insulin also contained protein substances, because his colorimetric tests had shown that protein was present. It soon turned out that ABEL was right. But it was not until 1936 that DAVID AYLMER SCOTT, who had joined the Toronto team, was actually able to prove that insulin crystals were protein salts formed from such metals as zinc, cobalt, cadmium or nickel.

D. A. SCOTT posed a different question. He wanted to find out whether it would be possible to replace the insulin injections, which often had to be given several times daily, with a delayed preparation. In 1934 research began in Toronto, under the direction of SCOTT, to extend the effectiveness of insulin by combining it with zinc. In 1936, a Danish research team led by HAGEDORN proved that the action of insulin could be extended when it was combined with "fish roe". The number of injections could be reduced from four a day with the oldstyle insulin to two. In the same year SCOTT and FISHER showed that protamin could extent effectiveness when added to insulin containing zinc: with the new protamin-zinc-insulin which was now produced, one injection daily generally sufficed (see also KERR, BEST, CAMPBELL and FLETCHER).

The crystallization of insulin brought the elucidation of its structure very much to the fore. In 1955, after ten years of research FREDERICK SANGER (b. 1918) finally succeeded in breaking down the structure of insulin in various types of animal as a combination of two polypeptide chains with respectively 21 and 30 amino-acids which were linked by sulfur bonds. In 1958 SANGER was awarded the Nobel Prize for Chemistry for this work. The analysis of the structure held out the hope that the insulin molecule might eventually be synthesized or at least partially synthesized.

In the early sixties three groups of researchers were working on the problem of synthesizing insulin: the group working with HELMUT ZAHN (b. 1916) at the Wollforschinstitut der Technischen

Hochschulen in Aachen, a team working with PANAYOTIS G. KATSOYANNIS (b. 1924) in the Biochemistry Department of the University of Pittsburgh and a team of Chinese research workers at the Biochemistry Institute of the Academia Sinica in Shanghai. The first two teams succeeded almost simultaneously and independently of one another, through separate synthesis of the A and B chains and their combination in obtaining synthetic insulin, although it was not very effective; by 1965 the Chinese team had succeeded in purifying it so much that it was obtainable in crystals (MEIENHOFER et al., 1963; DU YU-CANG et al., 1965). Just then news came from the research laboratories of Ciba-Geigy in Basel that one working party (SIEBER et al.) had succeeded in producing a total synthesis of human insulin with the formation of disulfide bonds which permitted a far greater yield of effective insulin.

If it looked at first as if the introduction of insulin to the therapeutic armoury had largely solved the problem of diabetes, it soon became clear that insulin treatment created a whole range of pathologic, biochemical and clinical problems that research would have to solve. In 1967 RACHMIEL LEVINE (b. 1910) discussed these problems. In 1924, two years after insulin entered the medical armoury, WILHELM FALTA (1875–1950) reported on a patient with rapidly progressive diabetes who even with 150 units of insulin – a very high dose at the time – failed to show any improvement. The same preparation was fully effective with another patient. In the same year and the year after, further observations of a strange *resistance* appeared (POLLAK; MAHLER and PASTERNY; STRAUSS; ARNETH; ESCUDERO; UMBER and ROSENBERG; TSCHERNING). Soon news of such cases multiplied, and by 1965 FRIEDRICH MEYTHALER (1898–1967) and HORST KOTLORZ had collected 323 relevant passages in the literature (WOLFF, 1968; KERP et al.; LARCAN), FALTA, the first to observe the phenomenon, already believed that, in the case he was treating, insulin was unable to affect the necessary organs and assumed that there was some sort of counteraction in the bloodstream. From this he concluded that there must be cases of diabetes that were not due to an insufficiency of the islets mechanism and the production of insulin, but to a metabolic disorder in some other part of the organism. This theory gained greater credence when it was found that a healthy person required only 32 to 40 units of insulin daily, an amount that the depancreatized patient needed in order to maintain carbohydrate metabolism and that was designated the "physiologic daily dose".

Among other causes, the most important has finally proved to be the formation of neutralizing antibodies of the IgG type (KERP et al.; FEDERLIN). The discovery of these antibodies resulted from observations by FRANZ DEPISCH (1894–1963) and R. HASENÖHRL in 1928 when they found in animal experiments that the serum contained a factor that weakend insulin, and from the first reports on insulin allergies made in the same year by LOUIS TUFT (b. 1898), who chiefly described urticarial eczema.

In 1924, shortly after insulin therapy was introduced and insulin-induced hypoglycemia became known, HARRIS SEALE (1870–1957) described five attacks of hypoglycemia that were not induced by insulin, in terms of a new clinical concept called *"hyperinsulismus"*. A year later, FRANZ JOSPH LANG (b. 1894) found that these disorders were caused by multiple adenoma in the pancreas, and in 1926 SHIELDS WARREN (b. 1898) was able to cite as many as 16 cases of pancreatic adenoma from writings on the subject, to which he was able to add 4 cases observed by himself (ROGERS, WILDER et al., OTT and SCOTT, HOWARD et al.).

The post-insulin era finally reverted to BERNARD's notion of a *"mid-brain diabetes" ("Zwischenhirndiabetes")* which found further supporters (STRIECK, BERG), while the experiments made from 1924 onwards by BERNARDO ALBERTO HOUSSAY (1887–1971) to discover a diabetogenic source in the pituitary were confirmed in 1937 by YOUNG's experiments in which he managed to produce permanent diabetes through protracted daily injections of extracts of anterior pituitary lobe (SCHUMACHER, 1961, p. 26). While these new findings created new problems, the question of the mutual influence of the endocrine glands, which has exercised diabetic research since then, does not fall within the scope of this historical survey.

Therapy

A special *diabetic diet* was undoubtedly one of the foremost therapeutic measures, even before the age of insulin. Even before it was recognized that diabetes was a disorder of carbohydrate metabolism, various kinds of diet had been recommended. A change to a diet decided purely pragmatically, which was nevertheless very effective, did not come until JOHN ROLLO (d. 1809), a Scottish physician, who, in 1797, had achieved good results with a meat diet, made his recommendation (MARBLE; ANDERSON; BECKENDORF). He gave a particularly detailed account of the case of Captain MEREDITH of the Royal Artillery, who became diabetic at the age of 34, and who was very obviously overweight. His diet consisted of a breakfast and supper of milk mixed with lime-water and bread and butter, while his dinner consisted of pudding made of fat and blood and mature, preferably rank pork. In this way he had – without being conscious of it – excluded carbohydrates almost entirely from the diet. The patient of course lost a great deal of weight and felt extremely well. A second patient was less cooperative and therefore died at the age of 57, 19 months after treatment was begun, mainly – as ROLLO pointed out – because during his last three months he indulged in such things as apple pudding, sugar in his tea, and wine.

The *"meat diet"* was used well into the 19th century, although gradually it was considered wiser not to cut out all carbohydrates, and patients had a certain amount of carbohydrate added to their diet, even though that caused some glycosuria. This kind of diet was initiated in the middle of the 19th century, mainly by ADOLF NIKOLAUS VON DÜRING (1820–1882) and RUDOLF EDUARD KÜLZ (1845–1895). The latter even distinguished between harmful and harmless carbohydrates and found that levulose, inulin, inosit, mannite, and lactose, as well as some root vegetables like celery, comfrey, etc. caused no deterioration of the metabolic condition. But it remains true that many specialists did recommend a carbohydrate-free diet with a lot of meat and fat (DICKINSON; PAVY; SEEGEN; R. SCHUMACHER, STEPP).

There was also the *"milk cure"* advocated by KÜLZ WILHELM WINTERNITZ (1835–1917) on the basis of experience, and, in 1902, KARL VON NOORDEN'S famous oats cure (R. SCHUMACHER; STEPP), while WILHELM FALIA developed his *"cereal diet"*. In 1911, LEON BLUM (1878–1930) recommended a varied *"wheaten flour"* treatment.

APOLLINAIRE BOUCHARDAT'S (1806–1886) observations led him to a different conclusion for he noticed that during the siege of Paris in 1871, his diabetic patients improved, which he rightly ascribed to the scarcity of food. His motto, *"mangez le moins possible"* became the gospel of several generations of diabetics. GUGLIELMO GUELPA (1850–1930) in particular, who regarded diabetes as a form of auto-intoxication which he tried to improve through cutting back on food, and NAUNYN were in favour of fast-days and intensified the treatment by prescribing purgatives on top of a very sparse diet (SCHUMACHER, 1961, p. 15). In 1914

Frederick Madison Allen introduced a strict so-called *"starvation diet"*, in which a period of complete fasting – until there was an improvement in the diabetic metabolic condition – was followed by a regime of under-nourishment, which did raise life expectancy in the pre-insulin age, but brought patients to a state of near inanition, as can be seen from a number of pictures of diabetics in the pre-insulin era.

To prevent these symptoms of undernourishment, Karl Petrèn (1868–1927) advocated a veritable *"fat diet"* (Wilder), with, as its chief feature, a drastic reduction of proteins. The carbohydrates were restricted to leaf vegetables, and in spite of its lack of balance, the diet did enable diabetics to work and allowed diabetic children to grow more or less normally (Newburgh and Marsh).

Besides these, a series of now obsolete diets were also recommended, like-, to mention just one – the so-called *"potato diet"*, advocated in 1902 by Adolph Mosse (1852–1936), which – and from what we know today this is hardly surprising – had to be dropped rapidly because of its devastating side-effects and its after-effects on diabetic metabolism.

All these diets had a common purpose, namely to prevent the dreaded mortally dangerous coma or at least to delay it for a time. It was some time before it was considered possible, with the help of insulin, to allow patients a balanced diet with an adequate calorie content. Since then, myriads of works and articles have appeared on this subject, far too many to allow a wider survey of theories on the nutrition of diabetics in the framework of this introduction. Admittedly no single comprehensive historical work on this subject has appeared to this day (cf Knick; Magnus-Levy). A comprehensive 18-page bibliography up to the year 1961 is in Joseph Schumacher's "Index zum Diabetes mellitus" (Schumacher, 1961, pp. 374–392).

Oral Treatment of Diabetes

Besides efforts to improve insulin production, attempts have been made ever since the discovery of insulin to find another chemical substance that will reduce blood sugar. Johannes-Hermann Otten (b. 1932), in a detailed thesis, has listed the various preprarations that have been tested in this connection, and Loubatieres from Montpellier, who discovered that certain sulfonamides have blood-sugar reducing properties, has brought out a comprehensive report in a number of languages, with a detailed bibliography, on the detection of antidiabetic action in this type of substance. OTTEN's account suggests that, besides mercury, copper, lead, manganese and iron compounds, cobalt and nickel salts as well as sodium bicarbonate (so popular in the 19th century), mineral water, and even carbolic acid, lactic acid, and glycerine and finally, shortly after it was introduced, sodium salicylate – which has recently again been recommended for diabetes (SCHWEIS-HEIMER; CREUTZFELDT and SÖLING, p. 200 seq.) – were used, as were numerous secret remedies. A number of drugs were tried after CASIMIR FUNK (1884–1967) and CORBIT claimed, in 1923, to have produced an effective diabetes treatment from yeast cells (BRUGSCH; ALZONA and ORLANDI). In the same year COLLIP isolated a blood-sugar reducing substance from various plants, naming it *"glucokinin"* (BERTRAM, 1928), and in the post-war period a number of Polish and Hungarian authors claimed similar properties for blood-sugar reducing alkaloids, "vicamin" (HANO; KALDOR and SZABO). Similar claims were made for reserpin (NADEL; NEUGEBAUER and LANG; KUSCHE and FRANTZ).

However, the statement made in 1928 by FERDINAND BERTRAM (1894–1960) remained true until the Second World War:

> "All attempts to replace parenteral insulin therapy with equivalent oral methods must be judged a failure."

The view expressed in 1925 by FRIEDRICH UMBER (1871–1946) that

> "All earlier efforts, whether worthy of interest or not, to improve the metabolism of diabetics by medicinal methods have become outdated since the introduction of insulin", seems to mark the end of such attempts.

Similarly experiments with so-called *guanidin*, which were found in 1918 by C. K. WATANABE greatly to reduce blood sugar, were brought to a close. But every single one of his experimental animals had died, since the resulting hypoglycemia could not be reversed by the administration of glucose. Views on the effectiveness of guanidin differed: loss of insulin through stimulation of the vagus, respiratory problems with increased intake of glucose through the muscular system, and a rise of anaerobic glycolysis were mentioned (OTTEN, 1966, p. 46). One thing, however, was certain: the toxic and the blood-sugar reducing doses lay close together, and ERICH FRANK (1884–1957) was the first to try to produce guanidin derivatives that would be more easily tolerated.

The first preparation in this series was *agmatin – guanidinobutylamin –*, synthesized from herring sperm. From 1926, onwards this preparation and *galegin* underwent clinical tests and they were marketed for a short time (FRANK, NOTHMANN and WAGNER, 1926, FRANK, 1928; REINWEIN and MÜLLER, 1927; SIMONET and TANRET; SLOTTA and TSCHESCHE; STAUR, 1928). *Synthalin A* and its improved version *Synthalin B* were *diguanidins* that were used until 1945 although not easily tolerated and highly toxic.

Attempts were made to replace diguanidins with *biguanids* which seemed better tolerated (HESSE and TAUBMANN; SLOTTA and TSCHESCHE). But in 1956 GEORGES UNGAR (b. 1906), LOUIS FREEDMAN and SEYMOUR L. SHAPIRO renewed research on biguanid in the United States, and, starting in 1956 a number of preparations underwent extensive clinical tests (POMERANZE, FUJIY and MOURATOFF; KRALL and CAMERINI-DAVALOS; BRADLEY). In 1958, HELLMUT MEHNERT (b. 1928) and WALTER SEITZ (b. 1905) introduced treatment with *silubin* in Germany.

Considerably earlier – that is in 1942 – work was begun that led to the discovery of the blood-sugar reducing properties of certain *sulfonamide compounds*, an achievement regarded as a major breakthrough in the history of diabetes. It was the introduction of oral sulfonamides in the treatment of diabetes that at last made it possible to treat diabetes patients – especially the increasing number of elderly patients – gently, without recourse to insulin, thus dramatically changing the whole approach to diabetic treatment.

In 1926/27 three research teams, in Switzerland, Italy and the United States, proved, entirely independently of each other, that colloidal subur, when dissolved and given orally, reduced blood sugar and glycosuria in diabetics, eliminated ketonuria and raised the alkali reserve (BÜRGI and GORDONOFF; CAMPANACCI and BALDUCCI; FÖLDES; OTTEN, 1966, p. 42). In 1930, on the basis of these observations, which, however, did not remain uncontested (BERTRAM, 1928), and, spurred on by the works published from 1926 on by FRANK, NOTHMAN and WAGNER on the subject of di-guanidin preparations, C. L. RUIZ, L. L. SILVA and L. LIBENSON, three Argentinians, tested the effect of a thiouric derivative, 4-or 5-methylthioinudiazol, on the blood sugar of rabbits. They found an incontestable hypoglycemic effect, but their findings did not lead to any further investigations, although in 1941, in Italian, LUCIO SAVAGNONE from Palermo, also reported on the blood-sugar reducing properties of certain sulfonamide derivatives.

From 1935 onwards, as a result of research by GERHARD DOMAGK (1895–1964), these had come to be regarded as particularly effective chemotherapeutic agents and become part of the pharmaceutical armoury. In 1941, JOSEF KIMMIG (b. 1909) synthesized a new sulfonamide, with the test number VK 57, which had been tested by his teacher, JOSEPH VONKENNEL (1897–1963) on patients with gonorrhea. This preparation was ceded to the Rhône-Poulenc company under the test designation 2254 RP and was tested there by DANIEL BOVET (b. 1907) and PIERRE DUBOST, but they did not publish their report until 1944 (LOUBATIÈRES, 1969). Round about that time, when a typhus epidemic broke out in the Montpellier region as a result of wartime conditions, MARCEL JANBON and his collaborators decided to try the new preparation on the patients in the isolation hospital of the medical faculty of Montpellier. But convulsions and a comatose condition – hitherto unknown side effects of sulfonamides — were observed, and three patients died though it was not possible to ascertain the cause of death immediately.

JANBON then turned to LOUBATIÈRES, who was also working in Montpellier and who had been investigation the efficacity of new insulin preparations since 1938. As early as 13 Juni 1942 he established that one single oral administration of Thiodiazol derivatives brought about an astonishing, steady reduction lasting more than 24 hours, in the blood sugar of healthy dogs. LOUBATIÈRES immediately realized the far-reaching significance of this result repeated his experiments and proved that the reduction in blood sugar was not due to a falsification of the blood count caused by some chemical changes in the blood but to a direct effect on the pancreas, results subsequently obtained through sophisticated research being very similar to those he had obtained with insulin preparations.

LOUBATIÈRES at once surmised that sulfonamide released endogenous insulin, and, on 30 June 1942, just a few days after the first experiments, he proved that sulfonamide had no effect whatsoever on depancreatized dogs. So, on 3 July 1942, JANBON and his collaborators reported the severe side effects they had observed to the Montpellier "Société des sciences médicales et biologiques"; the report appeared in the same year in the "Montpellier médical", a scientific journal albeit with a predominantly local readership (JANBON, CHAPAL, VEDEL and SCHAAP; JANBON, LAZERGES and METROPOLITANSKI). In this they also briefly referred to current animal experiments to explain the mystifying incidents, without however mentioning LOUBATIÈRES by name (LOUBATIÈRES, 1969, P. 1185).

On 11 November 1942, when the German army occupied the hitherto unoccupied part of France, LOUBATIÈRES was able to continue his experiments only with the greatest difficulty in a makeshift laboratory in the Chemical Institute. His second report on them, made in 1944, was handed to his chief, LOUIS HÉDON (b. 1895). Owing to war-time circumstances, this work did not appear in print until 1946. But at a congress of French-speaking psychiatrists and neurologists held in Montpellier from 28 to 30 October 1942, that is, shortly before the German troops marched in, LOUBATIÈRES and his Montpellier colleagues had delivered two lectures in which reference was made to the hypoglycemic effect of the sulfonamide preparations they had tested. Then, on 14 Oktober 1944, LOUBATIÈRES lectured to a session of the "Société de Biologie" in Paris, at which BOVET and DUBOST also reported on their research, on the results of the experiments he had been undertaking since 1942 (LOUBATIÈRES, GOLDSTEIN, METROPOLITANSKI and SCHAAP; JANBON, CHAPAL and VEDEL). On 18 November 1944, in a further lecture to the same assembly, LOUBATIÈRES named a number of other thiodiazol derivatives which had similar hypoglycemic effects.

LOUBATIÈRES established subsequently that the effect of the preparation on diabetics was due to stimulation of the B-cells in the pancreas and not apparently – as had been mooted by others – to idiopathic damage to the A-cells (HOLT, HOLT, KRÖNER and KÜHNAU).

In Europe, and especially in Germany, owing no doubt to the end of the war and the difficult post-war conditions, the work of the Montpellier school and in particular LOUBATIÈRES' reports remained unnoticed, except in the U.S.A. wherein 1946 KO KUEL CHEN (b. 1898), ROBERT C. ANDERSON and NILA MAZE, pursuing a report by JANBON and LOUBATIÈRES, did a further test on a thiodiazol preparation and also observed its hypoglycemic effect. In 1947, JEAN LABARRE and JEAN REUSE were able to confirm the findings, as did CLAUS VON HOLT (b. 1925) in Germany in 1948.

Whereas OTTEN stated in his thesis that the sulfonamide preparation identified as a hypoglycemic substance by LOUBATIÈRES was not used on human beings until after another sulfonamide derivative, sulfonyl urea, had been used therapeutically in Germany with some success (OTTEN, 1966, p. 61), LOUBATIÈRES indicated that as early as 1942 and 1946, in collaboration with JANBON, he had treated three patients with the thiodiazol preparation. In the case of a 30-year old woman with benevolent diabetes and furuncles the blood sugar content dropped continuously from 220 to 70 mg-%, although the sulfonamide had no effect in the case of two girls of 14 and 18.

But it was not until 1955, that LOUBATIÈRES mentioned the effect of thiodiazol derivative on human diabetes in a publication.

Meanwhile, by chance, the hypoglycemic effect of vertain sulfonamide derivatives, became known in two places in Germany. In 1951, sulfonyl urea, *loranil,* synthesized by ERICH HAACK (1904–1968) had to be withdrawn because of obscure side effects despite its efficacity against infections. About the same time, HELLMUTH KLEINSORGE (b. 1920) began experimental and clinical tests on a product synthesized in 1929 by HAACK at the instigation of CARSTENS, N_1-Sulfanyl-N_2-butylcarbanid with the experimental designation CA 1022. He established an unambiguous hypoglycemic effect, which was actually regarded as an undesirable side-effect, so that the Heyden company decided not to put the compount on the market until more light had been shed on the subject. That is why his interesting findings were not published straight away. It was not until the 5 Oktober 1955, in Bad

Homburg, at the 18th session of the German Society for Digestive and Metabolic Illnesses that KLEINSORGE reported on his interesting observations, based on trials involving 94 patients and 10 physicians. On 11 May 1956, he published a detailed account of his work in the "Deutschen Medizinischen Wochenschrift".

In a project undertaken in 1953 after they moved to the medical research laboratories of C. F. Boehringer & Sons in Mannheim, HAACK and his collaborators again synthesized the substance with which KLEINSORGE had undertaken the first clinical tests (HAACK; ACHELIS; HAACK and HARDEBECK). This preparation, experimentally designated BZ 55, low doses of which could attain a wide blood spectrum, was first tested by KARL JOACHIM FUCHS on some pneumonia patients in the 1st internal ward of the Auguste-Victoria Hospital in Berlin-Schöneberg. Fuchs noticed odd side-effects. In tests on himself he found *"notable tiredness, sweating, hunger, trembling, and a certain sense of euphoria"*, which immediately made him think of hypoglycemic effects. In fact, laboratory testing showed considerable hypoglycemia. Thus a number of side-effects involving unusual symptoms of the central nervous system could be put down to a gradual development of hypoglycemia. This raised the possibility of using substance BZ 55 in treating diabetes, and FUCHS and his teacher HANS FRANKE (1909–1955) actually succeeded in achieving a definite improvement in 50 diabetic patients, some of whom were under observation for a whole year. On the basis of animal experiments made by others (SUTHERLAND and DE DUVE, FERNER, 1948; CREUTZFELDT, 1955; HOLT and HOLT 1954), the two men admittedly still thought that the preparation must owe its effect to inhibition of the A-cells and glucagon.

In their very first work, FRANKE and FUCHS already mentioned LOUBATIÈRES results in animal experiments, which he had published in 1946. As soon as the first findings of FRANKE and FUCHS became known, BERTRAM, ELINOR BENDFELDT and HELMUTH OTTO (b. 1925) in Hamburg undertook the examination of 82 patients with diabetes mellitus of varying duration and degress of severity.

Here, however, we must mention that, from 4–7 September 1955, at the 22nd session of the German Pharmaceutical Society, ACHELIS, HAACK and HARDEBECK first made public their animal experiments with BZ 55, while in Bad Homburg on 5 October 1955, at the 18th session of the German Society for Digestive and Metabolic Illnesses, BERTRAM already reported over 100 diabetiv cases that had been treated successfully with BZ 55.

At the beginning of 1956, BZ 55 was marketed as *nadisan,* resp. *invenol,* while in the German Democratic Republic the substance previously designated CA 1022 became *oranil.* A product with similar effects synthesized by Hoechst with the test designation D 860 was N-4-methylbenzol-sulfonyl-N-propyl-carbamide. The preparation made by the Boehringer Mannheim company was given the abbreviation *carbutamid,* while that of Hoechst Dyeworks was called *tolbutamid.*

As early as August 1955, six German clinics combined to pool their results on the new test preparation D 860. Shortly before that, GUSTAV EHRHART (b. 1894) had reported on animal experiments, in an introduction, HELMUT MASKE (b. 1921) had summarized the experiments made so far on oral blood-sugar reducing substances. MASKE emphasized that LOUBATIÈRES thought that sulfonamide stimulated insulin secretion. Finally MASKE mentioned similar research done by VON HOLT and his team in 1954, which has been dealt with above. On the basis of these first field studies, MASKE stated:

"There can be no doubt that in a group of mainly elderly diabetics insulin can be replaced wholly or partially with BZ 55."

D 860 became especially popular in America, where it was quickly admitted because of its lack of adverse chemotherapeutic effects and the insignificance of its side-effects. From September 1956 it was marketed in Germany as *rastinon* by Hoechst Dyeworks, as *artosin* by Boehringer & Sons, Mannheim, and as *orabet* by VEB Heyden Chemical Works.

In 1960, finally, a further sulfonamide derivative, *glycodiazin* (2-benzol-sulfonamido-5-methoxy-ethoxy-pyrimidin) was tested jointly by two companies, Bayer and Schering and in 1964 the preparation was put out with the trade name Redul. Over 13,000 diabetics were tested before the substance was made available commercially (GUTSCHE; MEILER). A few years later, in 1966, the two companies, Boehringer and Hoechst, succeeded in discovering a product that was two hundred times stronger than the original tolbutamid, which has been available since 1969 as euglucon 5, with the generic name *glybenclamid* (AUMÜLLER et al.: QUABBE and KLIEMS, RAPTIS, RAPTIS et al., GERHARDS et al., SCHWARZ et al.), while between 1967 and 1972, Hoffmann-La Roche introduced a further sulfonylurea derivative, *glibornurid* (glutril) to diabetes treatment (DUBACH and BRÜCKERT, GUTSCHE, BEYER et al., KRALL, SELL and SCHÖFFLING, CORDES, BEYER, SELL, HAUPT and SCHÖFFLING, LORCH, GEY and SOMMER).

In conclusion we can say that LOUBATIÈRES' first reports on the blood-sugar reducing properties of sulfonamides released a deluge of works which even the diabetes specialist cannot hope to take in. The explanation of the way these oral diabetic medicines work, not only the sulfonamide but also the biguanid kind, raises new problems and questions. The possibilities and limits of oral diabetes therapy are now more fully understood and although the principle reiterated by JOSLIN of *"triple therapy"*, with *"insulin, diet, and physical exercise"* has been enriched by the addition of oral therapy, it cannot be replaced by these preparations.

We must also mention the latest development, *glisoxepid*, which was made available jountly by Bayer and Schering in 1974 as *"pro-diaban"* (PULS et al., SCHÖFFLING et al.; SCHÖFFLING [Pbl]).

Future Outlook

We introduced this historical account of the way in which understanding of diabetes and its treatment developed with the statement by the Greek physician Aretaeus of Cappadocia: *"Diabetes is a mysterious illness"*, and we decided to plan our survey not in the usual chronological manner but to use a kind of *"hour-glass"* view. Thus we have treated in turn the periods of *clinical observation*, diagnostic *clarification* through anatomic and *pathologic findings* and *biochemical discoveries*, bevor dealing with the therapeutic aspects including the *discovery of insulin, diet therapy* and the *treatment of diabetes by oral means.*

But if it was thought in 1921 that the discovery of insulin provided the basis, the gauge so to speak, for all knowledge of the subject, we must admit today that the production and use of insulin were merely the waist of the *hour-glass* through which, for a short time, all the diverse results of research and experiment were channelled. Soon it was realized that the three directions which diabetes research was taking, *clinical expericence, anatomy* and *pathology*, and *biochemistry* raised fresh questions and that insulin was by no way the final stone in the edifice as had been thought in the 'twenties.

It was insulin therapy that made survival possible, especially for youthful diabetics, previously often doomed, and the prolongation of their lives brought to light new complications of the disease which could hardly have been observed before. Although the dreaded, mortally dangerous diabetic coma became increasingly rare, other chronic sequels cam increasingly to the fore or indeed first came to be recognized as such. In 1875 THEODOR LEBER (1840–1917) and in 1890 JULIUS HIRSCHBERG (1843–1927) were the first to assemble the hitherto scattered published findings on *eye disorders of diabetics* (FISCHER) – the first clear case of retinopathy in a patient with glycosuria had been described by HENRY DEWEY NOYES (1832–1900)in 1869; similar cases were noticed in 1855 by EDOUARD VON JAEGER (1818–1884), and in 1858 by LOUIS AUGUSTE DESMARRES (1810–1882) and EUGENE BOUCHUT (1818–1891), but they attributed the eye troubles to secondary nephritis since they had also found albuminuria (FISCHER), and the full extent of this complication did not become apparent until our own time.

It was not until 1936, however, that the American pathologist PAUL KIMMELSTIEL(b.1900) together with CLIFFORD WILSON, examined the symptoms of albuminuria with edema, as well as with hypertonia, azotemia and retinopathy as sequels of chronic *diabetic nephropathy* and as a syndrome, since named after those who first described it (PAYNE and POULTON; LAIPPLY et al.).

It was really only this association that led research workers to consider the *vascular system of diabetics* (SCHUMACHER, 1961, p. 29 seq.), and soon it was seen that there was a significant connection between diabetes and coronary disorders and disorders of the peripheral arteries. Proceeding from these clinical findings, pathologists gained an interesting insight into the changes in the structure of the vessel walls some of which could be helpful in diagnosis.

It was the discovery of insulin that led to intensive research into the mechanism of its production in the islets of Langerhans and its secretion from them, a matter that is also closely connected with the question of the effect of oral antidiabetic drugs.

The biochemical researchers who thought in 1921 that isolating the hormone responsible for carbohydrate metabolism clarified all problems of diabetes soon had to admit that insulin also affected the *metabolism of fats* and *proteins,* so that today it is debatable whether diabetes is caused primarily by a disorder of metabolism.

It is precisely insulin treatment, which has proved so tremendously successful in individual cases and has not only prolonged the lives of millions of diabetics but enabled them have to fulfilled existence, that has led – because of the greater life-expectancy of diabetics – to an *explosive increase* in cases of diabetes (CONN), because diabetics frequently marry other diabetics, if only because they share the same diet, and produce diabetic children or children susceptible to diabetes accordingly. This is closely connected with the problem of timely *recognition of latent diabetes* and *prophylaxis* before it declares itself.

The idea that the discovery of insulin might solve all questions connected with the *"mysterious sickness" was a delusion,* and it was not until our generation that the hour-glass shape of diabetes research became recognized. No one can say today whether in future the widely divergent forms of modern diabetes research will come together a second time through a fresh spectacular discovery or whether generations of diabetes specialists, pathologists, statisticians and biochemists will have to content themselves with scientific progress made in stone at a time, building up an edifice of which the final shape can only be guessed at today in its barest outlines.

Let us recall the statement made in the 1st century A. D. by the Roman physician SCRIBONIUS LARGUS that *"medicines are the hands of the gods"*. He whom the gods favour may have the chance to grab the young god of good fortune, the *"Kairos"*, by his proverbial forelock as he sneaks past; but the gods often slip away from man's grasp, and no mortal knows why. For all medical researchers and above all specialists in diabetes, the old first aphorism from the Corpus Hippocraticum still remains true:

"Life is short, art is long, the right moment soon speeds past, experience deceives, judgement is difficult!"

Literatur

(Auswahl aus dem medizinhistorischen Schrifttum)

ALLAN, F.N.: Diabetes before and after insulin. Med. Hist. (Lond.) **16**, 266–273 (1972).

AMMON, R.: E.E.J. Lesser's Beitrag zur Insulin-Forschung. Medizinische Nr. 12, 397–398 (1954).

ANDERSON, F. J.: John Rollo's patient. J. hist. Med. **20**, 163–164 (1965).

BAQUET, R.: Les conseils aux diabétiques d'Apollinaire Bouchardat. Maroc méd. **51**, 250–253 (1971).

BARACH, J.H.: Historical facts in diabetes. Ann. med. Hist. **10**, 387–401 (1928).

BECKER, V.: Paul Langerhans – 100 Jahre nach seiner Doktorarbeit. Dtsch. med. Wschr. **95**, 358–362 (1970).

BERG, A.: 40 Jahre Insulin. Münch. med. Wschr. **104**, 1–3 (1962).

BERG, A.: Die Entwicklung der Lehre vom Diabetes bis zur Gewinnung des Insulins. Münch. med. Wschr. **104**, 807–815 (1962).

BEST, C.H.: The discovery of insulin. Proc. Amer. Diab. Ass. **6**, 87–93 (1947).

BIBERGEIL, H.: 50 Jahre Insulin. Rückblick und Ausschau. Dtsch. Gesundh.-Wes. **27**, 721–728 (1972).

CAMPBELL, W.R.: Paul Langerhans 1847–1888. Canad. med. Ass. J. **79**, 855–856 (1958).

CAMPBELL, W. R.: Anabasis. Canad. med. Ass. J. **87**, 1055–1061 (1962).

CHEYMOL, J.: A propos de »la découverte de l'insuline« par Banting et Best il y a cinquante ans. Bull. Acad. Méd. (Paris) **155**, 836–852 (1971).

COLLIP, J.B.: Reminiscences on the discovery of insulin. Canad. med. Ass. J. **87**, 1045 (1962).

DEROT, M.: La découverte de l'insuline. Vie méd. Nr. spécial **52,** 13–22 (1971).
DRÜGEMÖLLER, P., NORPOTH, L.: Wege und Irrwege der deutschen Insulin-Forschung. Dtsch. med. Wschr. **78,** 919–922 (1953).
EBSTEIN, E.: Zur Vorgeschichte des Coma diabeticum. Wien, klin. Wschr. **25,** 885–886 (1912).
EBSTEIN, E.: Zur Entwicklung der klinischen Harndiagnostik. Leipzig 1915.
EBSTEIN, E.: Aus der Geschichte der Zuckerharnruhr mit besonderer Berücksichtigung der Bauchspeicheldrüse. Arch. Verdau.-Kr. **33,** 215–226 (1924).
EBSTEIN, E.: Die Toxintheorie des Diabetes mellitus. Dtsch. med. Wschr. **26,** 170–171 (1900).
FEASBY, W.R.: The discovery of insulin. J. Hist. Med. **13,** 68–84 (1958).
FEDERLIN, K.: 50 Jahre Insulin. Dtsch. med. J. **23,** 612–617 (1972).
FISCHER, F.: Einst und jetzt: Die Historische Entwicklung der Retinopathia diabetica. Münch. med. Wschr. **96,** 1287–1289 (1954).
FISCHER, F.: Der erste Fall von Retinopathia diabetica. Wien. med. Wschr. **107,** 969–972 (1957).
FLECKLES, L.: Die Geschichte der gangbaren Theorien vom Diabetes, von Willis 1674, bis Pavy 1864. Dtsch. Klin. **17,** 89–93 (1865).
FLETCHER, A. A.: Early clinical experiences with insulin. Canad. med Ass. J. **87,** 1052–1055 (1962).
FRANK, L.L.: Diabetes mellitus in the texts of Old Hindu medicine (Charaka, Susruta, Vagbhata). Amer. J. Gastroent. **27,** 76–95 (1957).
GEMMILI, C.L.: The Greek concept of diabetes. Bull. N. Y. Acad. Med. **48,** 1033–1036 (1972).
GIACOMETTI, L., BARSS, M.: Paul Langerhans. A tribute. Arch. Derm. **100,** 770–772 (1969).
GOLDNER, M.G.: History of insulin. Ann. intern. Med. **76,** 329 (1972).
GOLDSTEIN, A.: To the history of diabetes mellitus hereditarius and prophylaxis. Koroth **5,** 713–715 (1971).
GRMEK, M.D.: Examen critique de la genèse d'une grande dêcouverte: »La Piqûre diabétique« de Claude Bernard. Clio med. **1,** 341–350 (1965/66).
GROEN, J.J.: Discovery of insulin told as a human story. Israel J. med. Sci. **8,** 476–483 (1972).
GUTSCHE, H.: Diabetes mellitus – zwei Jahrzehnte orale Therapie. Ther. Ber. (Bayer) **46,** 22–26 (1974).
HAMARNEH, S.: Arabic historiography as related to the health professions in mediaval islam. Sudhoffs, Arch. Gesch. Med. **50,** 2–24 (1966).
HARMSEN, E.: Zur Entdeckung des Glykogens vor 75 Jahren, Münch. med. Wschr. **79,** 1075 (1932).
HARMSEN, E.: Victor Hensen, der deutsche Entdecker des Glykogens. Med. Welt **8,** 1783–1784 (1934).
HAZARD, R.: Un précurseur oublié dans la découverte de l'insuline. Moniteur pharm. **25,** 2607 (1971).
HENSCHEN, F.: On the term diabetes in the works of Aretaeus and Galen. Med. Hist. (Lond.) **13,** 190–192 (1969).
HOFFMANN, J.P.H.: Die Geschichte des Diabetes mellitus. Med. Diss. Düsseldorf 1960.
HOLSCHER, H., KENDE, R.: Diabetes. Aus der Geschichte seiner Erforschung und Behandlung, Stolberg 1971.
HORNOR, A.A.: History of insulin. Ann. intern. Med. **76,** 330 (1972).
JAMES, T.: History of diabetes. S. Afr. med. J. **44,** 1344–1345 (11970).

KALBFLEISCH, K.: Diabetes. Sudhoffs Arch. Gesch. Med. **42**, 142–144 (1958).
KENEZ, J.: Zur Frühgeschichte der Insulin-Forschung. Münch. med. Wschr. **114**, 2003–2006 (1972).
KING, L.S.: Empiricism, rationalism and diabetes. J. Amer. med. Ass. **187**, 521–526 (1964).
KLOPPE, W.: Paul Langerhans (1847–1888) und seine Berliner Dissertation (1869). Dtsch. med. J. **20**, 581–583 (1969).
KLOPPE, W.: Die Zuckerkrankheit – historisch betrachtet. Diabetiker **20**, 252–254 (1970).
KNICK, B.: Zur Geschichte der diätetischen Behandlung der Zuckerkrankheit. Therapiewoche **23**, 905–911 (1973).
KORP, W., ZWEYMÜLLER, E.: 50 Jahre Insulinbehandlung an der Wiener Kinderklinik – das Schicksal zuckerkranker Kinder aus der ersten Insulinära. Wien. klin. Wschr. **85**, 385–390 (1973).
LACEY, A.H.: The unit of insulin. Diabetes **16**, 198–200 (1967).
LAUSCH, E.: Diabetes. Siege, Hoffnungen und immer neue Rätsel. Weinheim: Verlag Chemie 1971.
LEBENSOHN, J.E.: The semicentenary of insulin. Amer. J. Ophthal. **72**, 1155–1157 (1971).
LEIBOWITZ, J.O.: Maimonides on the incidence of diabetes. Israel J. med. Sci. **2**, 714 (1966).
LEIBOWITZ, J.O.: The concept of diabetes in historical perspective. Israel J. med. Sci. **8**, 469–475 (1972).
LEICKERT, K.H.: Insulin-Vorläufer – ein historischer Abriß. Erste Diabetes-Behandlungs-Versuche mit Pankreasextrakten. Arzneimittel-Forsch. **25**, 435–442 (1975).
LESKY, E.: Etappen in der Erforschung des Diabetes mellitus. Öst. Ärzteztg. **24**, 2373–2375 (1969).
LEVINE, R.: History of etiology of diabetes mellitus. Arch. Path. **78**, 405–408 (1964).
LEVINE, R.: Insulin. The biography of a small protein. New Engl. J. Med. **277**, 1059–1064 (1967).
LIPPMANN, O. v.: Zur Geschichte des diabetischen Zuckers. Chem. Z. **29**, 1197–1198 (1905).
LOUBATIÈRES, A.: Zur Geschichte der Entdeckung der oralen Antidiabetica. In: Handbuch des Diabetes mellitus. Hrsg. v. E.F. PFEIFFER, Bd. 2, S. 1179–1197. München: Lehmann 1969.
MAGNUS-LEVY, A.: Diabetikerdiäten der Vorinsulinära. Bull. Hist. Med., Suppl. **3**, 161–169 (1944).
MAIWALD, K.H.: Johann Peter Frank 1745–1821. Sein Beitrag zur Kenntnis des Diabetes mellitus. Ther. Monat (Boehringer Mannheim) **10**, 14–20 (1960).
MAJOR, R.H.: Johann Conrad Brunner and his experiments on the pancreas. Ann. med. Hist. **3**, 91–100 (1941).
MANI, N.: Die Entdeckung des Glykogens durch Claude Bernard. Z. klin. Chem. **2**, 97–128 (1964).
MANI, N.: Die historischen Grundlagen der Leberforschung. II: Die Geschichte der Leberforschung von Galen bis Claude Bernard. Basler Veröff. Gesch. Med. Biol., Bd. 21. Basel-Stuttgart: Schwabe 1967.
MANN, R.J.: Historical vignette „honey urine" to pancreatic diabetes: 600 BC-. 1922. Proc. Mayo Clin. **46**, 56–58 (1971).
MARBLE, A.: John Rollo. Diabetes **5**, 325–327 (1956).

MARTIN, E.: Problèmes de priorité dans la découverte de l'insuline. Schweiz. med. Wschr. **101**, 164–167 (1971).

MEINDL, R.: Zur Geschichte der Zuckerharnruhr. Med. Diss. Göttingen 1948.

MELLINGHOFF, K.H.: Georg Ludwig Zuelzers Beitrag zur Insulinforschung. Med. Diss. Düsseldorf 1971 und Düsseldorfer Beitr. Gesch. Med. H. 36, Düsseldorf: Triltsch 1971.

MINKOWKSI, O.: Die Lehre vom Pankreas-Diabetes in ihrer geschichtlichen Entwicklung. Münch. med. Wschr. **76**, 311–315 (1929).

MIROUZE, J.: Histoire du coma diabétique et de son traitement. Vie méd. Nr. spécial **52**, 25–35 (1971).

MÜLLER, R.F.G.: Die Harnruhr der Alt-Inder, Prameha. Sudhoffs Arch. Gesch. Med. **25**, 1–42 (1932).

MURLIN, J.R., KRAMER, B.: A quest for the anti-diabetic hormone 1913–1916. J. Hist. Med. **11**, 288–298 (1956).

MURLIN, W.R.: History of insulin. Ann. intern. Med. **76**, 330 (1972).

MURNAGHAN, J.H., TALALAY, P.: John Jacob Abel and the crystallization of insulin. Perspect. Biol. Med. **10**, 334–380 (1967).

MURRAY, J.: The search for insulin. Scott. med. J. **14**, 286–293 (1969).

MURRAY, J.: Insulin. Credit for its isolation. Brit. med. J. **1969 II**, 651–652.

MURRAY, J.: Paulesco and the isolation of insulin. J. Hist. Med. **26**, 150–157 (1971).

NOTELOVITZ, M.: Milestones in the history of diabetes – a brief survey. S. Afr. med. J. **44**. 1158–1161 (1970).

NOTHMAN, M.M.: The history of the discovery of pancreatic diabetes. Bull. Hist. Med. **28**, 272–274 (1954).

ORTH, H.: Die Antiken Diabetes-Synonyme und ihre Wortgeschichte. Janus **51**, 193–201 (1964).

OTTEN, J.H.: Die Geschichte der oralen Diabetestherapie. Med. Diss. Freiburg/-Breisgau 1966.

OTTEN, J.H.: Zur Geschichte der oralen Diabetestherapie. Med. Klin. **63**, 22–25 (1968).

PAPASPYROS, N.S.: The history of diabetes mellitus. 2. Aufl. Stuttgart: Thieme 1964.

PATON, A.: Notes for a history of diabetes mellitus. Brit. J. clin. Pract. **15**, 37–39 (1961).

PAVEL, I.: Zur Frühgeschichte der Insulin-Forschung. Münch. med. Wschr. **115**, 729–730 (1973).

PESTEL, M.: Le cinquantenaire de la découverte de l'insuline. E. Gley, précurseur de F. J. Banting et C. H. Best. Nouv. Presse méd. **1**, 1527–1528 (1972).

POREP, R.: Der Physiologe und Planktonforscher Victor Hensen. Med. Diss. Kiel 1970 und Kieler Beitr. Gesch. Med. H. 9, Neumünster 1970. S. 76 f.

POREP, R.: Der Prioritätenstreit um die Entdeckung des Glykogens zwischen Claude Bernard und Victor Hensen. Med. Mschr. **25**, 314–321 (1971).

POULET, J.: Le diabète avant la découverte de l'insuline. Vie. méd. Nr. spéc. **52**, 5–10 (1971).

PRATT, J.H.: Zur Geschichte der Entdeckung des Insulins. Sudhoffs. Arch. Gesch. Med. **38**, 48–57 (1954).

RECKENDORF, H.K.: Medizinische Konzeption und Therapie. Die Behandlung des Diabetes mellitus zu Beginn des 19. Jahrhunderts durch John Rollo. Ther. Monat (Boehringer Mannheim) **21**, 17–19 (1961).

ROSEMANN, R.: Zur Entdeckung des Glykogens vor 75 Jahren. Münch. med. Wschr. **79**, 1367–1368 (1932).
SALOMON, M.: Geschichte der Glycosurie von Hippokrates bis zum Anfang des 19. Jahrhunderts. Dtsch. Arch. klin. Med. **8**, 489–582 (1871).
SCHADEWALDT, H.: Das Pankreas in der Geschichte der Medizin. In: Pathogenese, Diagnostik, Klinik und Therapie der Erkrankungen des exokrinen Pankreas. Hrsg. v. N. HENNING, K. HENKEL und H. SCHÖN, S. 1–46. Stuttgart: Schattauer 1964.
SCHADEWALDT, H.: Die Geschichte des Diabetes. Allergie Immun. Forsch., Bd. 2, S. 9–22. Stuttgart: Schattauer 1968.
SCHIRMER, A.M. Beitrag zur Geschichte und Anatomie des Pankreas, Basel 1893.
SCHMIDT, F.: Insulin-Herstellung in Deutschland durch einen Mecklenburger Landapotheker. Pharm. Z. **117**, 1195–1196 (1972).
SCHNEIDER, T.: Diabetes through the ages: a salute to insuline. S. Afr. med. J. **46**, 1394–1400 (1972).
SCHUMACHER, H., SCHUMACHER, J.: Einst und Jetzt: 100 Jahre Diabetes mellitus. Münch. med. Wschr. **96**, 517–521, 581–588 und 601–604 (1956).
SCHUMACHER, J.: Index zum Diabetes mellitus. München–Berlin: Urban und Schwarzenberg 1961.
SCHUMACHER, J.: Geschichte des Diabetes mellitus bis zur Insulin-Ära. Dtsch. med. J. **22**, 707–715 (1963).
SCHUMACHER, R.: Die Carl v. Noorden'sche Haferkur, ihre Weiterentwicklung und ihr Einfluß auf die Diättherapie des Diabetes mellitus unter Berücksichtigung ihrer heutigen Bedeutung. Med. Diss. Freiburg/Breisgau 1963.
SEALE, H.: Banting's miracle. The story of the discovery of insulin. Philadelphia: Lippincott 1946.
SECKENDORF, E.: Kurze Geschichte des Diabetes mellitus. Med. Welt **5**, 1443–1445 (1931).
SPIEGELHOFF, W.: Die Geschichte der Pankreaserkrankungen. Med. Diss. Düsseldorf 1937.
STAHL, J.: La découverte de l'insuline. Strasbourg méd. **12**, 871–879 (1961).
STEIN, P.: Prioritäten und Prioritätsansprüche ums Insulin. Gesnerus **31**, 107–112 (1974).
STÖCKER, W.: Zur Geschichte des Diabetes mellitus. Therapiewoche **16**, 1077–1082 (1966).
STÖCKER, W.: 50 Jahre Insulin. Therapiewoche **21**, 2444–2450 (1971) und Pharm. Z. **116**, 1667–1671 (1971).
STÖCKER, W.: Der Prioritätenstreit um das Insulin. Therapiewoche **21**, 3464–3467 (1971) und Pharm. Z. **116**, 1764–1765 (1971).
STRIKER, C.: Famous faces in diabetes. Boston: Hall 1961.
STRIKER, C.: History of insulin. Ann intern. Med. **76**, 329–330 (1972).
TEE, G.J.: On Sami Hamarneh's Review of „Der Diabetestraktat" 'Abd al-Latif al-Bagdadi's. Isis **64**, 232 (1973).
THIES, H.J.: Der Diabetestraktat 'Abd Al-Latif al-Badadi's. Bonner Orient. Stud. NS Bd. 21, Bonn 1971.
VEITH, I.: Four thousand years of diabetes. Modern Med. **39**, 118–125 (1971).
VOSS, H.: 100 Jahre Langerhanssche Inseln, Anat. Anz. **125**, 333–335 (1969).
WOLFF, G.: Abriß der Geschichte der Zuckerkrankheit. Med. Mschr. **7**, 253–254, 527–529 (1953); **9**, 37–41 (1955).

WOLFF, G.: Zucker, Zuckerkrankheit und Insulin. Eine medizin- und kulturhistorische Studie. Remscheid-Lennep: Dustri 1955.

WOLFF, G.: Die Entdeckung des Insulins vor 35 Jahren durch Banting und Best. Med. Mschr. **10**, 468–470 (1956).

WOLFF, G.: Zur Geschichte der Harnzuckeruntersuchung. Ther. Monat (Boehringer Mannheim) **7**, 321–323, 838–846 (1957).

WOLFF, G.: Der Zuckerstoffwechsel – eine biographische Studie. Med. Mschr. **12**, 766–774 (1958).

WOLFF, G.: Beiträge berühmter Studenten zur Erforschung des Zuckerstoffwechsels. Münch. med. Wschr. **102**, 1203–1208 (1960).

WOLFF, G.: La découverte de l'insuline. Med. Hyg. **29**, 1102 (1971).

YOUNG, F.G.: Claude Bernard and the discovery of glycogen. Brit. med. J. **1957 I**, 1431–1436.

ZANDER, K.: Zur Begriffsbestimmung des Diabetes mellitus. Med. Diss. Freiburg/Breisgau 1972.

ZIMMERMANN, O.C.: Die erste Beschreibung von Symptomen des experimentellen Pankreas-Diabetes durch den Schweizer Johann Conrad Brunner (1653–1727). Med. Diss. Basel 1944 und Gesnerus **2**, 109–130 (1945).

Aus: *Handbuch der Inneren Medizin, hg. v. H. Schwiegk, Teil 2 a, Berlin ²1975, S. 1–44*

Diabetes, Sugar Consumption and Luxury Through the Ages

A question Posed by History

by ERICH EBSTEIN

Hans Ullmann published an article in this review (1928, No 3) entitled "The Increase in Diabetes – a Question of Nutrition?" In his interesting study he shows that increased sugar consumption and an increase in mortality from diabetes go hand in hand with a rising standard of living and cultural development.

In this connection with this discussion *Ullmann* has asked me whether there was any evidence from earlier times about sugar consumption on the one hand and "food culture" on the other.

In antiquity, only honey was known; the first news of sugar-cane came to Europe in 327 B.C., at the time of Alexander the Great's Indian campaign, when it was reported "that a peculiar kind of reed grows in India that produces a sort of honey without the aid of bees". (Cf *Lippmann,* History of Sugar, Leipzig, 1890, and do. in Abhandlungen und Vorträge. Leipzig 1906, p. 261–274 and 326–334.)

We must remember that the Roman author *Celsus,* whose writings on the art of healing are one of our main sources for Greek and Alexandrian medicine, lived at the time of Julius Caesar (100–44 B.C.) and the Emperor Tiberius. He has a short passage (Liber IV, 27, 2) about "excessive elimination of urine", which must refer to glycosuria, without using the term "diabetes" which is found for the first time in *Aretaeus* (2nd century A.D.). *Aretaeus* called it a mysterious illness and knew nothing of its etiology.

Today we distinguish between an endogenous and an exogenous starting-point for the development of diabetes.

When we examine the question in a historical context we can no longer claim that we have proof that (or whether), at times of great luxury with a high consumption of honey, sweet wines, cocoa and chocolate, doctors diagnosed more diabetes mellitus more frequently. We must, however, agree that it is possible that in such periods of "high living" alimentary glycosuria occurred.

As long as it is impossible to prove that sugar really is a more likely cause of diabetes than starches are, we cannot establish a direct relationship between sugar consumption and diabetes.

Here we might mention that at the time when *Celsus* was writing his medical work, there were pastry-cooks and shops in Rome, and in Caesar's time a love of good food was universal. Banqueting caused such an increase in the price of gourmet foods that Caesar legislated against it. All kinds of fruit were preserved in honey, whose conserving properties were well known (see *Lippmann* 1890, p. 15 seq.).

It is interesting to note that, as early as the 5th century, Indian physicians knew about the sweetness of diabetic urine, either through tasting it or because they had noticed that it attracted insects (*Erich Ebstein,* Zur Entwicklung der klinischen Harndiagnostik, Leipzig 1915). We also know that around 500 A.D. sugar cane was brought from India to Persia and that the first mention of solid sugar occurred in 627 A.D., when the Emperor Heraclius destroyed the palace of the King of Persia. The fact that sugar was listed among the royal treasures shows that it was still a great rarity at the time (see *Lippmann,* 1906, p. 262 seq.).

During the period after the conquest of Damascus (635), Jerusalem (638) and Syria (640), as the Arabs advanced triumphantly following their defeat of the Byzantine armies, a great deal was heard of the luxury and pomp found in the Middle East, and before long at the Ommayed court (see *Lippmann,* 1890, p. 110 seq.).

At that time (670) *Paulus Aeginita,* who lived in Alexandria, described diabetes at the "thirst sickness" (Liber III, 45).

Avicenna (980–1037), the Arab physician, who had personally observed cases of diabetes, knew of several kinds of sugar, e.g., dark sugar and cane honey, i.e., the juice of cane sugar. The 5th book of *Avicenna*'s established list of Arab medicines (650 remedies) mentions more than a hundred that were prepared with the aid of sugar (see *Lippmann,* 1890, 126 seq.).

Actuarius, who lived in Byzantium in the 13th century and described diabetes, also mentions sugar frequently in his writings, e.g., his account of the preparation of therapeutic rosewater by fermenting rose petals in a sugar solution (see *Lippmann,* 1890, 170 seq.).

In the course of the 14th century the taste for sugar and confectionery became a universal favorite, and everywhere sugar became the most sought-after and choicest of delicacies, so much that Florence, Bologna and other cities promulgated anti-luxury laws strictly regulating the supply and availability of even such items as pastry (see *Lippmann,* 1890, 225 seq.). So, for instance, at the beginning of the 14th century, for 200,000 inhabitants Milan had 1000 wine taverns, 400 bakers and 150 large inns.

Venice was the prinicpal centre of the sugar trade; its citizens became so much addicted to sugar, magnificent confectionery, and all kinds of food delicacy that in 1514 the Venetian senate again had to legislate against luxury. It forbade the gilding of sugar and sugar products, of fine marzipan and confectionery, and prohibited the consumption of all such sweetmeats; only plain sweetmeats and marzipan were permitted, and then only as dessert. But the law remained a dead letter (see *Lippmann,* 1890, 268 seq.).

Victor Trincavella (1476–1568) was practising in Venice at that time; in the course of 40 year's medical practice he had observed three cases of diabetes, but he was able to remember only two of them clearly. He attributed them to drinking ice-cold water during a high fever. He did not taste the urine, nor did he mention excessive indulgence in sugary foods as a possible cause.

The Nuremberg *Hochzeitsbuch* (Wedding Book) of 1485 also mentions a legal ban on the luxury of indulging in sugar and sweetmeats.

Jacob Sylvius (1478–1555) of Paris saw only one case of diabetes in the life and called it *"affectus rarus"*. In his work, *"Medicamentorum simplicium delectus"* (1562) he described, among other things, the preservation, candying and glazing of fruits and demonstrated the art of boiling sugar (see *Lippmann,* 1890, 272 seq.).

In a herbal of 1588 by *Tabernämontanus,* who was physician to the Elector of Speyer, the author said:

"So many seeds and fruits are covered with sugar, for banquets, nightcaps, and feasts that the disgusting over-indulgence makes us sick and spoils and shortens our lives; truly, since the beginning of the world there can't have been any worse excess and luxury than today" (see *Lippmann,* 1890, 287–289).

At the time of King Gustav I (Wasa) of Sweden (1496–1560), sugar was exported from Lübeck to Sweden: in a letter the King reproached his daughter, Katherine, Countess of East Frisia, claiming that she owes her ailing health to her over-indulgence in sugar when she was young, since this had damaged her stomach (see *W. Volz,* Beiträge zur Kulturgeschichte, Leipzig 1852, p. 216).

In 1535 *Charles Estienne* wrote: "Nowadays sugar is indispensable with food and drink, and there is a raging craze for it . . .; the best sugar comes from Spain, Cyprus, Rhodes, Candia, and Malta . . ."

Although, during this period of luxury *Paracelsus* prescribed the testing of urine samples, and talked in general of their *dulcedo* (sweetness), he made no connection between that and diabetes.

It is somewhat surprising that we first find an observation like the following in a "Histoire maccaronique de Merlin Coccaie (anonyn)", which appeared in Paris in 1606, and gave a deliberately exaggerated account of a sumptuous feast: "Tant sortes de vin ne se passèrent . . . dans les douces urines que Corse pisse" (see *Lippmann,* 1923, p. 211–213).

Thus sweet Corsican wine and sugar-containing urine are placed in direct juxtaposition. The writer, a certain *Folengo,* born in Venice in 1517, supposedly modelled himself on *Rabelais* (1483–1553), who mentioned sugar several times in "Gargantua" (see *Lippmann,* 1890, p. 274). Elsewhere, too, during the same period (*Salomon,* p. 34), diabetes was ascribed to drinking large quantities of wine.

We might mention that *Folengo,* from Venice, was a contemporary of the Venetian physician *Trincavella,* who had seen cases of diabetes mellitus.

As *Schelenz* has shown (Berl. Klin. Wochenschr. 1915, No. 23, p. 623–624), scurvy was regarded as a symptom of syphilis; indeed, in *Ray's* "Historia plantarum" (1686) both syphilis and scurvy were attributed to excessive indulgence in sugar, especially in Spain, less so in England.

The term "diabetic" seems to have been coined by *Marcello Donato* (d. 1600), who defined it thus: "A patient in whom liquid is eliminated unaltered through the kidneys is called diabetic by physicians." (*Max Salomon,* Geschichte der Gykosurie, etc., Leipzig 1871, p. 27).

The history of diabetes with special reference to the pancreas ("Geschichte der Zuckerkrankheit mit besonderer Berücksichtigung auf die Bauchspeicheldrüse") I have dealt with myself (Arch. f. Verdauungskrankheiten, vol. 32 [1923] p. 216–226).

It has been amply demonstrated that in times of penury, e.g., during the blockade of 1917, diabetes became a rare disease in Germany. Here I should just like to quote a phrase from *Friedrich von Müller*'s valuable work on the influence of wartime conditions on health in the German Reich (Münch, med. Wochenschr. 1920. Annex to No. 8, p. 245): "My well-to-do diabetic patients (and diabetes is an illness predominantly of the rich) have been revealed as extremely cunning hoarders thanks to their bank accounts, and a similar observations is found in a report by *Carl von Noorden*".

In this connection, we can learn a great deal from *Ullmann*'s edifying conclusion that a people's sugar consumption is a yardstick of their rising standards of living. Parallel with this is the increase in cases of diabetes. In times of penury, on the other hand, there is a decrease in sugar consumption and a corresponding decrease in cases of diabetes.

As we mentioned at the outset, *Ullmann* also agreed that it must remain a moot point "to what extent nutrition is an external factor that can be seen only as a triggering agent and if we can assume that there is always an endogenous disposition".

Lichtenfelt showed in his "Geschichte der Ernährung" (History of Nutrition), Berlin 1913, p. 102, that *per capita* sugar consumption had increased in every country. Of particular value in this connection are the sugar statistics for the period 1913/14–1926/7, compiled by *Rudolf E. Grotkass* (Magdeburg 1927; from the "Yearbook and directory of sugar factories"), which we should just like to mention here, as also the same author's essay on "Zuckerfabrikation im Magdeburgischen" (Sugar production in the Magdeburg district) in vol. 2 of the Magdeburg Wirtschaftsleben (1927).

Kurt Ritter, too, has shown in the same periodical (No. 17) that sugar consumption as a form of nutrition is relatively new in our latitudes and that it was regarded as a luxury until last century. In his work on the predictable increase in world sugar consumption and on the regions where sugar might be produced to meet the demand, in Die Deutsche Zuckerindustrie 1927 (Nos 14–17 and 19), *Grotkass* established that sugar consumption had doubled every 20 years since 1850.

The history of nutrition teaches us something about the consumption of sugar and honey and its possible connection with food practices, but the data for this are sparse and might perhaps be added to. Let us hope that these lines may inspire further research.

in: *Medizinische Welt* 49 (1928) 1840–1842

Antiquity

Diabetes

by KARL KALBFLEISCH

The following article was sent by K. KALBFLEISCH in 1943 to the editors of the *Philologischen Wochenschrift* (Leipzig), where it was due to appear among the "Communications". The text went to the printers and was arranged to be published in one of the volumes for the year 1944, but this year did not appear because of the emergency situation. However, reprints were produced with the title *Reprint from the Philologischen Wochenschrift 1944*. The author sent a few to friends and colleagues; the rest must have perished when KALBFLEISCH's house in Giessen was destroyed by bombs in December 1944. KARL KALBFLEISCH died at his home-town of Gelnhausen, where he had taken refuge, on 7 February 1946 at the age of 77. Obituaries by H.-G. GUNDEL appeared in the *Nachrichten der Giessener Hochschulgesellschaft* XX (1954), p. 165–178 and the Chronique d'Égypte XXVI (Brussels 1951), p. 460–467. As the *Philologische Wochenschrift* did not reappear after the war, another way had to be chosen to bring the article to general knowledge.
ANDREAS THIERFELDER, Mainz.

Anyone interested in the history of Greco-Roman medicine must often have asked how the name *diabetes* for the sugar disease is to be explained. As this is not dealt with very satisfactorily in the medical texts[1] available to me on this question and others closely connected with it, many may find the following remarks welcome.

Διαβαίνειν signifies "to stride (out)": *εὐ διαβὰς*, "far-striding", Hector slings a mighty stone M 458. *Διαβήτης* therefore means the two-limbed compass with which the mathematician METON worked (Aristophanes, *The Birds* 1003), but also the branched lifter, the double lifter or siphon through which the fluid to be removed, say wine from the cask, flowed (COLUMELLA III 10, 2 *per siphonem, quem diabeten vocant mechanici;* cf. HERON, *Pneumatica* I, 1–3). With this word, not yet used by HIPPOCRATES and his

[1] See especially MAX SALOMON, *Geschichte der Glykosurie von Hippokrates bis zum Anfange des 19. Jahrhunderts*, in the *Deutschen Archiv für klinische Medizin*, Vol. 8 (1871), pp. 498–582.

followers, according to the evidence of Soranus[2] the Herophilean, DEMETRIOS of Apameia in Bithynia (c. 100 BC, see RE IV 2847 f., No. 111) characterized the urinary flux in which the fluid taken is very soon excreted again.[3] The archaizing Ionic-writing eclectic-pneumatic physician ARETAIOS of Cappadocia,[4] a contemporary of GALEN, no longer understood this designation of the disease; his view was that the disease could well be explained by the fluid in the disorder using the body merely as a passage-way (*διαβάθρη*) to the outside. The disease was also called "hydrops in the champer-pot" or "diarrhea in the urine", or "thirst disease" on account of the associated persistent thirst.[5] This plurality of names shows that the disease attracted much attention and discussion, although it must have occurred very rarely; GALEN says in his text *Περὶ τῶν πεπονθότων τόπων*, which he wrote under Septimius Severus (193–199), therefore at the age of 60, that until then he had seen only two cases.[6] On the whole, the sugar disease as such was not known to the Greek and Roman physicians.[7] They were the less able to distinguish it from the (simple) urinary flux since, in the sugar disease too, there was often a great feeling of thirst which compelled the patients to take enormous amounts of fluid, so that often 6–8 liters were

---

[2] CAELIUS AURELIANUS Chron. III 8, 102: *Sed melius Demetrius Apameus ab hydrops discrevit eum qui sine dilatione potum liquorem per urinam egerit, diabeten appellans.* The Erasistrian APOLLONIUS of Memphis (RE No. 100, col. 149) had already used the comparison with a pipe (Caelius Aurel. elsewhere: *tanquam per fistulam transiens*).

[3] Cf. AETIUS XI 1,1 (cod. Vindob.): *κέκληται διαβήτης ἀπὸ τῆς πρὸς τοὺς καλουμένους διαβήτας ὁμοιότητος, οἵ τινες εἶδος σίφωνός εἰσιν* .

[4] ARETAIOS was greatly overvalued by SALOMON p. 493 as by HAESER (*Lehrbuch der Geschichte der Medizin* I 1875 p. 141 f.) and other recent physicians because his dependence on his precursors, especially Archigenes, was not noted: see MAX WELLMANN, *Die pneumatische Schule*, Berlin 1895, p. 23 ff. The passage listed above, Chron. IV 2 p. 66 Hude: *τῇδέ μοι δοκέει καλέεσθαι διαβήτης ἐπίκλησιν, ὁκοῖόν τι διαβήτης ἐών, οὕνεκεν ἐν τῷ σκήνεϊ τὸ ὑγρὸν οὐ μίμνει, ἀλλ ὅκως διαβάθρῃ τῷ ἀνθρώπῳ ἐς ἔξοδον χρέεται.*

[5] GALEN VII 81 Kühn: *ὁ καλούμενος ὕδρωψ είς ἀμίδα, τινὲς δὲ διαβήτην αὐτὸν ὀνομάζουσι ἄλλοι δὲ διάρροιαν εἰς οὖρα* cf. IX 597; also VIII 394, 13: *ἔνιοι δὲ διψακὸν ὀνομάζουσι.*

[6] VIII 394 Kühn: *τὸ πάθος . . . σπανιώτατον γιγνόμενον ἐμοὶ γοῦν ὤφθη δὶς ἄχρι δεῦρο* . See KURT BARDONG, *Beiträge zur Hippokrates- und Galenforschung*, in *Nachrichten der Akademie der Wissenschaften in Göttingen, Philol.-hist. Klasse*, 1942, p. 640.

[7] On the other hand, it seems to have been already known to the Indian physicians in the 5th century; see EDMUND O. VON LIPPMANN, *Abhandlungen und Vorträge zur Geschichte der Naturwissenschaften*, Leipzig 1906, p. 333 f.

drunk and excreted daily. Only in 1674 did the English physician Willis discover the sweet taste of diabetic urine. Thereafter, the sugar disease was distinguished as diabetes mellitus from the (simple) urinary flux or diabetes insipidus. In 1835 AMBROSIANI demonstrated the presence of sugar, already surmised earlier, in the blood of diabetics.

In the absence of insulin the so-called acetone bodies are formed and produce a severe toxic state termed coma. When the course is as pictured in ARETAIOS IV 2: "Long is the development of diabetes, long its incubation. But once it has matured, the sufferer has no longer to live, for then decline is rapid and death soon arrives,[8] then one may well deduce the sugary urinary flux, diabetes mellitus with coma ("Death usually follows within the first 12–24 hours", EWALD in Eulenburg, Real-Encyclopädie der gesamten Heilkunde III p. 807), yet simple urinary flux, diabetes insipidus, ist not to be excluded.

---

[8] ARETAIOS Chron. IV 2 p. 21 ff. Hude: *χρονίη μὲν ἡ τῆς νούσου φυή, μακρῷ κυΐσκεται κρόνῳ. βραχύβιος δὲ ὤνθρωπος ἦν ἡ πατάστασις τελεσθῇ· ὀξείη γὰρ ἡ τηκεδών, ταχὺς δὲ ὁ θάνατος.*

Synonyms for Diabetes in Antiquity and Their Etymology

by HERMANN ORTH

The history of ancient terms in modern terminology tends to begin when they confront us for the first time as conceptually and linguistically established terms in the old literature. Their history within antiquity is then sealed, the name undergoes no further change, the old concept attached to it has usually undergone the most changeable of fortunes. This is partly to be ascribed to the ignorance and caprice of later physicians, but very often the narrow precision of technical terminology attached to our terms requires that the general meaning almost always associated with the Greek word in ancient medical science be narrowed down to suit modern terminologic needs. Thus, research in the special history of the terms customarily begins with the first appearance of a technical word in the ancient literature and restricts itself to the investigation of its conceptual aspect.

Thus, the need is to review the first historical paragraph and to note that the old term did not arise suddenly as the inspiration of a Greek physician, like Athene from the head of Zeus, but emerged from a primal concept and primal name to undergo a maturing development, not uncommonly long and with various paths, until it appears as a finished technical term of a Greek author. Of this paragraph, so informative for medical history, we know nothing. We would only be able to say something if the ancient literature had been completely preserved. Sadly, this is not the case; precisely the most important part for our task, the literary legacy of Alexandria, has been almost entirely lost.

We might, then, have had to relinquish an important part of our terminologic research had not conscientious and historically minded physicians of late antiquity quoted on occasion from the lost texts of the Alexandrian doctors and bequeathed us valuable information on historical questions, among them the history of the development of the old terms.

Later quotations from disease descriptions stemming from the old Alexandrians and their schools allow us now to make this rare contribution to the etymology of diabetes synonyms. Four of the synonymous names of one medical school that have become known to us in this manner fell into disuse even during antiquity. Only the name "diabetes", the inspired linguistic creation of an Alexandrian-trained doctor, has survived the ages to become a universal term.

When new observational and intellectual findings limit or overthrow the validity of existing views, new concepts are advanced whose linguistic embodiment follows hard on their heels. Concept formation is a logical process, dependent only on the nature and worth of the new knowledge, but nomenclature is an art and a matter of the gift for appropriate formulations.

The impulse to the construction of an Ur-diabetes concept came from the observation thast many of the disease pictures formerly regarded as hydrops were incompatible with the valid symptomatology of hydrops. The old medicine saw as the main symptoms the agonizing thirst, the avid drinking, the accumulation of fluid in the abdominal cavity and body tissues, as well as the almost entire failure of passage of urine.[1]

As CAELIUS AURELIANUS (6th century AD) writes in his chapter on hydrops,[2] the Alexandrian APOLLONIUS of Memphis (second half of the 3rd century BC) observed a clinical picture deviating from traditional hydrops in which no fluid accumulation occurred, and the urine was excreted *sine retentione* (without accumulation) and *sine dilatione* (without delay) "as if running through a water-pipe", *(alium dixit fieri hydropem cum retentione, ut si quid biberit, sine dilatione tanquam per fistulam transiens egeratur, ejus autem quem retentione fieri dixit, secundum plurimos tres esse differentias affirmat).* The two names of APOLLONIUS for this disease, soon termed 'diabetes', are: *hydrops sine retentione (sc. urinae)* and *hydrops sine dilatione (sc. urinae emissionis),* the first of the six transmitted synonyms. CAELIUS AIRELIANUS also reports[3] that DEMETRIUS of Apamea (second half of the 2nd century AD), also of the Alexandrian school, had found a better expression to dinstinguish the new disease from true hydrops, calling it 'through-passer' *(diabetes). (sed melius Deme-*

---

[1] For the pathology and symptomatology of the hydropic disorders, cf. Cassius Felix cap. 76 *'ad hydropicos'* and *Caelius Aurelianus* morb. chron. lib. III, cap. VIII: *'de hydrops'.*

[2] *Cael. Aurel.* m. chr. III, 8, 101

[3] *Cael. Aurel.* m. chr. III, 8, 102

trius Apameus ab hydrope discrevit, eum qui sine dilatione potum liquorem per urinam egerit, diabetem appellans).

These two quotations by CAELIUS from APOLLONIUS and DEMETRIUS are the only evidences of the pathology and symotomatology of an Ur-diabetes, if it may be so called. Without these, we would have known nothing about its origins in Greek medicine. CAELIUS fortunately anticipated his own chapter on diabetes which, as was wont with this author, must have contained valuable contributions to the history of the disease, but which was sadly lost. DEMETRIUS contributed nothing to the concept of Ur-diabetes and adopted APOLLONIUS's concept, yet he clarified it through a happy linguistic formulation. Thereby, the agonizing thirst and avid drinking are common to hydrops and the new disease, but the latter runs its course, not only without fluid accumulation, but also – and this is of pathognomic – importance – with immediate excretion of the latter, as it were during the actual drinking. This process of 'passing through', not clearly specified by APOLLONIUS, was expressed by DEMETRIUS with his 'diabetes'[4] in inspired fashion.

The symptom-triad of pathologic thirst, drinking and immediate excretion characterizes the nature of the Ur-diabetes, a concept that has not changed throughout antiquity and beyond. But we must not omit to note that only end-states of untreated diabetes mellitus – not seen by us for many a day – and of diabetes insipidus can be so characterized. None of the old physicians has depicted the process as shortly and impressively as CASSIUS FELIX:[5] The disease, he writes as a true methodologist, "is called through-passer by the Greeks because, in fact, immediately after drinking the fluid is immediately evacuated again through the urinary tract because of the porosity of the internal organs as if it were pouring through an empty space" *(et appellatur a Graecis diabetes, siquidem mox potione accepta per urinales vias raritete membrorum interiorum descendat tamquem per inania feratur).*

For over two centuries the literature now gives no further information about the history of the three Alexandrian synonyms. We do not encounter the two oldest again at all, and diabetes only again with ARETAEUS and GALEN, but on the basis of later sources we can reliably reconstruct the fate of the Ur-

[4] The Greek inventor of the name would have said "through-passer" if he had spoken German. He must have been clear in speech and thought.

[5] *De medicina* cap. 46

nomina. ARETAEUS speaks exclusively of diabetes;[6] GALEN writes about it in his comprehensive chapter on kidney diseases[7] and uses mainly this name, but does not commit himself to this and does not reject other traditional names. For him, the linguistic aspect of the terminology is less important than the medical task: "Should one now call the disease diabetes, thirst disease or urinary flux? We should not rack our brains over a suitable name, but seek a path to recovery from the sick part of the body or the symptoms present. It seems to me even to be a kidney disease, what some doctors call 'hydrops in the chamber-pot' *(hýderos eis amída)*, others the 'through-flow in the urine' (diárrhoia eis oúra), others the 'through-passer" *(diabētēs)* and yet others the 'thirst disease' *(dípsakos)*. But so far I myself have only seen twice patients with immoderate thirst and therefore avidly drinking, as if what is drung is quickly excreted again in the urine while they were drinking it."

The Ur-nomina of APOLLONIUS do not appear again in GALEN's recital of the synonyms applicable at his time. They must have been repeated subsequently, although the understanding of the Ur-concept by ARETAEUS and himself did not alter. But a medical school based on the Ur-concept and the Ur-name seems to have elaborated the clumsy terms of APOLLONIUS and to have attempted a clearer linguistic definition of the essence of the concept. The derivation of the 'dropsy in the chamber-pot' and the 'through-flow in the urine' from the Ur-names cannot be denied. In the 'dropsy in the chamber-pot' even the excretion finds its due regard and verbal fall-out. The existence of a *hydrops sine retentione* and *sine dilatione* is an unqualified postulate for the formation of the new name. The accord with the origin of the disease (the hydrops) is not to be ignored, but the new nomenclatory emphasis ('in the champer-pot') lies here on the excretion itself and the path it follows. The next name, 'through-flow* in the urine', shifts the emphasis on to both directions and makes it more meaningful. Reference to hydrops as the origin of the disorder is now lacking; the excretory pathway is designated even more clearly, if possible; and the speed of the process finds an obvious expression in the comparison with *diarrhoia* (dysentery).

---

[6] Aretaei *acut. morb. lib. II,* 2 *de diabete*

[7] GALEN: *de locis affectis,* lib. VI cap. III, cf. also Oribasii *synopsis ad Eusthatium* IV cap. 32

* The German *Durchfluss* of course means "diarrhea".

ARETAEUS, GALEN and their posterity decided on what was known to be the longest recognized name for diabetes, which prejudiced nothing. With it, medicine offered a fourth field of meaning to the Greek homonym *diabetes,* with its original meaning of divergence and transmission, already designated by 'Circle', 'Chambermaid's plumbline' and 'Fluid siphon'. The final name compresses the thirst-slaking and immediate excretion of the drink in the urine into one, summarizes the facts about the designatory word, and therewith confirms the long-concluded development of the ancient term, at least as an expression of a sensorily perceptible process. The word is the pattern of a completed technical term from the nomenclatory bases of ancient medicine and has lasted well because of this and because of its precision. In any case a better one was not to be found. It best expresses what the ancients understood under their six synonyms.

Whereas the *nomina* of APOLLONIUS and their elaborations no longer emerge in the literature, after GALEN, the one first named by him as *dipsakos,* the thirst disease, appears together with diabetes in his medical successors as a solitary synonym. As the literary transmission fails in the 2nd century AD, and the expressly unscientific (as opposed to scientific) 'through-passer', understandable by every layman, obviously became a firm and unequivocal synonym for GALEN, there remains only the supposition that the term stemmed directly or indirectly from Alexandrian medicine and stood there, even if not as *dipsakos,* then under another scientific name and an otherwise interpreted pathologic concept, for a clinical disorder with agonizing thirst and insatiably avid drinking.

Now, we are somwhat orientated about the Alexandrian epoch of Greek medicine by the books of the two first Latin-writing authors. Celsus, as an ecyclopedist of the Greek, predominantly Alexandrian, theses, mentions neither *diapsikos* nor a Latinized name for it and does not write about any clinically similar disorder. But the Roman physician SCRIBONIUS LARGUS, in chapter 105 of his *Compositiones medicamentarum* produced in 47 AD, a *vitium stomachi*[8] that gives us an indication as to the source of

[8] *os ventriculi,* esophageal orifice, lowest part of the esophagus in which, by the agreed opinion of Greak physicians of all periods the cause of the thirst was to be sought. Cf. Galeni de loc. aff. lib. VI cap III and Aretaeus *de curatione diab.* lib. II, cap. 2

the lay 'thirst disease'. SCRIBONIUS writes: "There is a disorder of the stomach that proceeds with dryness, feeling of heat at the stomach mouth, and as it were an insatiable and unquenchable thirst. The Greeks called it *enkausis* (burning) because it dries up all the juices of the stomach mouth. We know of patients who have drunk up whole jugs full of water[9] without in the least quenching their thirst" *(est stomachi vitium quod cum siccitate et ardore eius et irrequiebili ut ita dicam et inexstinguibili siti contingit. encausin Graeci vocant ab eo quod exsiccat omnem stomachem humorem. scimus quosdam urnas aquae bibisse neque ideo sitim aliqua ex parte exstinguisse).*

SCRIBONIUS expressly emphasizes that the name and concept of *encausis* stemmed from the medicine of Alexandria and therefore of Greece. In short, impressive fashion he describes the clinical aspects and pathogenesis and refers to his knowledge of cases in the ancient literature where enormous amounts of fluid were drunk. And finally, because according to the Greek pathology the cause of the *enkausis* is to be sought in that part of the body which the ancients opine to be the site of the morbid thirst and drinking, it may be assumed, not without weighty grounds, that *dipsakos* has been the popular term for the scientific *enkausis* and has persisted for 700 years alongside the scientific diabetes on account of its plastic expression and general intelligibility, whereas scientific but clumsy technical terms have vanished with outgoing antiquity. Which disease should probably be called the thirst disease by doctors and all laymen if not the *enkausis* of Scribonius, with its unbelievably high amounts drunk, so impressive to the laity, and the general medically recognized dogma and topic of thirst in the stomach? That *dipsakos* was equivalent to *diabetes* in GALEN's time is as little doubtful as its synonymity with the 'hydrops in the chamber-pot' and the 'through-flow in the urine'.

The existence of the ancient term *enkausis* raises problems of terminology, to be answered only with every reservation because of the paucity of tradition. Retrospectively, we may regard the term as diabetes in the modern sense. Certainly, GALEN's period considered it as identical with the ancient diabetes. But was it in the medical school that this name was created? Inseparably associated with the picture and concept of the ancient diabetes is the urinary flux, striking as to quantity and time of appearance. We omit its mention here. Assuming the complete-

[9] A jug *(urna)* held 10 liters!

ness of SCRIBONIUS' quotation, this is not remarkable. We have available a series of disease descriptions to be regarded as diabetes – certainly in the modern but not in the ancient sense – which were designated with other names in antiquity. CAELIUS AURELIANUS[10] reported such a characteristic disease picture in the 6th century AD. None satisfy the requirements of the ancient diabetic triad and all omit one or other of the three cardinal symptoms or fall entirely out of frame like the *Decipiens*. In the case of the *encausis* the excretion is not mentioned, and it is not easy to show that it belongs to this series of diseases, incompatible with the model of the ancient diabetes but acceptable by us today as diabetic disorders. Yet it is slightly probable. I find the following interpretation more acceptable. No ancient medical school could avoid recognizing the immoderate thirst and avid drinking as general symptoms of disease, but the position was otherwise with the recognition of a strinking fluid excretion as a morbid symptom. In view of the abnormally high amount of drink – SCRIBONIUS speaks of "whole jugs" each of about 10 liters content – it could still be considered as obvious and physiologic and disregarded by a school of physicians in the derivation of a concept and a name. But this does not at all mean that this school was unaware of the ancient concept of diabetes. Very probably it was aware of it, but could not or would not accept it in the usual scientific controversies and therefore expressed its opinion of the physiologic nature of the urinary flux by advancing a new concept and name, that of *encausis*. This seems to have no great recognition and duration after GALEN no longer acknowledged it as debatable.

Summary

'Diabetes' has not been the only name for the ancient medical general concept. It was preceded and accompanied by five synonyms, none of which survived antiquity.

As the sources stand, it is the Alexandrian physician, APOLLONIUS of Memphis, who must be credited with the scientific endeavor of having abstracted from the general concept of the ancient hydrops the Ur-form of the later diabetes and established it as an independent disease. The new concept still possessed the agonizing thirst and avid drinking which were characteristic symptoms of the old hydrops, but differed from it in the absence of fluid accumulation in the body and scanty passage of urine; the

---

[10] morb. chron. lib. III cap. VII. 91

patient immediately excreted the drink again. This observation was reflected in the new names: *hydrops sine retentione* (sc. *urinae*) and *hydrops sine dilatione* (sc. *urinae emissionis*), which, in their author's conception, characterized the new disease as a triad of pathologic thirst, drinking and rapid excretion. This concept did not alter throughout antiquity.

A century later, without impugning the concept, the Alexandrian DEMETRIUS of Apamea took a closer look at the name and gave expression with his diabetes (through-passer) to the immediate urinary flux, often appearing even during drinking, a characteristic fact that APOLLONIUS had clearly not adequately emphasized.

The new term was adopted by ARETAEUS, likewise by GALEN, who made preferential use of it but did not reject the conventional synonyms of his time, the 'hydrops in the chamber-pot', 'through-flow of the urine' and 'thirst disease'. The first two of these synonyms are the easily recognizable scientific elaborations of APOLLONIUS's names within one school of physicians, but the 'through-flow of the urine' did not achieve completion and does not appear in the urine after GALEN. Only dipsakos (thirst disease) was still preserved by GALEN's unoriginal medical successors and compilers, AETIUS,[11] ALEXANDER[12] and PAULUS.[13]

The source of the generally intelligible name dipsakos, plainly standing for diabetes, was to be demonstrated. The word was very probably to be attributed to the *enkausis stomachi* described by Scribonius Largus as the cause of the burning thirst in the Greek pathology. It was without doubt a depiction of the diabetic thirst and drinking and, like so many disease descriptions of the Greek physicians, a diabetes under another name. This concept must have already been generally disseminated before GALEN, which is why the good and generally intelligible term of 'thirst disease' must have been adopted in place of the no longer significant name of *enkausis*.

The Ur-diabetes concept of APOLLONIUS with the diabetic triad of morbid thirst, drinking and rapid excretion specified not only the linguistic form of all diabetes synonyms but also the symptomatology up to the end of antiquity. An amplification of the clinique and classification of the Ur-diabetes did not take place. What ARETAEUS and GALEN observed and wrote in this context has no place in an etymologic study.

[11] *libri medic.* III, cap. 1

[12] *de diabete* lib. XI, cap. 6

[13] *libri medic.* III, cap. 45, 10

in: *Janus 51 (1964) 193–201*

News, Notes and Queries

On the Term Diabetes in the Works of Aretaeus and Galen

by FOLKE HENSCHEN

The word diabetes comes from the Greek verb διαβαίνω(diabaino) which means I go or I run through; and διαβήτης (diabetes)the thing the fluid runs through, that is a siphon or a waterpipe. The term diabetes seems to have been introduced into medical nomenclature by Aretaeus (Hirsch 1883, Reed 1954, etc.).

Aretaeus' description of the disease runs, according to Francis Adams' translation of 1856 (pp. 338–9), as follows:

> Diabetes is a wonderful affection, not very frequent among men . . . The course is the common one, namely, the kidneys and the bladder; for *the patients never stop making water, but the flow is incessant, as if from the opening of aqueducts.** The nature of the disease, then, is chronic, and it takes a long period to form; but the patient is short-lived, if the constitution of the disease be completely established; for the melting is rapid, the death speedy. Moreover, life is disgusting and painful; *thirst, unquenchable; excessive drinking,* which, however, is disproportionate to the large quantity of urine, for more urine is passed; and *one cannot stop them either from drinking or making water.* Or if for a time they expire. *Thirst, as if scorched up with fire* . . . But if it increase still more, the heat is small indeed, but pungent, and seated in the intestines; the abdomen shirvelled, veins protuberant, general emaciation, when the quantity of urine and the thirst have already increased; and when, at the same time, the sensation appears to me to have got the name *diabetes* as if from the Greek word *διαβήτης (which significies a siphon)*, because the fluid does not remain in the body, but uses the man's body as a ladder (διαβἄΰρη), whereby to leave it.[1] They stand out for a certain time, though not very long, for they pass urine with pain, and the emaciation is dreadful; nor does any great portion of the drink get into the system, and many parts of the flesh pass out along with the urine.

In his book on the *Therapeutics of chronic diseases* (Bk. II, Chap. II, 485–6) Aretaeus writes about the cure of diabetes: '. . . in diabetes, the flow of the humour from the affected part and

---

* The italics are mine, F.H.

[1] Altogether, this interpretation is so unsastifactory, that I was almost tempted to alter the text. It is possible, however, that διαβαΰρη is faulty, and that we ought to read διαβήτη.

the melting is the same [as in dropsy], but the defluxion is determined to the kidneys and bladder . . . In the latter disease [diabetes] the thirst is greater; for the fluid running off dries the body . . . For the thirst there is need of a powerful remedy, for in kind it is the greatest of all sufferings; and when a fluid is drunk, it stimulates the discharge of urine . . .'

Galen speaks about diabetes in several of his writings. As no good English translation is available, I have used Renander's Swedish translation in the following: In the book *On the localisation of diseases* Galen says: 'I am of the opinion that the kidneys too are affected in *the rare disease which some people call chamber-pot dropsy, other again diabetes or violent thirst. For my own part I have seen the disease till now only twice when the patients suffered from an inextinguishable thirst, which forced them to drink enormous quantities; the fluid was urinated swiftly with a urine resembling the drink.'* Further down he discusses thoroughly 'The mechanism in diabetes,' but this chapter is scarcely of special interest in this connection. He summarizes the results in the following words: 'Diabetes is a genuine kidney disease, analogous to voracious appetite.'

When Galen says that some people call this disease chamber-pot dropsy,[2] and others diabetes, this seems to indicate without doubt that he has adopted the term introduced by Aretaeus, although he omits to mention the name of the author who first used it. It seems to me that this utterance could perhaps contribute to the settlement of the important problem, not yet solved, concerning Aretaeus' place in the history of medicine, whether prior to, at the same time as, or after Galen.

Aretaeus, and, as I suppose, after him Galen gave the striking name 'diabetes' to the characteristic disease which they had observed and described. However, what was the real nature of the disease they called 'diabetes'? It seems that this question has not been discussed seriously up to now. Subsequent authors seem to have assumed, without any reservations, that the 'diabetes' of these two classical authors has been our 'diabetes mellitus'. Aretaeus and especially Galen, accentuate the great rarity of the disease and the enormous thirst. These two characteristics seem to me to be very remarkable circumstances, favouring my suspicion that the 'diabetes' of these two authors does not corre-

[2] The term 'hydrops ad matulam' was still known, to nineteenth-century clinicians and Hooper's *Medical Dictionary* refers from this term to 'diabetes'.

spond to our 'diabetes mellitus'. We must not forget that Galen had a very large practice in Rome at the time of the emperors; and it seems feasible to assume that diabetes mellitus was a very common disease in the capital of the world with its luxurious life. But Galen says frankly: 'For my own part I have seen the disease till now only twice; the patients suffered from an inextinguishable thirst which forced them to drink enormous quantities.'

This accentuating of the rarity of the disease and the enormous thirst directed my thoughts some time ago to another interpretation of the Greek physician's expressive word 'diabetes'. Could they perhaps have seen some cases of the rare diabetes insipidus? Of course, there is nothing to prove this, and it is possible to bring the statements of the Greek authors into agreement with modern experience. They may have observed and described some of those relatively rare cases of diabetes mellitus with exceptionally intense thirst. Such relatively rare cases have fascinated them, they have described them in their writings, whereas all other cases of diabetes mellitus without conspicuous thirst have escaped them and the limited diagnostic capacity of that time.

Numerous works of later Greek, Roman and Arabic authors follow more or less slavishly Galen's writings, and a disease called 'diabetes' is described in the same terms as in his works. Also medieval authors quote Galen who made no annotation of the sweet taste of the urine. This is the more remarkable, as it was a routine diagnostic method to taste the patient's urine!

As is well known, it was only in 1674, that the sweet taste of the urine was described by the great Thomas Willis. In this desease, he says, the urine is quite different from all the patient's drinks but also from all body fluids, 'being exceedingly sweet as if there had been sugar or honey in it'. Thereafter more than one hundred years elapsed until Matthew Dobson in 1776 showed that the sweet taste of the urine depended on sugar, which he prepared from the urine of diabetics.

The sweet taste of the urine of diabetics is said to have been noticed for the first time in India and possibly in China too, many centuries before our era. According to Gotfredsen, Huang-Ti's famous textbook *Nei Ching (Canon medicinae)* contains a description of a disease which cannot be any other than diabetes mellitus.

Hirsch says in 1883 that the earliest statements on diabetes mellitus are to be found in Sushruta's *Ayur-Veda* where

Hessler's translation runs: 'Mellita urina laborantem quem medicus indicat, ille etiam incurabilis dictus est'. (When the doctor states that a man suffers from honey urine, he has also declared him incurable.) In another passage with a detailed description of the disease one reads: 'Dulcis fit urina, sudor et phlegma' (sweet is the urine, the sweat and the phlegm).

Concerning the supposed discovery of sweet urine in India the very critical Gotfredson says: (translation from the Danish original) 'The Indians are usually said to have been the first in world medicine to have had an idea about diabetes; they are said to have discovered that the urine tastes sweet and will be secreted in copious quantities. They know that the sufferer's (prameha), main symptom is abundant water secretion. There are 20 subdivisions of this prameha; in two of them, sugar urine (iksumeha) and honey urine (madhumeha) the urine has a sweet taste. Among numerous secondary symptoms there are noted: sweet taste in the mouth, thirst, loss of appetite, vomiting, drying, and boils. As a further symptom it is also stated that the urine will be sucked up by ants and other insects.' However, it is never mentioned that the doctor tastes the urine and Reinhold Müller who has exposed the whole problem to a careful analysis on the basis of the original writings, has not found any positive proof that the Indians knew of the sweet taste of the urine in diabetes.

If Müller is right, how then shall we regard the 'discovery' of ancient Indian medicine that has attracted such attention and has been mentioned by so many authorities and has been called 'the crown-jewel of the Indian healing art' by Fåhraeus?

However, this question belongs to the history of Indian medicine, and has little to do directly with my original question: the import of the term 'diabetes' in the works of Aretaeus and Galen: Does their term 'diabetes' mean diabetes mellitus or, at least in certain cases, diabetes insipidus?

References

ARETAEUS, THE CAPPADOCIAN, *The extant works,* ed. and trans. by Francis Adams, London, 1856.

FRANK, L. L., 'Diabetes mellitus in the text of old Hindu medicine', *Amer. J. Gastroenterol.,* 1957, 27, 76.

GALEN, *Om sjukdomarnas lokalisation,* trans. by A. Renander, Stockholm, 1960.

GOTFREDSEN, E., *Medicinens Historie,* 2nd ed., Copenhagen, 1964.

HIRSCH, A., *Handbook of Geographical and Historical Geography*, 3 vols, London, 1883–1886.
MÜLLER, R., 'Die Harnruhr der Alt-Inder', Arch. Ges. Med., 1932, 25, 1.
REED, J. A., 'Aretaeus, the Cappadocian', *Diabetes*, 1954, 3, 1.

in: *Opuscula Medica 13 (1969), S. 190–192.*

Aretaeus the Cappadocian

His Contribution to Diabetes Mellitus

by EUGENE J. LEOPOLD

Among the medical authors of the early days of the present era, two names readily come to mind, those of Celsus and Galen. The works of these masters of medicine have left a deep impression, which has lasted even unto this day. Somewhere, either between these two, or contemporaneously with the latter, lived and wrote another medical scholar, of whom it has been said that "He left descriptions of disease not excelled, until his day and for a long time thereafter, for completeness of description and clarity of thought." This was said of Aretaeus, the Cappadocian. Neuburger introduces him with these words: "Ideal and reality meet in this epoch in the masterpieces of a much discussed author, of whom we know with certainty, only that he lived in one or the other of two periods, yet left work which exerted great effect on succeeding ages."

As early as the third century B.C. Greek physicians and midwives began to wander to Rome. Among these early disciples of the Hippocratic art, many were lured to Rome by the spirit of adventure and the opportunity for riches, for the art of healing was well rewarded in Rome at that time. The Hippocratic teachings at first were well received, but soon fell into disrepute because few of its disciples were worthy of emulation. Archagathas, 219 B.C., because of his skillful treatment of wounds, rose to high honors. When he ventured out of his field, the repair of wounds, and essayed major operations of other types, his recklessness in cutting soon brought upon him the derisive title "Carnifex" and upon Greek physicans much disfavor. It was Asklepides of Prusa (b. ca. 124 B.C.) trained in rhetoric, philosophy and medicine, the friend and companion of Lucius Crassus, Mark Antony and Cicero, who finally implanted in Rome true Hippocratic medicine, which now, through the teachings of a master, quickly supplanted the Roman medicine founded largely on mystery and superstition. A century later we come to Celsus and Pliny, the younger. Comparatively little is known about Aretaeus; even the exact period of his activity is in question. He mentions no medical authorities except Hippocrates, and is not named by any contemporaries. In fact, the first record of him is found in the writings of Aetius of Amida, who lived in the sixth century. He quotes him frequently by name. Medical writers who lived about the time when Aretaeus was active were Celsus and Galen. Celsus (30 B.C.–30. A.D.) in all probability preceded Aretaeus, but no mention of the prolific compiler is found in the works of the Cappadocian. Galen (b. 131 A.D.) was either a contemporary colleague or lived after him. There is great similarity to be found in the writings of Galen and Areteaus. Both use Hippocrates as a model and have a partiality for the philosophy of Plato. They show a better knowledge of anatomy than do any known writers of the period. Both display marked similarity in their therapy. They describe various types of the pulse in almost the same terms. Philologists point out that they differ in one striking manner. Galen wrote in the Greek of his day, the Attic Greek of Xenophon. Aretaeus' known works are in Ionic Greek, which was used by Hippocrates but which was long out of common usage when he wrote. This difference may, or may not, mean that they were contemporaries. It seems to have been a rather common practice for writers of that period to have used one form of Greek in some of their writings and another in other works. Lucian, the satirist and Artian (100 A.D.) did it. Aretaeus quotes only Homer of all the poets and he wrote in Ionic Greek. Galen quotes the later dramatic poets who wrote mainly in Attic Greek. With his great respect for Hippocrates, it seems that Aretaeus may have used the Ionic style in conformity to a rather common practice of physicians and historians of that period to copy Hippocrates and Herodotus, who wrote in Ionic Greek. Whatever be the reason, it presupposes upon the part of our author a careful and thorough study of the language of a past age.

That Aretaeus and Galen do not mention each other cannot be taken as evidence that they were not known te each other. They may have been rival practitioners. Rivalry was quite common among medical men of the age. Or, we may be dealing with another example of a custom quite common a short time before, in the age of Quintilian, when it was uncommon for living writers to quote any of their contemporaries by name, probably because they felt it was impossible to form an unbiased opinion on their work ("sine angor aut studio"). Dioscorides, the founder of Materia Medicae and the elder Pliny were contemporaries, the former a prolific writer and the later a great compiler. Both wrote many works and often discuss the same subjects, but neither names the other. It may be that "the fame of him who dominated medical thought, for fifteen centuries, as did Aristotle, the schools," Galen, overshadowed our author. Considerations of this kind make it seem probable that Aretaeus lived during the first half of the second century and in Rome.

Aretaeus is always described as "The Cappadocian." This suffix indicates that he was a native of Cappadocia which was, at his time, one of the far eastern provinces of the Roman Empire. Previously, in the days of Herodotus, Cappadocia was a large country extending from Mt. Taurus to the borders of the Euxine Sea, and from the lower Halys River (R. Kizil Irmak) to the Euphrates. It was an independent kingdom until it was conquered by the Persians during the reign of Alexander the Great. They divided it into satrapies, one on the coast of the sea, Pontus, and an interior one, Cappadocia. In 17 A.D., the latter was conquered by the Romans and it became a province of the Roman Empire.

We know nothing of the education of Aretaeus; in fact our knowledge of the man himself is so slight that we cannot say definitely where he received his education. It is thought that he studied at Alexandria and that he spent some time in Egypt. He mentions that country by name and describes some diseases as being common there. When he came to Rome we do not know, but he is familiar with the better known wines of Rome of the second century, the Falernian, the Fundian and the Sequine and recommends them. His use of the Ionic dialect and the fact that he places the major emphasis on the pneuma, place his time in the second century. This is borne out by his emphasis on the "Pneuma", the spirit, the doctrine of the Pneuma goes back to Hippocrates, but it did not become the basis of a School until much later. Athenaeus of Sicily (ca. 50 A.D.) may be regarded as the founder of the Pneumatic School, which added the pneuma to the four elementary qualities of the older schools and made it the source of life. Disease was due to some change of the pneuma. The bright light of the Pneumatic School was Archigenes of Apamea (100 A.D.), a well known physician during the time of Trajan. He brought the School to its greatest heights. Arataeus is classed as a member of the Pneumatic School. Some discussion has arisen as to the place due Aretaeus in medicine, because of the similarity which has been noted between his works and some fragments of the writings of Archigenes found sometime ago. Wellman believes the latter to be the source of much of the material which has been ascribed to Aretaeus. But, most all medical historians agree with Neuburger when he says "No one Grecian author after Hippocrates of whom we know, reaches the heights of Aretaeus, and no work in the whole literature approaches closely the true Hippocratic spirit in description of disease and viewpoint of Therapeutics as do these books of the Cappadocian." Whatever the future may bring to light as to which one, Aretaeus or Archigenes borrowed from the other, the classical and clear descriptions of disease and the uncomplicated and conservative therapy which have come down to us under the name of Aretaeus, place the author upon true Hippocratic heights. These show a mind undisturbed by conflicting systems and schools, unwilling to sacrifice itself to fanciful theories or indulge in useless speculations, yet giving clear, concise pictures of disease and its treatment based upon sound thought and great experience.

It seems strange that these classical presentations of disease which we now have, should have been so little known or quoted during a period of more than one thousand years. In explanation, Adams points out that the medical writings of Roman authors after the second century, for a period of several centuries, show little indication of any research on the work of former ages. Whatever the reason, we find the first trace of our author in the works of Aëtius of Amida, physician to Justinian I (527–565), who quotes Aretaeus frequently. Alexander of Tralles, who lived about the same time, knew the writings of Aretaeus. So did Paul of Aegina (625–690). All of these were compilers and systematizers of the medical knowledge of the preceding ages. Following this group, there pass almost a thousand years during which no trace is to be found of Aretaeus. In this long period, Roman medicine was barren. The Arabian School rose and declined. But this School drew its knowledge of the medicine of Greece and Rome from the compilations of Aetius, Alexander of Tralles, Paul of Aegina and Oribasius. It did not go back to the original sources. Wigan believes the fame of Archigenes, the bright light of the Pneumatic School, perhaps overshadowed our author. Likewise, the School of Salernum was founded and passed its period of fame. Bologna and Montpellier and other universities were increasing the knowledge of anatomy and physiology and dissecting human bodies. Yet there is no trace found of the Cappadocian.

The art of printing was invented about the middle of the fifteenth century. It greatly aided that great rebirth of knowledge, which we call the Renaissance. So we find the earliest printings of the authors of antiquity appearing about the beginning of the sixteenth century. The first edition of the Works of Aretaeus was published at Venice in 1552 by Junius Paulus Crassus. It is in Latin and in the preface of the volume, the editor states that it "is a translation into Latin of an old and worm-eaten book written in Greek, which accidently has fallen into my hands." He does not give the title of the book but continues: "the margins of the pages of the old book had many notes written in Latin on them by former possessors, not in Greek as was the text." Several chapters of the old book were missing from Book II on the Treatment of Chronic Diseases. The translation was made by a scholar and was evidently based upon material now unknown. He, however, did not have the advantage of the several Codices which have come to light since then. This edition was reprinted at Paris in 1554 by Wm. Moriel and James Putanus and at Frankfort in 1587 in the Medicae Artis Principis edited by Henricus Stevenus from the work of an unknown author.

The "Edita Princeps," the first edition in Greek, was published at Paris in 1554. It was edited by Jacobus Goupylus and printed by Adrian Turnebaum, the famous printer to King Henry II of France. It was based upon a Greek manuscript in the Royal Library at Paris, and contains the chapters missing in the Crassus' edition. It is a very finely put up edition, but suffers from faulty punctuation and the addition of many conjectural readings which sometimes make the text almost impossible to understand. In the same year, Goupylus brought out a Latin edition, based upon the Crassus volume above mentioned. In 1581, Crassus edited a revised edition in Latin, which contained the chapters missing in his first edition. It was printed by Peter Pernam.

The first Greek-Latin edition to be published was edited by George Heinisch and printed at Augsburg by Augustus Vindelicorum in 1603. It is based upon three old Codices, the Venetum, the Bavaricum and the Augustaeum. It is not a very good edition. However, the next Greek-Latin printing is quite different. It was edited by John Wigan, dedicated to Dr. Freind, the friend of Dr. Richard Meade, and printed by the Clarendon Press at London. It is based upon two manuscript Codices, one in the Vatican Library at Rome and the other, the Harleyean, in the Bodleian

Library at Oxford. Because of its careful printing and its full notes and emendations, it is a most excellent edition, although marred somewhat by numerous text errors. Boerhaave tells us that only 300 copies of the book were printed.

The next edition was published under the direction of the famous Dr. Hermann Boerhaave, edited by Johann van Groenwald, and printed by Janson Van der Aa at Leyden in 1731 and reprinted in 1735. It is an edition in Greak and Latin, the former based on the Wigan edition and the latter on the Goupylus edition of Crassus' publication of 1581. Besides the text, it contains the complete Commentaries of Peter Petit, doctor of Paris (b. 1662). These were written about 1692 and Adams states that "one can scarcely overrate the value of his contribution" since they are "the most ingenious and judicious labors ever expended on an ancient author, not excepting that of Foes on Hippocrates." Besides these Commentaries, the book contains an Index to the Greek text made by Maittaire, a famous classical scholar of the time; an Appendix, "Variae Lectonis," of the various editions and Codices; Conjectures and Emendations by Daniel William Trilleri on the Leipzig edition of 1728; and finally, a Latin Index to Diseases and Drugs. Beorhaave had already edited editions of Hippocrates and Galen and was preparing to edit Aretaeus when he received "from that famous and renowned Richard Meade," a copy of the Wigan edition of Aretaeus. Of the many other editions of the Works of Aretaeus which have appeared since the edition of 1735, I should like to mention but two. The first is the Greek-English edition of Francis Adams, published by the Sydenham Society in 1856. It is an excellent work, especially as the English translation makes it available to many more readers. I am indebted to this edition for much of my material. The other is an elaborate and excellent edition by the Danish philologist, Karl Hunde, published in Greek-German, as a part of the monumental "Corpus Medicorum Graecorum" by Teubner in Leipzig in 1923.

The works of Aretaeus which we now posses are comprised in four books, "De causis et signis Acutorum Morborum" (On causes and signs of Acute Disease), "De causis et signis Diutunorum Morborum" (Chronic Diseases) and four books of Therapy of Acute and Chronic Diseases, each in two books. There are fifty chapters on Causes and Signs and forty-three on Therapy; the treatment of cholera, mania, paralysis, phthisis, empyema, dropsy and colics are missing, but the descriptions of these diseases have come down. Besides these books, Aretaeus mentions works on fever, on surgery, on gynecology, on prophylaxis and on pharmacy, of which no trace can be found.

He treats of many conditions, but especial emphasis should be placed on his description of pleurisy, with empyema, pneumonia and phthisis, the paralytic states, tetanus, epilepsy with its preceding aura, hysteria, cholera, certain affections of the throat (diphtheria), jaundice, edema, gout, ischialgia, leprosy, diabetes and various intestinal, hepatic and vesicular diseases. Of all of these he has left masterly descriptions. Of course these terms do not always mean for him that which we understand by them today. His chapters may indicate symptoms, groups of diseases or an entirely different concept than we have today. Heart disease is discussed by him under "Syncope". "De Jecoris" includes several diseases of the liver and likewise kidney diseases are "De Renum acutis affectibus."

What views did Aretaeus hold? He believed the body was made up of humor, spirit (pneuma) and solid constituents and that health and life depended upon the proper interplay of these constituents. He recognized four humors, the same as did Hippocrates, the blood, the phlegm, the light bile and the dark bile. Blood is formed in the liver from the food taken. The phlegm is secreted by the brain and descends to the other organs. Light bile comes from the liver, while black bile is made by the spleen.

To him, the heart was the most important organ of the body. "What other organ is more important?" he asks. It is the site of animal heat and of the spirit (pneuma), the source of respiration and of life. It draws the pneuma from the lungs, which are dependent upon the heart. The aorta arises from the heart and lies to the left of the vena cava in the body. It (the aorta) carries out the pneuma to the other organs. The veins carry the blood to all parts as nutriment.

The liver is the point of origin of the veins. It is composed largely of blood; it produces blood and bile. Inflammations of the liver produce jaundice, caused by the obstruction of the bile ducts.

The lungs are of spongy texture and without feeling. The pain of Pneumonia is due to the covering membrane being affected.

The kidneys are true glands which contain cavities, like a sieve, for the collection of urine. They are connected by two tubes, one on either kidney, with the bladder. He describes two short, broad veins leading from each kidney, which carry matter to the liver and give the appearance that the kidney is suspended from the liver (renal veins emptying into vena cava, opposite the liver?).

The stomach is the domain of pleasure and disgust by aiding good digestion and promoting good spirits. Some digestion occurs in the colon, which is the fleshy part of the intestine.

The spleen is the strainer for the blood. Jaundice from it gives a dark green color to the skin. It is a sieve. Frequently it becomes enlarged; rarely does it suppurate. In marshy regions it is especially affected.

The uterus he describes thus:

In the middle of the flanks of women lies the womb. It is like an animal for it moves itself hither and thither, also obliquely to the right or left, either to the spleen or liver and it is subject to prolapse. In a word, it is erratic. It may be suddenly carried upwards, compressing the lungs, heart, diaphragm, liver, intestines and obstructing breathing and speech.

The brain is the site of sensation and the source of the nerves and the phlegm. Blood is the nourishment of the body, the food of all parts, the heat of all parts. It is the food of inflammation and must be removed in that state. Yet he is emphatic that blood must not be wasted and practiced bleeding most conservatively.

Various causes, some curious, are assigned for diseases. Cold and wet affect the respiratory tract. Climate plays an important part in causation; the dry air of Egypt causes throat disease; wasting, loss of flesh, causes anasarca and phthisis. Food, faulty in quantity and quality may produce angina, apoplexy, dropsy, dysentery, inflammation of the liver. Excess of wine causes angina, apoplexy, inflammation of the liver, paralysis and madness. Cantharides may cause an inflammation of the bladder or dropsy. The catheter may do injury to the bladder. A wound may cause tetanus, which is a very painful condition, rapidly fatal with spasms. A part of his description is as follows:

Tetanus is an exceedingly painful, spasmodic affection following a wound, blow, abortion, or exposure to cold, and proving quickly fatal. It begins in the muscles and tendons about the jaws, extending thence to the whole frame. The convulsions bend the body backwards so that the head is lodged between the shoulder-blades (opisthotonos), or forward (emprosthotonos), or extended out straight. In all cases the jaws are locked so firmly that they can only with difficulty be pried apart. If the teeth be forcibly separated and liquid be forced into the mouth, it is not swallowed, owing to the contraction of the fauces, but is squirted out or held in the mouth, or regurgitated through the nostrils. The face is congested and variously distorted, the eyes are fixed or rolled about, the cheeks and lips are tremulous,there is grinding of the teeth, the jaws quiver, there is subsultus of muscles and there is a painful sensation of suffocation. The urine is retained or passed voluntarily.

A disease may arise from another disease. Suppression of urine causes the formation of calculus. Phthisis arises from damp and cold air. From a cough may come pneumonia, an ulcer of the lung or hemorrhage of the lung. Empyema follows pleurisy and especially the pleurisy of pneumonia. Disease of the liver may result from dysentery. Abortion may be followed by prolapsus and tetanus. Paralysis may result from gout. He knew the seventh day crisis of pneumonia and the meaning of rusty sputum. He describes the characteristic differences between arterial and venous hemorrhage. He pointed out that care must be taken in diagnosing the affected side of the face in facial paralysis and said that by noting "the difference between the two sides in laughter, speaking or winking of the eyes, the true state becomes evident."

Aretaeus stands out among the writers of the period, neurologically and psychiatrically. He devotes several chapters to Epilepsy and describes the aura. "The paroxysm of Epilepsy is preceeded by circular flashes of purple or black, or it may be of all the colors of the rainbow, or by peculiar sounds, or by a bad smell, or by manifestations of irritability or anger, or by a feeling of dread, as of an attack of a wild beast." This is followed by contractions, first involving the thumbs and great toes and rapidly extending to the head, when the patient falls suddenly as if struck with a piece of wood or with a stone, and indeed this impression of having been maliciously struck down may remain after recovery, especially in first attacks.

When the affection has become habitual, patients realize from the seizure of a finger or other part that a convulsion is coming on and call upon those present to bind or stretch such part. By such means the attack may be postponed for a time. With the fall the patient becomes unconscious, the hands are clenched, the limbs are stiff or are dashed hither and thither, the head is drawn forward so that the chain rests on the chest, or backward, or to one or the other shoulder. The lips are compressed or drawn apart, or stretched sideways over the teeth as if smiling. The tongue protrudes from the mouth, incurring the risk of being badly bitten, the eyeballs are rolled inwards, the eyelids for the most part wide apart showing the white and quivering, the cheeks are congested, the eyebrows frowning. Soon the whole countenance becomes livid and swollen, the vessels of the neck-are distended, the patient moans and makes gutteral noises as if he were being throttled, foam issues from the mouth, and there is erection of the genitalia. As the attack draws to a close there are unconscious discharges of urine, semen and feces, and the patient lies pale, torpid, heavy and exhausted. At length he rises up, the paraoxysm being ended.

The chapter on the Etiology of Apoplexy has been lost, but there is one on the cure of apoplexy. He differentiates between the apoplexy of the old and that of the young. In the former, he recommends bleeding from the affected area, but not too much blood should be removed less one weaken the patient. One should not delay bleeding either, since it may save a life. He discusses paresis, paralysis and paraplegia in addition to apoplexy. The essential of all is the loss of sensation, loss of motion and feeling. Paraplegia affects an arm or leg by loss of motion. Paralysis causes only loss of motion. The rare loss of sensation, he says, should be called Anaesthesia.

Very interstingly he says that, when the paralysis is spinal, it is on the same side as the lesion and when it is in the brain, it is on the other side (crossed paralysis) and he knows that the nerves cross soon after leaving the brain.

Melancholia occurs:

When in the course of a chronic disease, the black bile rises up to the diaphragm, which produces anger, sadness and great depression. The individuals are called melancholic because bile is synonymous with anger and black bile means strong, raging anger. Some fear to be poisoned, others are misanthropic and seek seclusion. Still others show a suspicious nature and finally are those who lose all desire to live.

In masterly fashion, he gives the bearing of temperature, of position in life, of occupation, of suppressed secretions (humors) on the origin of various mental diseases. The effect of these diseases on nutrition and health in general, he depicts faithfully. But, he does not mention the use of psychic therapy which Celsus used.

That he used the stages of physical diagnosis, becomes evident in the descriptions of disease which he has left. The notation of various types of breathing, of the fullness of the veins in heart disease, of the color of the skin in various affections and many other instances show that he made a careful inspection of his cases.

He noted enlargements of the liver and spleen and states that the boundaries of the enlarged liver may be outlined by the hand, applied with slight pressure to the abdomen, which sinks down in empty space at the end of the liver. He felt the enlarged spleen and says it was not tender to touch. These are a few examples which show that he used palpation.

Apparently he used percussion at times, for in his description of tympanites, he says, "The abdomen, when tapped, sounds like a drum, nor does the air shift its place when the patient changes his position. This is not the case, if fluid be present."

The evidence that he anticipated Laennec by some 1600 years, seems fairly clear. Hippocrates spoke of "Rhomgbi" or râles, which he heard in pneumonia, phthisis and empyema. Aretaeus uses the same term in his chapter on Asthma, which includes several diseases having dyspnea in common. Apparently the faithful student also ausculted the heart. In the chapter "On Syncope", where he discussed various conditions of the heart, this passage occurs:

But the stomach is neither the origin or the seal of life; and yet one would be injured by atony thereof, for food which proves injurious to the heart, does not hurt the stomach itself, but, by it the heart; since those dying in such cases have symptoms of heart affections, namely, pulse small and feeble, *bruit of the heart* with violent palpitations, vertigo, fainting, torpor, etc.[1]

Notice that he does not lay especial stress on the bruit, but mentions it mixed with other symptoms. This would seem to indicate that it was nothing unusual to him. Since heart murmurs are rarely heard at any distance from the heart, it would appear that Aretaeus placed his ear on the chest over the heart and ausculted the heart.

To therapeutics, Aretaeus devotes two books, containing forty-three chapters, quite in contrast to Hippocrates, who has very little to say on treatment. He used many drugs, acids, alkalines, emetics, purgatives, stomachics, diuretics, astringents, hemostatics. Local treatments practiced are leeches, cups, friction, massage, gargles, cataplasms, fomentations, blisters, ointments and baths. The catheter and the cautery are mentioned frequently. Venesection plays an important rôle and is used in almost every disease which he mentions. But, he always cautions to regulate the amount drawn by the strength of the patient. The more severe the disease, the greater the urgency to bleed.

[1] De Causis et Signis Acut. Morb. Book II, chap. III.

Especially in the diseases in which the brain is involved, is bleeding indicated. Cupping is frequently recommended in place of venesection, "because it does not weaken the patient." Both the dry and the wet cups are used. The former are recommended especially in Pleurisy. He mentions forms of venesection not known to us today, from the lingual veins in protracted throat affections, from the veins of the forehead, the pulse, the ankle, the pubes and the base of the hand. But the usual site is from the vessels which we use now.

Purgatives hold second place in his therapy. The strongest are the hiera of aloes, hellebore and elaterium. Hellebore is the best and often efficacious when other remedies fail. Enemata were used, one type to remove fecal matter and another to affect withdrawal of the humors from the head, face and neck, in quinsy. Blistering the head with cantharides and trephining are recommended in diseases of the brain.

Taking individual diseases and symptoms, pleurisy is treated by dry cupping to the back, the shoulder or the hypochondria. Medicines, which attenuate the fluids and promote expectoration, such as brine with vinegar or honey or mustard moistened with honey water, are advised. The chest is to be covered with wool moistened with oil, natron and salts. Ligatures applied to all the extremities, help to stop the bringing up of blood, but unwashed sheep's wool, moistened with a liquid such as auster wine, is to be applied to the part from which the blood flows. But more important than any of these are the things to be taken by mouth. These are of three kinds, those that act by contraction or compression of the vessels, those that coagulate the blood, and those that dry up the blood. In cardiac disease, venesection is advised, but not too much less syncope be produced. The instructions on diet and drink are especially full in this chapter.

Diet is of great importance in epilepsy, no flesh food being allowed. In fact throughout the books on therapeutics, great emphasis is placed on the manner of life, the careful regulation of living, exercise, massage, baths and diet. He prefers mild drugs but when energetic action is needed, he does not hesitate to advise radical measures. Of great interest is the fact that Aretaeus does not feel himself released from the duty of the physician when dealing with incurable disease, even though he has nothing to offer but sympathy and consultation. How far he has traveled in this from the teachings of the Hippocratic School.

Aretaeus' place in the history of diabetes mellitus is based on the fact that he gave to the disease its name. Celsus in "De

Medicine" writes of a disease in which the overflow of urine is greater than the fluid intake, which causes emaciation and endangers life. He gives directions for treatment which vary according to whether the urine is thin (low specific gravity) or thick (high specific gravity). Whether this disease is diabetes mellitus is open to doubt.

Aretaeus names his disease "Diabetos." He goes a step further when he insists, as he does, on the part which thirst plays in the symptomology. I give you his description of Diabetes.

Diabetes, Which Is The Excessive Flow Of Urine

The affection called Diabetes is a wonderful but fortunately rather rare disease. It consists of a liquefaction of the flesh and bones into urine. As with Hydrops, the cause is of a wet and cold nature. The kidneys and bladder, the usual passageways of fluid, do not cease emitting urine and the outpouring is profuse and without limit. it is just as though the aqueducts were opened wide. The development of this disease is gradual (chronic) but short will be the life of the man in whom the disease is fully developed. Emaciation proceeds quickly and death occurs rapidly. Moreover, life for the patient is tedious and full of pain. The desire for drink grows ever stronger, but no matter what quantity (of fluids) he drinks, satisfaction never occurs, and he passes more urine than he drinks. He cannot be stopped either from drinking or from urinating. For if he be restrained even for a short time from drinking, the mouth becomes parched, the body dry and they feel as though all their viscera were being consumed by a raging fire. They despair of all and death occurs shortly amid a burning dryness, thirst as if caused by a burning fire. But, if the patient holds his urine for a time, no pain can be greater. The loins, the hips and the scrotum swell. When they pass urine again, they pour out the collected fluids, which have become heated, into the bladder and the swellings disappear. But, if the disease be fully established, recognition is easy. But, if it is still approaching, the patients have a dry mouth; the saliva is white and frothy as though they were thirsty, but the thirst is not yet fully developed; a heaviness in the hypochondiac region, a feeling of hot or cold passing from the stomach to the bladder is, as it were, the beginning of the approaching disease. They pass a little more urine than usually and have some thirst, but it is not yet severe. But, when the disease develops a little more the heat, though slight, is biting and is felt in the viscera, the abdomen develops folds, the veins stand out, and the body grows small when the urination and thirst have increased. And when the disease is at its height, they urinate constantly. From this fact, the disease has derived its name, "Diabetes," meaning "siphon." For fluids do not remain in the body, but use the body only as a channel through which they may flow out. Life lasts only for a time, but not very long. For they urinate with pain and painful is the emaciation. For no essential part of the drink is absorbed by the body while great masses of the flesh are liquified into urine.

The cause of the disease may be that some one of the acute diseases may have attacked these parts of the body and left behind in the crisis, some malignant poison. Also, it is not improbable that at times the cause may be some pernicious poison from one of the diseases which affect the bladder and kidneys; just as if one be bitten by a Dipas (Adder), a like symptom follows. For the bite of the Adder causes an unquenchable thirst in man. Though he drinks copiously, his thirst is not satisfied and his bowels crave drink. But, if he feels pain, due to the distention of his viscera and feels uncomfortable because of the amount of water he has drunk, if he restrains himself from drinking for a time, the thirst recurs and he drinks again copiously. The evil of the affliction is that thirst and drink eventually increase one another. There are other cases, which do not pass urine nor cease their desire for drink. These, because of the unsatiable thirst and the distention of the belly by fluids, burst open suddenly.

The Treatment of Diabetes

The disease, Diabetes, which is the excessive flow of urine, is a type of Hydrops, with which it has in common appearance and causation. It differs only in the location from which the fluids escape. For, in Ascites, the peritoneum is the site of the collection of the fluids and they have no escape, but accumulate there continuously. But, in Diabetes, the flow of humor is indeed the same and likewise the emaciation, but the water passes to the kidneys and bladder and is thus voided. In Ascites, this occurs only when the patient is so fortunate as to recover from the disease. This is well, if the cause be explained and not only the burden be lightened. For in Diabetes, the thirst is greater and the overflow of fluid drys up the body.

But the remedies for stopping the melting are those which are of value in Hydrops. But, there is a need of a real medicine for the thirst, which is of all types of pain, the greatest. If fluid be taken, it causes urination and the urine carries off with it many parts of the body which have been liquified. Therefore, what is needed, is a medicine to control the thirst. For the thirst is great and the desire to drink is unsatisfiable. No amount of drink can stop the thirst. Therefore, we must direct treatment towards the stomach, which is the site of the thirst. When you have purged the body with Heira, use Epithemus (local application), made of Nard balsam, Mastic, Dates and raw Quinces. Especially good as a lotion is the juice of Quinces with Nard and Oil of Roses. A plaster of the pulp of Quinces with Mastle and Dates is useful. Also a mixture of these with wax and a salve of Nards is good for moistening. Likewise, and as a plaster, use the juice of Acacia and of Kytinus Hypocistis (astringent). Furthermore, the water used to drink should be that which has been boiled with many fruits. As food use milk, and with it use cereals, starch, groats and gruels, a stringent wine, undiluted, as a tonic for the stomach. If it be little diluted, it aids in emptying and dispersing the other humors, for they cause the thirst. In fact wine, which is at the same time astringent and cooling, acts equally because of its transforming and cooling properties, while a sweet wine, just as does blood, increases strength because it forms blood. In the same way various medicines are used, Theriaca and Mithridatica, and those obtained from the rind of the autumn fruits (which the Greeks call "Opwram") and all others which are useful in Dropsy. Likewise the whole diet and mode of life a that which is prescribed in Dropsy.

Unfortunately we cannot say what the treatment of dropsy was, since that chapter is missing. Some five hundred years later Hindu medical authorities wrote of the "Madhu Meha" or honey urine and the Arabs knew and treated diabetes mellitus. Just as were lost for more than a thousand years the writings of Aretaeus, so sugar disappears from the literature for the same length of time to be refound by Thomas Willis (1612–75).

The opinion has been expressed by no lesser student of the history of medicine than Dr. Osler that, "I doubt very much whether Corvisart in 1800 A.D. was any more skillful in recognizing a case of pneumonia than was Aretaeus in the second century A.D. When one has read the pages of this old master, one cannot help but be impressed greatly by the scholarly presentations of disease which he has left us."

References

1. NEUBURGER, M. Geschichte d. Medizin. Stuttgart, Enke, 1906, Vol. 1.
2. WUNDERLICH, C. Geschichte d. Medizin. 1859.
3. GARRISON, F. History of Medicine. Ed. 4, Phila., Saunders, 1929.
4. OSLER, W. Evolution of Modern Medicine. Yale Univ. Press, 1913.
5. ARETAEUS. Works. London, Sydenham Soc., 1856.
6. ARETAEUS. Works. Leyden, 1735.
7. ILBERG, G. Aretaeus, *Ztschr. k. d. ges. Neurol. u. Psychiat.*, 86:227, 1923.
8. CORDELL, E. Aretaeus. *Bull. Johns Hopkins Hosp.*, 20:371–377, 1909.

in: *Annals of Medical History 2 (1930), 424–435.*

India and China

Epistemological Fashions in Interpreting Disease

The Deleterious Effects of Western Terminology on the Application of the Scientific Tradition of Chinese Medicine (illustrated by the case of diabetes mellitus vs. sitis diffundens [hsiao-k'o]) *

by MANFRED PORKERT

I. The Linguistic Problem

Our use of the term 'fashion' will surprise all those brought up in the belief that the gathering and interpretation of scientific data is a strictly logical affair, subject only to the rules of reason and unaffected by any accidents of temper or talent. The fact is that precisely the latter, too, decisively condition the development of all scientific theory just as of any other product of culture.

This raises serious problems when the exchange of scientific assets between the members of different linguistic or even cultural groups is to be achieved.

Such exchange, as a rule, entails inflections of the ideas transmitted. Whether these inflections are slight or drastic depends upon a number of factors, most of which escape precise definition – e. g. the cultural gradient between donor and receiver, the catholicity of the respective idioms, the momentary scientific or political prestige of the idiom of origin, etc.

In the end, there is little difference between the problem of transmitting complete theories or systems and that of the transmission of single technical concepts. Consequently, to develop the problem involved, it is apt and more convenient to examine the principal alternatives for the inter-idiomatic communication of single technical terms viz.

1. Terminological loans

The foreign designation is taken over together with a new object, technique or method.

---

* This paper was presented at The First International Symposium (1976), Division of Medical History of the Taniguchi Foundation

2. Semantic imitation

The new object . . . is designated by a term chosen on the basis of certain similarities of the new object to familiar objects or procedures.

3. Phonetic imitation

The new terms is chosen on the phonetic resemblance of an indigenous term to a foreign designation, thus extending the meaning of the indigenous word to encompass the new even though possibly utterly unrelated concept.

4. Translation

After a more or less thorough rational comprehension of the new object or technique an entirely new term is coined from etymological elements of the indigenous idiom.

The literature of all times as well as the far-flung and intensive intercultural communication of this present age provides abundant evidence showing that any of these alternatives may be adopted by one individual or by a whole social group; also that each alternative has its specific advantages and drawbacks. Thus

– *Terminological loans* have the advantage of congruence with the term in the idiom of origin, hence facilitate the communication with other linguistic groups; however they contribute little to (or even impede) the integration of the new term to the existing conceptual system.

– *Semantic or phonetic imitations* do facilitate the integration of the new concept; but, on the other hand, they are prone to alter, deflect or deform the original idea, adding to or subtracting from its meaning.

The same danger at an even higher degree obtains for *translations* which, if chosen on the basis of defective information, may thoroughly transform or vitiate the original concept. On the other hand, congenial and successful translations consummate the integration of the hitherto foreign concept into its new setting to a degree which no other procedure can achieve.

Throughout history, the predominance of any language for political or economic reasons, leads to diffusion of its vocabulary into other idioms, not always enhancing but sometimes lessening their expressiveness. Greek, Latin, Chinese, Sanskrit, Arabic, English, to lesser degrees French, German, Spanish and Russian have played or are still playing such roles in their respective spheres and ages. And, as stated, the considerations just summarized for the interlinguistic transmission of single concepts and terms may be extended without restrictions to the transmission of complete theories and systems of philosophy or science.

There occurs loan, imitation, translation, each of which is liable to be as much motivated by intellectual or political fashions as by a clear rational purpose.

An example in point and central to this study is the adoption of the causal and analytic method by medicine in China and Japan. This adoption occured (and still occurs) at the expense of the indigenous body of systematized knowledge. It started in the 19th century and was prompted solely by the then overwhelmingly impressive achievements of Western science and technology (including medical science and technology) and precisely not by any kind of critical assessment or comparison of the rationale of either Chinese or Western medicine. This adoption momentarily may have been a great stimulus to the intellectual development in China and Japan; yet, on the long run, it inavoidably impedes and endangers the continuity of a mature scientific tradition.

II. The Epistemological Issue

1. Preliminaries

The criteria of exact science

If there is universal agreement that what is termed the technical and scientific revolution of recent times has been brought on by the remarkable development of only a few disciplines, notably physics and chemistry, a precise question as to the essential premises of this science is wont to sollicit confused and contradictory responses even from scientists. Consequently, it may be useful to recall that these essential criteria are

1. positive experience,
2. univocality of statements,
3. stringent rational integration (systematization) of empirical data.

Also it should be noted that, by contradistinction, other criteria such as notably
- the causality nexus,
- controlled experiment,
- quantification of data constitute

accidental criteria whose application is limited to some specific disciplines or fields of research only.

2. The compliance of Chinese medicine with the essential criteria of exact science

A pertinent albeit general appraisal of Traditional Chinese Medicine suggests that it conforms on the whole to the essential criteria of exact science as enumerated.

Ad 1.: There is practically no controversy about the fact that Chinese medicine is based upon positive empirical data, upon close and skilful observation of natural and social phenomena. (Admission of this is implicit even in the most dilettante accounts of Chinese medicine appearing today in the Far East and in the West, and which label Chinese medicine an "empirical medicine".)

Ad 2.: Univocality of statements, as any close examination of Western physics or chemistry will reveal, is solely and exclusively achieved by the expression of data *with reference to conventional standards*, in this instance to the c.g.s.-systems and its derivatives.

Chinese medicine, as, by the way, all Chinese science, achieves similar univocality by referring its data to the *Yin-yang-* and *wu-hsing-*(Five Evolutive Phases) conventions and their technical derivations. (We shall revert to this point below, limiting us here to the apodictic statement that there is absolutely no evidence in Chinese medical literature prior to its contact with the West (in the 19th century) that in *medical contexts yin* and *yang* and the five. E.P.s were ever meant *as anything else*. The qualification of the *yin-yang* and the *wu-hsing* as "principles" or "philosophical principles" is the gratuitous invention of Western brains [in the same vein as the translation of *wu-hsing* by "five elements"]. It is characteristic of an obscurantist and pseudo-scientific trend in certain Western disciplines to whom Indian yoga, Japanese zen, Persian sufi-ism and Chinese medicine form just one ill digested hodge-podge of "wisdom of the East". It is a matter of great regret that in the imitative enthusiasm not a few

Far Eastern authors have started to rehash this insipid interpretation, thus again adding grist to the mill of Western faddists and setting in motion a vicious circle.

Ad 3.: The pervading impression that everyone with any degree of familiarity with the original sources of Chinese medical literature receives is of the sophistication [not over-sophistication] and stringent systematization of collected data. And yet, even with these arguments granted, the fundamental dissimilarity of Chinese and Western medicine looms all the more baffling. Indeed, certain seeming contradictions can only be resolved through a clear understanding of the polarity of Chinese and Western science.

3. The polarity of Chinese and Western science

After what has just been stated, if we use the term "polarity", we do not do so because the expression may be *en vogue* in certain contexts. Rather are we motivated by its strong and basic implication, namely polar statements are mutually exclusive, at the same time mutually perfectly complementary.

Polarizing filters perfectly shut off light of one plane of oscillation, letting pass that of all other planes with different intensities. Any scientific method and its concomitant terminology produces effects similar to that of a polarizing filter: it gives unimpeded passage to cognate data, more or less modifies most other information and hermetically precludes directly polar statements.

It is well to keep in mind these effects when we are faced with the fact that today throughout the world, and including China and Japan, practically everybody making a claim to a scientific opinion on Chinese medicine has, to start with, been thoroughly inculcated the essentials of *Western* medicine. This fact, by itself, would suffice to explain why modern medical authors either flatly are at a loss to conceive any scientific system different from yet at a par with Western medicine; or, if they suspect that there might be more to Chinese medicine than some drug and acupuncture recips, why they experience extreme difficulties in substantiating such a hypothesis.

Why should this concern us? Because to the extent that in recent times the exact sciences of the West implement their criteria for heuristic methods of unprecedented stringency and effectiveness, there is increasing evidence showing that precisely these criteria and truly scientific methods are really applicable and produce impressive results only within a few clearly defined sections of medical endeavour – leaving others on the level of protoscientific empiricism. Every physician has been taught that the specificity of diagnoses and therapy as well as the precision of prognoses is in direct proportion to the rational elaboration, hence to the scientific stringency of any statement. Consequently, in his daily practice, he is constantly reminded of the steep gradient existing in Western medicine between very precise and very vague statements. But he will lack the leisure as well as the intellectual tools to explain this gradient. This leads us to the question of the limitations of the specific method of Western medicine, causal analysis.

4. Causal analysis and its limitations

Everybody is aware that not each and every object or effect may be completely perceived from a single vantage point or out of one single perspective. And surely this truth applies not only to particular professions such as e.g. astronomers, who are obliged to erect their observatories in the Northern as well as in the Southern hemisphere and in favourable climates, but to absolutely every scientific discipline. It also applies to heuristic methods and to epistemological modes. Thus in order to perceive and control substratum, matter, soma, causal analysis is required. Causal analysis implies that all relations of an observed effect to other simultaneous effects are consciously severed or suppressed (*analyein* = to losen, to resolve) and the relation to its cause is explicitly established. Causes axiomatically precede[1] their effects in time, hence, by definition, lie in the past. Past effects constitute materialized effects, hence matter.

Inversely, causal analysis confines positive perception and control to subtrative, material, somatic objects. Not even the most judiciously chosen real vantage point will let our eyesight (or the perception of instruments invented to boost their power) let us take in all the things that may be seen; similarly, no single mode of cognizance – which also implies a finite cognitive horizon – will enable us to perfectly perceive all cognizable effects. The limiting factor of the significance (and applicability) of caus-

[1] Concerning the mistake of the extension of the law of causality during the 19th century cf. the next section but one.

al analysis is what – from the vantage point of human perception – appears as the decrease of the homogeneity of substratums. This homogeneity of substratums appears to be greatest in elementary particles whence we observe a steady decrease as we proceed from these in the direction of atoms, molecules, cells, tissues of primitive and higher organisms, animals, human beings, social, political, cultural communities, planetary and galactic system . . . The various informations that any text book gives e.g. on the oxygen atom is not merely the result of the observation of one single and particular oxygen atom; rather is it based upon the observation of a statistical number of such atoms.

This procedure will yield statements of a probability almost equal to 1 because of the high homogeneity of the atoms, in other words as a consequence of the fact that the oxygen atoms involved show practically no significant individual differences. Similar consequences apply to other phenomena, with the evident restriction that a decrease in homogeneity (= increasingly significant individual differences) will reduce the stringency, the probability, hence the positive quality of statement based upon causal analysis.

Due to the continuous decrease of the homogeneity of substratums, the limit of significance of statements based upon causal analysis is evidently situated in the center of the scale occupied by biological phenomena – where human medicine exercises its functions. In other words, in the vicinity of this borderline, causal statements approach and finally attain the average probability of all aleatory procedures. Or, put still differently, the greater the differentiation and complication of biological organisms (= decrease in homogeneity), the less probability attaches to inferences drawn from the observation of one single individual as regards the reactions of all others; the less stringency also attaches to statistical data obtained from the observation of a large number of similar individuals if used to prognosticate in detail individual and specific changes. In brief, the stringency and significance of statements based upon causal analysis show a clear decline in the field of human physiology; and they fade away into utter indetermination when psychic or social phenomena are involved.

5. *Inductive[2] synthesis and its limitations*

The fact just described that statements based upon causal analysis will completely lose all stringency and significance is by no means tantamount to a complete fadeaway of stringent rational statements bearing on the phenomena concerned; after all, causal analysis is not the only mode of cognizance, not the sole perspective permitting the rational expression of positive statements on reality.

In order to perceive and control functions, movement, dynamic or psychic phenomena, inductive synthesis is required. Inductive synthesis implies that agents actually inducing effects in each other are consciously maintained or assembled (*syntithinai* = to put together). Induction implies the simultaneous presence of agent and effect (and perception). Present effects constitute dynamic effects, functions, movement.

Inversely put, inductive synthesis confines positive perception and control to dynamic, functional effects or phenomena. Needless to insist, just as causal analysis, inductive synthesis has its natural and axiomatic limitations. The significance of statements based upon inductive synthesis out of the human cognitive perspective appears to be limited by the stability of functions, in other words by the relative duration within which a given function is maintained in the same quality or direction. This stability of function appears as being great in galaxies and shows a continuous decline in planetary systems, cultural, political, social communities, human individuals, higher and lower animals . . . In other words, the stability of function varies in inverse proportion to the homogeneity of corresponding substratums.

In practice, this theorem establishes the complementary validity, significance and applicability of causal analysis and inductive synthesis: to the extent that the positive quality of statements based upon causal analysis decreases, that of statements based upon inductive synthesis increases – and vice versa.

At this juncture we should have little difficulty in realizing that thematical overlapping of the positive results of causal analytic science and inductive and synthetic science may occur only in a small central area, that, consequently, aside from this, both *will furnish equally positive and significant data on utterly different aspects of reality.*

---

[2] Our use of the terms "inductive, induction, inductivity" in publications of the past one and a half decades derives from and extends the meaning these terms have in electrodynamics.

6. *The consequences of the causal and analytic polarization of Western medicine*

The concrete and practical evidence of the arguments just developed is ubiquitous and compelling. If nevertheless, up to now, the leading authorities in Western medicine have not acted upon it, this neglect is not due to mere sluggishness or the existence of better insights, but above all to the blinding effect of a historical conjunction.

Western medicine is no exception to the rule that medicine at all times and in all climates was and is an essentially practice oriented discipline. Consequently, three centuries or ten generations have passed until the powerful challenge of Descartes' philosophy and Vesalius' investigations led to consistent efforts and decisive advances: only during the second part of the 19th century did Western medicine accomplish the transition from the stage of protoscientific empiricism to science in the modern and narrow sens – by consistently applying causal analysis in a number of pertinent subdisciplines. This endeavour, led by men like Ehrlich, Koch, Pasteur, Virchow . . . to name but a few, produced unprecedented changes in health care: control of infectious diseases, extension of the statistical life expectancy, drastic reduction of infant mortality – all this essentially carried by the development of anatomy, histology, microbiology and bacteriology, physiology, surgery.

Such medical innovation and the concomitant effects were in the 19th century and apparantly still are to many physicians today such an overwhelming experience that it made (makes) them completely oblivious of fundamental changes in our scientific outlook that had taken place at the same time. By far the most decisive and far-reaching change was that physics, the pacemaker of exact science in the West, in the work of men like Faraday and Maxwell, departed from the unilateral fixation on causal analysis, according equal importance to inductive synthesis, thus paving the way for new and almost purely inductive disciplines like electrodynamics and nuclear physics.

By the turn of the century, Western medicine as described, and backed by the economic and political power of the Occident, victoriously spread across the globe. Medical science, in all civilized countries including China and Japan, came to be defined exclusively by the standards of Western medicine. Thus crisis becomes inevitable.

Today, two generations later, the symptoms are evident: Beside the solid success of Western surgery and control of bacterial epidemies, and increasing number of complaints and disorders with which physicians are faced in everyday practice receive only palliative or no treatment at all. The pressure on medicine to cope with these ailments *without any inquiry into the methodological premises of Western medicine* increasingly lowers the efficiency of almost all health care, producing more dangerous drugs, more complicated machines and greater frustrations in medical personnel and patients alike.

Public demand and the frenzied search for new remedies makes for the maintenance or the introduction of hoary or doubtful recipes of unproven efficiency. The recent craze of acupuncture applied in the West out of all context with its systematic origin borders on quackery.

Indeed, not the least bane due to Western medicine's infatuation with causal analysis is that it almost totally precludes any rational exploration of a scientifically relevant confrontation with the mature results of the Chinese medical legacy. This leads right to the core of the present discussion.

7. The message of Chinese medicine obscured by the fashionable use of Western terminology

The massive influx and acceptance of Western science and technology into China and Japan since the 19th century there gradually led to contempt for if not to outright ostracism of all traditional learning including medicine. (And, to be sure, this disdain, as we had intimated elsewhere,[3] was only to a small extent justified by real shortcomings of indigenous science; it was [and in fact still is] preponderantly motivated by the trauma and inferiority complexes in the wake of the political and cultural collapses following Western expansion into East Asia.)

In Japan the government flatly ruled that Western medicine constitutes the only scientifically acceptable and proven kind of medicine and consequently prerequisite to the training and to the licensing of every physician; in China (People's Republic, Taiwan, Hongkong, Singapore) the struggle between both systems is still on with the sympathies of the medical establishment

[3] Wenner Gren Symposium Proceedings, Burg Wartenstein Symposium no 53 (Toward the comparative study of Asian medical system); The intellectual and social impulses behind the evolution of traditional chinese medicine.

clearly going to "Western medicine" with its cosmopolitan and modern flavour.

In this situation the practitioners and advocates of traditional medicine fell to what they thought was the best expediency for convincing everybody of the value of the traditional craft; they tried to explain it in terms of Western medicine. The fate of homöopathy and a number of other empirical disciplines should have warned them! Traditional Chinese medicine produced a most miserable show when bereft of its scientific rationale and cast together with dozens of "ethno-medicines", with "empirical techniques of needle-pricking" – inspite of its "quite impressive inventory of medicinal herbs".

From what has been explained above it should be clear that those well intentioned native defenders of their medical heritage are in reality jettisoning and destroying what is directly required to close a gap in the system of universal medicine. This gap exists because of the hitherto unilateral development of scientific medicine in the West. And the mature fruit of China's traditional medicine may serve to close this gap because it has a similar rational sophistication as Western medicine and because it is complementary by its axiomatic basis. Prerequisite to the combination of both systems is

a) the strict abstention from pseudo scientific explanations of one system in the terms of the other;
b) the thorough and consistent appraisal of each system as a whole and in its own right;
c) the comparative empirical verification of accepted data.

The following section is an attempt to adumbrate what is at stake as well as an outline of the concrete methods employed.

III. Diabetes mellitus vs, Sitis diffundens (hsiao-k'o)

The disease today named *diabetes mellitus* has occurred since ancient times. Its increased incidence in modern times (it is expected that five percent of the population of the U.S. will eventually contract the disease) is apparently due to the higher life expectancy and more copious diets. (The corresponding modern Chinese term is *t'ang-niao-ping,* i.e. sugar-in-urine-disease.) In the system of *traditional* Chinese medicine most of the corresponding symptoms are subsumed under the designation *hsiao-k'o* i.e. *Sitis diffundens.*

1. Diabetes mellitus

As conceived by Western medicine, *diabetes mellitus* is an acute and chronic metabolic disorder characterized principally by hyperglycemia resulting from an absolute or relative deficiency of metabolically active insulin.[4]

"The lack of insulin results in deficient tissue utilization of carbohydrates, necessitating increased catabolism of proteins and fats to supply the energy needs of the body. The increased catabolism of fats leads to ketosis, while the hyperglycemia causes excessive loss of glucose through the urine (glycosuria). Thus arise the cardinal metabolic manifestations of diabetes: hyperglycemia, ketosis and glycosuria, sometimes terminating in death. In addition to these metabolic derangements, *diabetes mellitus* is also associated with widespread alterations in the blood vessels, kidneys, eyes, peripheral nerves and heart. Most of these vascular changes take the form of an accelerated aging process including augmented arteriosclerosis and degenerative changes in the small blood vessels. A major focus of investigation today involves the question of whether these vascular alterations (angiopathy) are directly related to the carbohydrate metabolic derangement, or whether the biochemical abnormalities and the angiopathy merely occur concomitantly, both being secondary to more fundamental derangements. Conceivably, an as yet unidentified metabolic derangement in the walls of blood vessels might occur along with, but separate from, the carbohydrate metabolic abnormality; diabetes might then represent a concurrence of separate, possibly related errors of metabolism. Hyperglycemia and acidosis have been effectively controlled as causes of death. The major challenge at the present time is to prevent the disabling and sometimes fatal widespread vascular changes. Thus the question of whether careful control of the hyperglycemia and acidosis can retard or prevent the development of the "vascular complications" of diabetes is one of the most controversial issues in medicine today (Reaven and Salans).

In other words, the characteristic symptoms of diabetes (hyperglycemia, ketosis and glycosuria) can be assessed without difficulty; also the immediate cause of these symptoms has been determined to be a deficiency of the enzyme insulin produced in the beta cells of the islets of Langerhans of the endoplasmic reticulum of the pancreas. Consequently, the appearance of the

---

[4] This and all subsequent quotations bearing on *diabetes mellitus* are taken from Stanley L. Robbins, M.D. "Pathology", Philadelphia 1967.

principal symptoms can be checked by the substitutive administration of heterologous insulin. This palliative measure is up to now the *ultima ration* of Western causal analytic medicine, its only recognized and predictable "therapy". For as regards the further causal etiology, due to the high complexity (= low homogeneity) of the substratum involved, the method of causal analysis leads to a large number of hypotheses of only slightly better than average probability.

To instance, a hereditary propensity for diabetes has been established. In the case of implied homozygosity (both parents having the disease) there is approximately "a 90 percent chance of this disorder occuring in the offspring. There is, however, still no adequate explanation for the failure of the disease to become manifest in most individuals harboring the inherited diabetic trait while some with the same inheritance are overtly diabetic.

"Most diabetics mysteriously remain totally unaffected for significant periods of their lives, despite the hereditary trait present from birth".

It is clear that in the consistent application of causal analysis, factors or causes beyond the simple failure of the beta cells in the islets of Langerhans must be looked for. Yet, "while we speak of an absolute or relative deficiency of metabolically active insulin as the cause of *diabetes mellitus*, there is still no precise understanding of the nature of this insulin lack. Moreover, in addition to the insulin lack, the growth hormone of the pituitary, the adrenal steroids and the thyroid hormone are also intimately related to the development of the diabetic state. Perhaps the most important of these is the anterior pituitary growth hormone or some factor closely related to it. This hormone inhibits the intracellular phosphorylation of glucose by blocking the action of hexokinase or some other enzyme in the Embden-Meyerhof pathway. In the experimental animal, the prolonged administration of growth hormone causes protracted hyperglycemia that eventually results in permanent diabetes by exhaustion and destruction of the beta cells of the pancreatic islets". Although these results look significant if seen in connection with the occurrence of the "growth-onset" diabetes *(diabetes mellitus juwenilis)* hitting children between eight and ten years of age, no diagnostic information is in sight, describing specific pathological mechanisms, insuring a clear prognosis, defining a safe course of therapy.

2. *Hsiao-k'o = Sitis diffundens*

The term of *hsia-k'o*, lit. "diffusion thirst" is first[5] encountered in chapter 13 of the *Chin-k'uei yao-lüeh,*[6] dealing with the disorders of micturition. It derives from the impressive symptom of micturition. It derives from the impressive symptom of thirst *(k'o)* accompanied by immediate and massive secretion of ingested fluid. This definition ("incessant thirst, much urine") also opens the eight paragraphs devoted to *sitis diffundens* in the *Chu-ping yüan-hou lun* of 610 (chapter 5).

In subsequent literature, *sitis diffundens* in addition to polydipsia, turgid urine, is characterized by polyuria, emaciation in spite of polyphagia, sweet flavour of urine. Moreover, the high incidence of ulcers in *hsiao-k'o* patients is noted.

Chinese medicine defines *sitis diffundens* primarily as an affection of the *oo. pulmonalis, stomachi* or *renalis.*

After what has been said above and explained in our Theoretical Foundations of Chinese Medicine, it should be clear that these orbs, notwithstanding a terminological resemblance, have hardly anything in common with the organs of Western medicine or their functions as postulated by Western physiology: the *o. pulmonalis* represents the structive basis of rhythm, time sense, temperature control and constitutes the first defence line against heteropathies; the *o. stomachi* actively regulates the assimilation of alien energies, and, more generally, the transformation, balancing and distribution of all forms of energy within an individual; the *o. renalis* stands for the inborn (constitutional) potentials, hence all potentiation of energies, the capacity for directed emotions. [All autonomous nervous functions postulated by Western medicine and the respective regulations resort to this.]

To consider their principal symptoms and their diagnostic interpretation, clinical medicine, depending upon whether respectively the symptoms of polydipsia, polyphagia or polyuria are most strikingly in evidence, distinguishes an upper, middle and lower variety of *sitis diffundence: Shang hsiao-k'o, Chung hsiao-k'o, Hsia hsiao-k'o.*

a) *Diffusio superior (Shang hsiao)*

Symptoms: Permanent thirst and polydipsia, dry mouth and

[5] Second Hand time, consequently 2nd century A.D.

[6] The mentions in the *Nei-ching Su-wen* are not conclusive; as far as historical precedence is concerned at least the chapters 69 and 72 in which mention of the term occurs, constitute section interpolated during the Tang.

parched tongue; normal feces yet increased quantity of urine and frequency of micturition; deep red colour of tip and borders of the tongue; thin, yellow coating of the tongue; *pulsus exundantes et celeri.* The harassing thirst, dry mouth and tongue are indicative of *ardor orbis stomachi,* or in conjunction with the redtipped or red bordered tongue, of *ardor orbis cardialis,* transmitting its *calor* to the *o. pulmonalis.* Consequently, the structive energy of the *o. pulmonalis* is impaired and the active liquids of the *o. pulmonalis* are available in insufficent quantity. The increased frequency and quantity of urination is likewise due to this mechanism: the inner glare *(ardor)* induces thirst; the drink ingested to quench this, however, due to the impaired function of the *o. pulmonalis,* cannot be condensed and assimilated into body liquids but instead, is immediately excreted. The red tip and borders of the tongue, the thin and yellow coating of the tongue, the *pp. exundantes et celeri* are all concurrent symptoms of *calor vigens* and of *repletio.* The therapy of this *diffusio superior* must concentrate a) on *refrigeratio caloris,* dissipation of heat and glare, b) on stimulating the production of active juices *(chin).*

b) *Diffusio mediana (Chung hsiao)*

Symptoms: This middle variety has the principal symptoms of overactive digestion and permanent hunger; emaciation, obstipation; tongue coating is yellow and parched; *pp. lubrici et repleti.* Overactive digestion and permanent hunger on the one hand, obstipation on the other is indicative of *vigor caloris sinarteriarum splendoris yang* (i.e. of the conduits of the *oo. stomachi et intest. crassi*) and of ensuing dissipation and evanescence of the structive potentials. The emaciation is likewise a result of the *vigor caloris orbis stomachi* dissipating the structive energies and potentials, thus diminishing the sustentation of the flesh (which is the *perfectio* of the *o. lienalis,* the inner orb to the *orbis stomachi*). The symptoms of the tongue and pulses concur with this. The therapy of this disorder consists a) in *refrigeratio caloris orbis stomachi,* and in dissipation of glare; b) in the sustentation of the structive energies.

c) *Diffusio inferior (Hsia hsiao)*

α) If induced by *inanitas yin* alone, the symptoms are; Polyuria with frequent micturition; urine is sweet in flavour and resembles a fatty emulsion; dry mouth and red body of the tongue; *pp.*

mersi, minuti atque celeri, copious urine here is induced by the diminished structive energies, by an impaired *yin renale* or, more generally, by a depressed and exhausted *calorium inferius* (corresponding to the *oo. renalis, vesicalis et intestinorum*); consequently, the structive potential of the *o. renalis* is insufficient to control and restrain the active energies. Indirectly, the sweetness and appearance like molten grease of the urine is also due to the same deficiency of the *yin renale* – whose active energy expanding in turn violates the *o. lienalis* (= *intima* of the *o. stomachi*) and which thus has its assimilating capacity affected so that the *ch'i frumentarium* passes on to the *o. renalis* (and from there into the *o. vesicalis,* the *species* of the *o. renalis*) insufficiently refined. The dry mouth, the deep-red tongue in company of *pp. mersi, minuti atque celeri* indicate an erratic *ignis ministri* (i.e. active energy of the *o. renalis*) due to *inanitas yin.* – The therapy of this condition consists in a *rigatio ch'i structivi* and a stabilization of the *o. renalis.*

β) If *inanitas* of yin and yang obtains, the aggravation of the aforementioned symptoms is evident from frequent and copious urination of urine like molten grease; sometimes the urge to micturate arises immediately after the intake of fluid; darkened complexion; impotence; withered-looking ear conch; pale tongue with white coating; *pp. mersi et minuti,* without force. These symptoms are partly congruent with those in the preceding paragraph. The urge to micturate immediately after the intake of fluid indicates the extreme exhaustion of the *yang renale.* The darkened complexion and the parched-looking ear conch indicate that the residual structive energy of the *o. renalis* stagnates and in the absence of sufficient active energy cannot spread. The impotente is also due to an *ignis ministri dilabens.* The symptoms of tongue and pulses corroborate the diagnosis of similar exhaustion of active and structive energies in the *o. renalis.* Treatment consists in *tepefactio* (cautious warming) of the active energy components and in *rigatio o. renalis.*

d) *Collateral Symptoms*

such as ulcus, impaired vision, deafness, night blindness, will, after proper diagnosis (involvement of the *o. hepaticus* or impairment of the *ch'i structivum*) necessitate complementary therapy (*rigatio o. renalis + suppletio o. hepatici,* draining of toxins, etc.).

The therapeutic prospects for the complete cure of the described conditions are good to very good. With the exception of terminal stages with extreme sugar levels in the urine and with concomitant complications including coma, all disorders are described as responding to drug treatment or moxibustion based upon careful diagnosis.

3. *Conclusion*

The immediate juxtaposition of the diagnostic accounts of *diabetes mellitus* and *sitis diffundens (hsia k'o)* should make perfectly clear a number of points, viz.

1. the utter impossibility of directly converting the statements of one system into those of the other; hence
2. the pseudoscientific nature of all attempts to combine elements of one system with elements of the other, e.g.
   a) the administration of Chinese drug or acupuncture prescriptions on the premise of a Western diagnosis or, more rarely vice versa;
   b) the criticism of elements of Chinese medicine on the premise of Western medical theory;
3. that the dogmatic monopoly of health care by one system necessarily totally obliterates (by rendering unintelligible) the data of the complementary system; irrespective of their scientific quality and therapeutic relevance.

Consequently, as the comparative data on *diabetes mellitus* and *sitis diffundens* instance, a number of former decisions and present rules in health policy stipulating the predominance of Western causal analytic medicine even in China and in Japan are evidently neither based upon a thorough and rational appraisal of the relative merits of Western and Chinese medicine nor dictated solely by the concern for more effective health care. Instead they are prompted by certain historical trends and irrational convictions, notably that of Western medicine representing science, Chinese traditional medicine representing empiricism and superstition. Clearly, today such convictions themselves must be classed as superstitions.

in: *Nihon Ishigaku Zasshi. Journal of the Japan Society of Medical History 23 (1977), 1–18*

The Urinary Flux of the Ancient Indians (Prameha)

(with Special Reference to the Carakasamhita)

by REINHOLD F. G. MÜLLER

In 1805, in Ceylon, the English physician DR. CHRISTIE treated an indigenous doctor for diabetes mellitus and obtained from him information about the traditional perceptions of that disease, *madu mehé* (honey urine) from the specialist text *Yoga Ratnakêre.* This last was represented as a 300 year old translation from the Sanskrit, ostensibly as a *Pāli* text. In the *Edinburgh Medical and Surgical Journal,* Vol. VII (1811), p. 296–298, CHRISTIE afterwards gave a review of the pertinent chapter on *pra mehé.*

In his historico-geographic pathology, AUGUST HIRSCH combined this report with the relevant section of the *Suśrutasaṃhitā,* on the express assumption that the source of the above-mentioned translation was to be found in this old medical work. And it is on this incident that has rested since the evidence of an extraordinarily early acquaintance with diabetes mellitus on the part of the Indians, one that has been regularly assessed as very noteworthy from the viewpoint of modern medicine.

The manuscript, which provided the first knowledge of Indian views on the *prameha,* is not accessible. *Yogaratnākara (Ānandāśrama,* Sanskrit Series 4, Poona 1900) contains the Sanskrit text, which, according to JOLLY (*Medizin,* 2) was published by an unknown author. Bh. SINH JEE, in his *History of Aryan Medical Science* (215), without further evidence, ascribes the book to the Jain monk *Nayanaṣekhara* from the year 1676.

There, in the section *mehanidāna,* the 20 individual diseases listed by CHRISTIE are briefly described, of which the first 10 are caused by *śleṣman* (mucus), the next 6 by *pitta* (bile) and the last 4 by *vāta* (wind).

The following table has been compiled to provide an overview and a path of approach to the traditions of ancient times.

	Christie 297–296	*Yogaratnākara, mehanidāna*	*Mā Mādhavanidāna, prameha- 7–17*	*Ga-Pu Garuḍapurāṇa, 159, 19–24, 2–5*
śleṣman:				
1.	*Udaka-*	*udaka-*	*udaka-*	*udaka-*
2.	*Ikshu-*	*ikṣu-*	*ikṣu-*	*ikṣu-*
3.	*Sura-*	*sāndra-*	*sāndra-*	*sāndra-*
4.	*Sandra-*	*surā-*	*surā-*	*surā-*
5.	*Pishta-*	*piṣṭa-*	*piṣṭa-*	*piṣṭa-*
6.	*Sukra-*	*śukra-*	*śukra-*	*śukra-*
7.	*Saikta-*	*sikatā-*	*sikatā-*	*sikatā-*
8.	*Sita-*	*śīta-*	*śīta-*	*śīta-*
9.	*Samairima*	*śanair-*	*śanair-*	*śanair-*
10.	*Alala-*	*lālā-*	*lālā-*	*lālā-*
pitta:				
11.	*Manjesta-*	*kṣāra-*	*kṣāra-*	*kṣāra-*
12.	*Rakta-*	*nīla-*	*nīla-*	*nīla-*
13.	*Nila-*	*kāla-*	*kāla-*	*kāla-*
14.	*Hariddra-*	*hāridra-*	*hāridra-*	*hāridra-*
15.	*Rala-*	*māñjiṣṭha-*	*māñjiṣṭha-*	*māñjiṣṭha-*
16.	*Ksahara-*	*rakta-*	*rakta-*	*rakta-*
vāta:				
17.	*Wasa-*	*vasā-*	*vasā-*	*vasā-*
18.	*Mudja-*	*majja-*	*majja-*	*majja-*
19.	*Hasta-*	*kṣaudra-*	*kṣaudra-*	*hasti-*
20.	*Madu-*	*hasti-*	*hasti-*	*madhu-*

Sourced and abbreviations: *Ca* = *Carakasaṃhitā*, large, double annotated edition of N. and B. Senagupta, Calcutta 1928/29; currently extends up to *indriyasthāna*; thereafter from the edition of *Narendranātha*, Lahore 1929, quoted. – Su = *Suśrutasamhitā*, ed. *Nānakacandra*, Lahore 1928 – *Va* = *Aṣṭāṃgahṛdaya*, ed. A. M. Kunte, Bombay 1925. (The *Astāṅgasaṃgraha* of the older *Vāgbhaṭa*, incidentally, is not available for borrowing from any public library in Germany.) – *Mā* = *Mādhavanidāna*, ed. *Cakradhara*, Lahore 1926. – *Ga-Pa* = *Garuḍapurāṇa*, ed. *Jīvānanda Vidyāsāgara*, Lahore 1890. On this last tradition, it should be noted that the sequence of the *prameha*-individual diseases begins at 159,2 with *hāridrameha* and reverts only later to the initially missing diseases with *udakameha* at 159, 19. This misplacement in the arrangement is very probably attributable to a mixing-up of loose pages, as also occurs elsewhere; Kirfel has already referred to this (Garbe Festschrift 107). This circumstance points to a late editorial period and throws a particular light on the continuance of this tradition thereafter. The doctrines in the *Ga-Pu* are conveniently of the *Dhanvantari* in the mouth, therefore arising from the same doctrinal system to which *Su* belongs.

Vā Aṣṭāṅgahṛdaya, nidāna- 10	Aṣṭāṅgasaṃgraha, *nidāna*- 10, 2	Su Suśrutasaṃhitā, *nidāna*- 6	Ca Carakasamhitā, *nidāna*- 4
udaka-	*udaka*-	*udaka*-	*udaka*-
ikṣu-	*ikṣu*-	*ikṣu*-	*ikṣu*-
sāṇdra-	*sāndra*-	*surā*-	*sāndra*-
surā-	*sūrā*-	*sikatā*-	*sāndraprasāda*-
pisṭa-	*pisṭa*-	*śanair*-	*śukla*-
śukra-	*śukla*-	*lavaṇa*-	*śukra*-
sikatā-	*sikatā*-	*piṣṭa*-	*śīta*-
śīta-	*śīta*-	*sāndra*-	*sikatā*-
śanair-	*śanair*-	*śukra*-	*śanair*-
lālā-	*lāla*-	*phena*-	*ālāla*-
kṣāra-	*kṣāra*-	*nīla*-	*kṣāra*-
nīla-	*kāḷa*-	*harideā*-	*kāla*-
kāla-	*nīla*-	*amla*-	*nīla*-
hāridra-	*hāridra*-	*kṣāra*-	*lohita*-
māṇjiṣṭha-	*māñjiṣṭa*-	*māñjiṣṭhā*-	*māñjiṣṭha*-
rakta-	*śoṇita*-	*śoṇita*-	*hāridra*-
vāsa-	*vasā*-	*sarpir*-	*vāsa*-
majja-	*majja*-	*vāsa*-	*majja*-
hasti-	*hasti*-	*kṣaudra*-	*hasti*-
madhu-	*madhu*-	*hasti*-	*madhu*-

The meaning of the special terms is translated here according to JOLLY, *Medizin* 83: 1. *udaka*- water; 2. *ikṣu*- sugar; 3. *sāndra*- viscous; 4. *surā*- brandy; *sāndraprasāda*- viscous decoction; 5. *piṣṭa*- porridge; *śukla*- white; 6. *śukra*- semen; lavaṇa- salt; 7. *sikatā*- sand; 8. *śīta*- cold; 9. *śanair*- gradual; 10. *lālā*- saliva; *phena*- foam; 11. *ksāra*- lyes; 12. *nīla*- blue; 13. *kāla*- black; *amla*- acid; 14. *hāridra*- turmeric; *lohita*- blood; 15. *māṁjiṣṭha*- madder; 16. *rakta*- blood; *śonita*- blood; 17. *vasā*- *fat; sarpir*- butter; 18. *majja*- marrow; 19. *kṣaudra*- honey; 20. *hasti*- elephant; *madhu*- honey.

Some errors of JOLLY are corrected in the table.

The separate elements of the prameha are listed once more as another, probably older, quotation from the *Carakasaṃhitā*. The group of the *pitta* and *vāta* is here, namely in the *Sūtrasthāna* 19, 12, identical with the above quotation. The first group contains the following series: 1. *udaka*, 2. *ikṣu*-, 3. *rasa*-, sāndra-, 5. *sāndraprasāda*-, 6. *śukla*-, 7. *śīta*-, 8. *śanair*-, 9. *sikatā*-, 10. *lālā*-.

In the foregoing table, the disease properties of the urine are listed according to key-words from different strata of Indian medicine. In the regular and, for the older periods, almost exclusively oral handing down of the texts the wording and the word order allow an apparently reliable conclusion as to the actual dependence of the separate traditions.

From these viewpoints it emerges that, apart from phonetic inflexions, the material brought forward by CHRISTIE contains anomalies. If, however, his parallel of the Sanskrit text of the *Yogaratnākara* is chosen as the starting-point for a retrospective assessment, a congruence with the *Mādhavanidāna* is conspicuous but not surprising, because the latest reputed special text on pathology dominated Indian medicine for the greater part. It may be conditionally inferred from this that the systematics of urinary irregularities is definitely confirmed at around 800. However, it is not too risky to transfer the duration of the rigid form of that text classification to the times of the second *Vāgbhaṭa*. For the demonstrated concordance also relates to the *Aṣṭaṇgahṛdayasaṃhitā* except for the last two designations which are interchanged, whereby *kṣaudra* (honey) is replaced by *madhu* (sweet). Only in the collections of the *Suśruta* and *Caraka* appear minor deviations which, after this example, may lead to the supposition that the relevant teaching program had not yet attained a definite form of transmission. However, this objection is significantly weakened by the same skeleton classification into three groups of the *doṣa,* the proportionate decrease in curability and the constant number of the subclassifications. In overview, a proportionately firmly outlined teaching tradition is thereby demonstrable up to that early epoch in which medical knowledge is comprehensible in its compartmental collections.[1]

The question whether the old Indian physicians had a knowledge of urinary sugar flux must be considered as somewhat misstated. For, in the pragmatic historical setting, it should not relate to merely a single observation without retrospective reference to a broad range of texts. This defect is not eliminated if a mass of material is collected as a specific selection. The aim which historical investigation often helps to induce, or at least for which it ensures a wider sympathy, remains dependent on

---

[1] The *Siddhayoga,* 35 (*Ānandāśrama,* Series 27) deviates from these texts. Variations from older periods are not known to the autor.

the problem posed and furthermore conceals the danger of material distortions. Against this lack of independence in the sense of an exactitude in science, protection can only be aimed at to a certain extent – and certainly not only in the present context – by clarifying as far as possible the sense of the texts regarding circumstances and origins. This path is so rarely adopted in Indian medical history that it often leads to unbroken ground and hence seems remote. However, the path must be ventured again and again if the scientific principle of historical research is not to be lost in romanticism, but rather witness the renaissance that Indian doctors now offer. Over the great extent of the materials of medical and other tradition in India a discontinuity or unevenness in many rudiments is unavoidable because no reliable general overview exists, or because the author's knowledge is inadequate. However, something may yet be gained by a scrupulous or critical approach. Here, the very first report on the matter gives us a hint.

CHRISTIE concludes his treatise: "Yet it is a curious circumstance, that the Indian physicians should have described so distinctly the sweetness of the urine in *madu mehé*, which had escaped the observation of both the ancient and modern physicians of Europe till the time of Willis." Therefore the investigation has proceeded since from the key-word: *madhu-meha* = sweet urine. Here, a taste attribute and a special feature of the human body is expressed.

As is well-known, "taste" plays a great part in Indian medicine, under the term *rasa* which already emerges as a technical term in the old traditions. The basic meaning of *rasa*, however, is that of a fluid, a form of which the *Su sūtra 15, 9* for instance is completely aware. Its various forms have only invaded anatomic and therapeutic territories with time. Moreover, the medical concept of taste was still not established when the *Sūtrasthāna* of the *Carakasaṃhitā* was compiled. The opening of the 26th section depicts the legendary assembly of the oldest authoritative physicians and their relevant doctrines, which enjoyed more or less validity until the clarification in the *Saṃhitā* text. *Caraka* (or his source author, *Agniveśa*) places the son of the *Atri* *(Ātreya)*, the *Punavarsu*, decisively in the mouth, as actually given by six *rasas*, namely: *madhura* – *amla* – *lavaṇa* – *katu* – *tikta* – *kaṣāya*, i.e., sweet – sour – salty – sharp – bitter – astringent. This so-called *Ātreya* system has achieved a certain superiority in the doctrines, which, partly brought about by skill, can be more or less incorporated with the other sections of the *Puna-*

varsu.[2] Of the other theories about the *rasa*, the first-listed and actually the oldest of the *Bhadrakāpya* recognizes only one type, which is not distinguished from water (sa *punarudakādananya iti*);[3] Punavarsu admits it with the acknowledgment that the starting-point of the six *rasa* is water *(teṣāṃ ṣaṇṇāṃ rasānāṃ*

---

[2] In the presentation to Garbe (Erlangen 1927) 157–162, Lüders showed from his records that the division into eight is older than that into six parts. However, the first was still accorded a certain validity *(Ca vimāna*-8,32; *yathā anyatrāṣṭau rasāh, saḍatra rasāḥ* or *ṣaḍanyatra)*; the special statements on the *rasa*, in *Ca sūtra*- 26 and *vimāna*-1 and also in Su sūtra- 40,42 recognize the classification into six, as occurs elsewhere with this property, e.g., in *Ca sūtra*-1,*43; śarīra*- 2,*3; Su sūtra*- 1,22; 14,*I*; 46, I, etc.

[3] The other divisions are: twofold through Śākunteya in the one *rasa*, with cutting *(chedanīya)* and calming *(upaśamanīya)* property. As a third, *Maudgalya* here appends a *rasa* with both the aforesaid properties *(śadhārana)*. The fourfold division through *Kauśika* arises from the mutations of *svādu, hita* and their two combinations (*svādu* counts as savory or sweet, *hita* as beneficial): The number five of the *Bharadvāja* corresponds in appurtenance to the so-called 5 elements: *bhauma-udaka-āgneya-vāvya-āntarikṣāḥ*. *Nimī* extends to six sections with *kṣāra;* as against this, *Agniveśa*, the authority, turns away from fluids in *Ca sūtra*- 26,*14; Kṣaraṇāt kṣārah nāsaraso dravyaṃ hi*, i.e., *kṣāra* turns away from fluids, it is no rasa, for it counts as *dravya*. The term *dravya* verbally expresses the property of a movement, as a gerundive or adjectival form of *dru*=run. The equation in *15: samanvite vā dravye* reinforces this opinion *(sam-anu-ita* = taken together) in the sense of the combination of several *rasa*, the statement being in *14*. When later *(20)* each *dravya* is designated as comprising 5 elements *(bhautika)*, this confirms the interpretation as substance, object or such. However, the meaning derived above is to be reckoned as the original and still used here, also supported by the present etymologic explanation. Science usually cautiously opposes such word definitions by the ancient Indians, but it cannot be denied that the resulting condition here is acknowledged in the medical texts. For *Su* repeats the explanation in an extension to operating conditions, where *ksāra* is derived from fluids or wounds *(sūtra*- 11, *3: tatra kṣaraṇāt kṣaṇanādvā kṣāraḥ)*. Thus, a contextual equivalence of *kṣāra* and *kṣara* must be assumed; and in this focus, the term *dravya* also keeps its literal meaning (cf. *Ca vimāna*- 8, *83*, where *kṣāra* is replaced by *drava:* cf. p. 18). *Dhāmārgava* then adds yet another, eighth, *rasa: avyakta*, whose nature is not explained in the text and is hard to define form the word formation. For 'ointment' *(añj)* already has a wide linguistic application in the Vedas; literally, *avyakta* would mean "the unanointed". As for a very probable dependent relationship of the 7th and 6th *rasa*, forms of different fluidity must be assumed, such as viscous and unctuous. Such a supposition accords with the fact that the last two *rasa* no longer met with unconditional recognition at a later date regarding the original concept as fluid and its development towards taste. Faced with such embarrassments, Indian medicine tends to conclude its taxonomy with a reference to innumerable *(aparisaṃkhyeya)* details. So also here, through *Kāṅkāyana*, who, as may be incidentally remarked, seems to have been the composer of the 9th song in *Atharvaveda* XI.

yonirudakam). Likewise, *Su* repeatedly emphasizes that *rasa* refers to water.

The *rasa* therefore appertain to water (*sūtra*- 42,1: *tasmādāpyo rasāh*) or: the actual water *rasa* (ibid: *khalvāpyo rasāḥ*). In accord with these views the treatment of water in *Su* begins with the indication that the drinkable heavenly water is a *rasa* not (yet) to be closely defined, imperishable, animating, refreshing, etc. (*sūtra*- 45, *1: pāniyamāntarīkṣamanirdeśyarasmamṛtaṃ jivaṇaṃ tarpaṇaṃ . . .)*[4]

The texts of the rasa are expanded many times in the special editions in *Ca* and *Su* and their combinations with other systems elaborated; this will not be discussed further here. The traditional text illustrations show that the original concept of the *rasa* does not correspond to an abstraction of sense perceptions, to which the modern term 'taste' points, but also to a physicochemical definition.[5] Such a development in the ancient Indian concepts is admissible only in the further course, obviously or mainly under the influence of the therapeutic aspects of the *rasa*. The basic concept is much more that of a fluid in physical or concrete form. And the basis of this conclusion is supported, not only by occasional fragments of text, but also by examples in the *Ca* and *Su* which appear emphasized as to form and content in the special treatises.

The orientation over "taste" is actually necessary in any investigation of sugar efflux in the urine. From the other documents there emerges an attitude to the theory of the three *dosa* which divides the disease into three main groups. Without more ado, it may be said that this technical term refers regularly to the triggering of the disease and its course, corresponding to the general literal meaning of *dosa* as blemishes. The relevant views

[4] The heavenly water actually corresponds to the rainwater in the text *āntarikṣam* (sic); this designation is linked with the old philosophy, cf. HERTEL, Abhdl. Sächs. Akad. Wiss. XL/2, 181–2, and refers to the 5th element (cf. the foregoing note). Besides the study by HERTEL, reference to *Indo-Iranischen Quellen und Forschungen, Vol. VI,* is most advisable for an understanding of the ancient outlook.

[5] The ancient Indians were naturally aware of the fact that, for instance, water to which salt was added assumed such a taste. This observation is even made the starting-point for didactic discussion in the *Chāndyoga-Upanisad* VI, 13. But the very emphasis on the value of this knowledge here shows an awkwardness in cognition theory alignment of the process which essentially distinguishes it from realistic modern conclusions.

therefore operate in the pathological, and not the physiological, field. Despite the great importance of this doctrine of the old scientific speciality, an exhaustive or generally conclusive conceptual clarification appears impossible. However, for the questions involved here it may be adequate to a certain extent if we agree to the combination of the *dosa* with the *raga*, as happens in *Su, sūtra*- 42, 1.

tatra madhurāmlalavaṇā vātaghnāh / madhuratiktakaṣāyāḥ pittaghnāḥ / kaṭutiktakaṣāyāh śleṣmaghnāḥ /

(From the *rasa* it is here learned:) There are sweet, sour, salty destructive *vāta;* sweet, bitter, astringent destructive *pitta;* sharp, bitter, astringent destructive *śleṣman.*

Incidentally, the physical phenomenon of the rasa is reflected at this place, somewhat in the form of a personal struggle. *Su* cites: *tatra vāyurātmaivātmā pittamāgneyaṃ śleṣmā saumaḥ iti*

The *vāyū* is there *ātman,* truly *ātman;* the *pitta* refers to *agni;* the *śleṣman* to soma.

The lexicographic meaning of *atman* is manifold, including: self, body, matter. In the old medical tradition, despite the frequent appropriate use of the *vāyu* system, there are rare express definitions of this technical term. Therefore a corresponding text passage may be quoted as a hypothetical parallel to the explanation which appears the more remarkable because it derives from a special treatment of the *vāyu:* in *Su, sūtra*- 1,4 this is termed *svayambhū,* i.e., formed through itself. The keyword used here (like verbally similar termṣ) points to old concepts of gods and the matural forces they incorporate, as also plainly in *Su, sūtra*- 6,1 and *nidāna* 1,4. If a contextual meaning of *ātman* is allowed for in from the *Ṛgveda,* then, in the text under discussion, *ātmaiva ātmā* may be approximated to *svayambhū* in the sense of matter, one's own body, self.[6]

As here Vedic views are used for specifying the meaning of *vāyu,* that derived from the prevailing explanations of the *Tridoṣa* text may seem surprising. However, this position is throughly justified because, in the three firmly-linked parts of the doctrine, the last two sections evidently arise from the Vedic sphere.

The *pitta* is related to *agni,* to fire, whose estimation occupies first place in the ancient Aryan concept of life. It may be noted

[6] Cf. *Die Medizin im Ṛg-Veda,* Asia Major 1930, 319, 329, 353. In *Ca vimāna*- 8, 32, for the diseases whose cause seems assigned to *vāta* and so-called supernatural beings, the keywords named are *vātādikṛtā bhūtakṛtāśca.*

incidentally that the linkage of *pitta* and *agni* is verifiable elsewhere[7].

If, finally, *śleṣman* is assigned to *soma,* this relationship also seems surprising according to the explanations of the *doṣa* hitherto, namely the connexion of "mucus" with the ancient Aryan intoxicating beverage, but the latter is what is acutally meant in the text. This is evidenced by the etymologic explanation of *śleṣman* in *Su, sūtra-* 21,3: *śliṣa āliṅgane.* The word śleṣman must thus derive from *slisa* (to embrace), which last word corresponds to an embrace *(āliṇgana).* How far this wordy or wordplay explanation is justified can be left to the expert. However, it is not only expressly and predominantly emphasized in the text, but also faithfully renders very old traditions of that god "to whom one ascribes his body".[8]

Originally, *soma* was considered as fluid heavenly fire. Which properties are here recognized for it in medical-theory are shown in *Su, sūtra-* 14,1 (end). In the description of the body juice, *saumya* and taijasa are named side by side. *Tejas* denotes heat, and the reference to *soma* is used circumstantially as a synonym, i.e., *saumya* in the sense of glow, corresponding to the original meaning. When Hoernle translates *saumya* as "cooling",[9] this meaning of cold is not safely derived from the immediate text, but is based only on an analysis of the *doṣa* mentioned in the original into *kapha* (= śleṣman) and *pitta* by the commentator *Ḍallana.*[10]

---

[7] Cf. the relevant places in *Su, sūtra-* 15, 21, 35, where the fireforms of the *pitta* are listed. The designations *āma-pakva* (like its derivatives *āmāśya-pakvāśya)* which also occur frequently in *Ca,* belong to the same field of Vedic influences. Some statements on the topic occur in *Janus* 1930, 196 ff. For the disease *vātikaṣaṇḍa, Ca* quotes fire in the meaning of *pitta, śarīra-* 2, 20; *vāyvagnidoṣād –.* However, these are only a few examples of the equation *pitta = agni,* provided from personal statements.

[8] HERTEL, Indo-Iranische Quellen und Forschungen VI, indes: *Sóma*

[9] The *Suçruta-Samhita,* 89–90 (Bibliotheca Indica, N.S. 911).

[10] *Nibandhasaṃgraha* 14,1: – *kimayaṃ saumyaḥ kaphavat athavā taijasaḥ pittavaditi saṃśayah/.* In *Su, śarīra-* 3,1, *saumya* and *āgneya* refer to an opposition of semen *(śukra)* and the woman's periods *(ārttava),* whose fire forms are demonstrable in the Vedas (cf. *Asia Major* 1930, 338–340) and whose double meaning corresponds to the ancient Aryan fire theory; we owe this exposition and explanation to Hertel. *Soma* has probably become "cold" fire through an assimilation to the moon and through the connexion of the latter with a fire disease, the *yakṣma.* The texts in the *Ṛgveda* apocrypha and the *Taittirīya-Saṃhitā* are readily accessible in translation by Hertel, *Indische Märchen,* 16–17, 345–357. This fire text still exists in India, not of course in European circles.

It would certainly be mistaken to derive a generally valid explanation of the *doṣa* from these separate if significant textual sources, although further examples are available.[11] Doubtless, however, this limitation demonstrates a linkage between the *Tridoṣa* text and old traditions.

Such connexions, henceforth scattered, will be drawn on when this treatise returns to discuss the actual topic. The disease is designated *prameha* and corresponds to the verb *meha, mih, migh,* i.e., to urinate. This expression already occurs in the *Ṛgveda* (IX, 74, 4), where the *sudānavaḥ* (the fine trickling: an apithet of the gods, chiefly the Storm Gods *marut*) who urinate *(mehanti) soma* which is named *amṛta* (immortal). In the medical texts, the guideword *pra-* (pre) is apparently restricted to a disease concept, and the simple form *meha* is also used in this sense. In the oldest medical traditions, *prameha* already appears with 20 variants under the grouping of *doṣa,* thus as a disease system of manifold pattern.[12] Transient forms are not known from medical text transmission.

Consequently, the three following old texts must form the startingpoint for the real investigation, and certainly with regard to the genesis of the philosophy of this disease.

Ca, here as always very detailed, deals with the important parts in verse form in *nidāna-* 4, *6, 8, 10.* The account in *Su* is very brief, in the style of a concise manual of a linguistically unbound kind *(nidāna-* 6, *4–6*). The account in *Vāgbhata (Vā)* is again in artistic form *(nidāna-* 10, *8–18),* in almost word for word agreement with *Mādhvanidāna,* prameha- *7–17.* To shape the presentation of the clinical picture in its signs, the 20 kinds of

---

[11] An (older) parallel to the *Su* (cf. *śarīra-* 6, 21) occurs in the main introductory statements in *Ca, nidāna-* 1, 3: *(-āgneyah saumyā vayavyāśca).* Here the three *doṣa* are not expressly mentioned, but only as emphasized by commentators *(Gaṅgādhara* and *Cakrapāṇi)* in an appendix to the large *Ca* edition. So as not to promote misunderstandings, it should be specially noted that they in no way deal conclusively with the impromptu references in the footnotes and more over the topics adduced.

[12] The Bower MS generally mentions no number, but "all kinds of urinary flux" *(sarvamehā)* in II, 604, 608, 942. Only in one place – *pramehāṃścaika(va) viṃsati(ṃ)* – are 21 quoted. The one *(eka), apparently emphasized, urinary disorder is referred to by* HOERNLE, in commentary 13 on his translation, as *madhumeha,* obviously assumed to be an irremediable diabetes. HOERNLE might have found support in this from the brief mention of *madhumeha* in II, 250, even if the special danger is not laid down in the text. The author seems to approximate the assumption that 1 with a remedy was added because, by Indian views, the zero at the end of a number generally meant incurability.

prameha are listed in the following table according to the key-words in *Ca*, with the respective code-words from the accounts in *Su*, *Vā* and *Mā* in the parallel column on the right.

If the listings given above are reviewed, a close, regular and content-wise combination of *Ca* with *Vā* and *Mā* emerges, whereas *Su* occupies a special position. Thereby appears in *Ca* the conjecturally oldest outcome, at any rate of that which achieved valued esteem in the later period.

Śleṣman.

1. *udakameha* (watery urinary flux).

a) transparent *(accah)* b) abundant *(bahu)* c) bright *(sita)* d) cold *(śīta)* e) odorless *(nirgandha)* f) water *(udaka)*	*Su* 1: *udakameha.* a) clear *(śveta)* b) painless *(avedana)* c) watery *(udaka-sadṛśa)*
	Vā and *Mā* 1: *udakameha.* identical with *Ca.*

2. *ikṣvmeha (sugary urinary flux).*

a) excessive *(atyartha)* b) sweet *(madhura)* c) cold *(sīta)* d) slightly mucous *(īṣat-picchila),* e) like cane-sugar juice *(kāṇḍekṣu-rasa-saṃkāśa).*	Su 2: *ikṣumeha* a) like cane-sugar juice *(ikṣurasatulya)*
	Vā and *Mā* 2: *ikṣumeha* a) like cane-sugar juice *(ikṣu-rasa iva)* b) excessive *(atyartha)* c) sweet *(madhura)*

3. *sāndrameha* (viscous urinary flux).

a) becoming viscous *(sāndri-bhū)* b) remaining overnight *(paryuṣita),* in a vessel *(bhājana)*	*Su* 8: *sāndrameha* a) turbid *(āvila)* b) viscous *(sāndra)*
	Vā and *Mā 3: sāndrameha* a) becoming viscous *(sāndrī-bhū)* b) remaining overnight *(paryuṣita)*

4. *sāndraprasādameha* (thick-sediment urinary flux).

a) sedimented (literally struck together: *saṃhan*, passive) b) gradually deposited *(kiṃcid-kiṃcid – prasad)*	*Su* 3: *surāmeha.* a) *surā*-like *(surā-tulya)*
	Vā and *Mā* 4: *surāmeha* a) *surā*-like *(surā-tulya)* b) transparent above *(upari-accha)* *c) thick below (adho-ghana)*

5. *śuklameha* (clear urinary flux).

a) clear *(śukla)*
b) gruel-like *(piṣṭa-nibha)*
c) repeated (or) immediate *(abhīkṣṇam)*

Su 7: *piṣṭameha*

a) hair-raising *(hṛṣṭa-roma)*[13]
b) *gruel-water (piṣṭa-rasa)*

Vā and *Mā* 5: *piṣṭameha*

a) also hair-raising *(samhṛṣṭaroma)*
b) gruel-like (piṣṭa, instrument)
c) thick like gruel *(piṣṭavat-bahula)*
d) clear *(sita)*

6. *śukrameha* (seminal urinary flux).

a) semen-like *(śukra-ābha)*
b) mixed with semen *(ṣukra-miśra)*
c) momentary *(muhur)*

Su 9: *śukrameha*

a) equivalent to semen *(śukra-tulya)*

Vā and *Mā* 6: *śukrameha*

as in *Ca* 6a and b.

7. *śītameha* (cold urinary flux).

a) excessive *(atyartha)*
b) sweet *(madhura)*
c) cold *(śīta)*
d) abundant *(bhṛśa)*

Su 0

Vā and *Mā* 8: *śītameha*

a) frequent *(subahuśas)*
b) sweet *(madhura)*
c) cold *(śītala)*

8. *sikatāmeha* (sandy urinary flux).

a) curdled urinary excrement *(mūrta-mūtragata, plural)*
b) small faulty constituents *(doṣa-aṇu)*
c) sand *(sikatā)*

Su 4: *sikatāmeha*

a) painful *(saruja)*
b) sand passed *(sikatā-anuviddha)*

Vā and *Mā* 7: *sikatāmeha*

a) Vā: dilute urine *(mūtra-aṇu)*, *Mā:* dilute curdled *(mūrta-aṇu)*
b) of sand type *(sikatā-rūpin)*

[13] *hṛṣṭa-roma* (*hṛṣ* = bristle; *roma* = body-hair) forms a common expression of the emotional affect already found in the *Ṛgveda;* the guide-word *sam* in *Vā* and *Mā* in the meaning of "together" was likely to depict an enhancement in this concept.

9. *śanairmeha* (slow urinary flux).

a) slow *(manda)*,
b) without rapid passage *(avega)*
c) with difficulty *(kṛoccha)*, a) and c) repeated
d) gradual *(śana)*

Su 5; *śanairmeha*

a) slow *(śana)*
b) with mucus *(sakapha)*
c) powder *(mṛtsna)*

Vā and Mā 9: *śanairmeha*

a) slow *(śana)*
b) ditto *(manda)* repeated

10. *ālālameha* (mucous urinary flux).

a) bound like threads *(tantu-baddha-iva)*
b) slimy *(picchila)*

Su 10: *phenameha.*

a) drop by drop *(stoka-stoka)*
b) slimy *(saphena; phena* = drops of spittle)

Vā and *Mā* 10: lālāmeha

a) mucus or spittle *(lālā)*
b) bound like threads *(tantu-yu)*
c) slimy *(picchila)*

Su 6: *lavaṇameha*

a) clear *(viśada)*
b) salt-like *(lavaṇa-tulya)*

Pitta

11. *kṣārameha* (caustic urinary flux).

a) caustic *(kṣāra)* with reference to the four sensory perceptions: scent, color, taste and feel *(gandha, varṇa, rasa, sparśa)*

Su 14: *kṣārameha*

a) caustic-like (kṣāra-pratima) fluid *(sru)*

Vā and *Mā* 11: *kṣārameha*

as in *Ca*

12. *kālameha* (black urinary flux).

a) bone-black color *(masī-* or *masīvarṇa;* also *ajasra*, probably referring to the color: fresh)
b) hot *(uṣṇa)*

Su 0

Vā and *Mā* 13: *kālameha*

a) black *(kāla)*
b) like bone-black *(maṣī-nibha)*

13. *nīlameha* (blue urinary flux).

a) like jay's wings *(cāṣa-pakṣa-nibha)* b) sour *(amla)*	*Su* 11: *nīlameha* a) frothy *(saphena)* b) transparent *(accha)* c) blue *(nīla)*
	Vā and Mā 12: *nīlameha* a) like blue *(nīla-ābha)*

14. *lohitameha* (red urinary flux).

a) smelling of meat *(visra)* b) salty *(lavaṇa)* c) hot *(uṣṇa)* d) red *(rakta)*	*Su* 16: *śoṇitameha* a) fiery-seeming *(śoṇita-prakāśa)*
	Vā and *Mā* 16: *raktamehe* a) smelling of meat *(visra)* b) hot *(uśṇa)* c) salty *(lavaṇa)* d) like red *(rakta-ābha)*

15. *māñjiṣṭhameha* (madder-red urinary flux).

a) madder-red watery seeming *(māñjiṣṭha-udaka-saṃkāśa)* b) abundant *(bhṛśa)* c) smalling of meat *(visra)*	*Su* 15: *māñjiṣṭhameha* a) madder-red watery-seeming *(māñjiṣṭha-udaka-prakāśa)*
	Vā and *Mā* 15: *māñjiṣṭhameha* a) like red water *(māñjiṣṭa-salila-upama;* cf. *Ca* 1 f)

16. *haridrameha* (yellow-root urinary flux).

a) yellow-root seeming *(hari-dra-udaka-saṃkāśa)* b) sharp *(kaṭuka)*	*Su* 12: *haridrāmeha* a) with burning feeling *(sadāha)* b) yellow-root *(haridrā)*
	Vā and *Mā* 14: *haridrameha* a) sharp *(kaṭuka)* b) like yellow-root *(haridrasaṃ-nibha)* c) burning *(dahat)* *Su* 13: *malameha.* a) sour *(amla)* refers to *rasa* and *gandha.*

Vāta.

17. *vasāmeha* (fatty urinary flux).

a) mixed with fat *(vasā-miśra)* b) fatty appearance *(vasā-bha)* c) repeated *(muhur)*	*Su* 18: *vasāmeha.* a) fatty appearance *(vasā-prahāśa)*
	Vā and *Mā* 17: *vasāmeha.* as in *Ca. (Vā* has *vasāṃ vā* instead of *vasābhaṃ)*

18. *majjameha* (marrow urinary flux).

a) marrow *(majjan)* *with urine (saha mūtreṇa)*	*Su* 17: *sarpirmeha* a) butter-seeming *(sarpis-prakāśa)*
	Vā and *Mā* 18: *majjameha* a) marrow-like *(majjan-ābha)* or b) mixed with marrow *(majjan-miśra)* c) every moment *(muhur-muhur); Vā* has *majjānaṃ* instead of *majāhaṃ*

19. *hastimeha* (elephant's urinary flux).

a) like an elephant in rut *(hastin-matta iva)* b) indefatigable *(ajasra)* passage of urine *(kṣar)*	*Su* 20: *hastimeha* a) like an elephant in rut *(mattamā-taṇga-vat)* b) passes after-increase *(anu-pravṛddha)* urine
	Vā and *Mā* 19: *hastimeha* a) as in *Ca* 19 b) as in *Ca* 19 c) without pressure *(vega-vivarjita)* d) with juice *(sa-lasīka)* und e) stagnant *(vibaddha)*

20. *madhumeha* (sweet urinary flux).

a) concentrated *(kaṣāya)* b) pale *(pāṇḍu)* c) dried *(rukṣa)*	*Su* 19: *kṣaudrameha* a) honey-juice-colored *(kṣaudra-rasa-varṇa)*
	Vā and *Mā* 20: *madhumeha* a) sweet *(madhu)*

The group of the *pitta* will be first selected here, because it needs to be discussed separately in the context of the sugar disease. In the field of medical theory about *pitta,* a reference to fire has first been demonstrated in the context of old (Vedic) attitudes to life. Naturally, there are no literal evidence in the *Ṛgveda.* It is quite understandable if the bile is not mentioned in these prize songs or in the sacrificial elements mentioned in them. It is otherwise in the *Atharvaveda* in which diseases and cognate evils play a greater role and where the term is used at two places. The first evidence in I, 24, 1 has not so far been unequivocally explained and is mentioned here only because it seems to point to the opposition between light and dark and a relation to the sexes, therefore in an orientation to the later special concept of *doṣa,* which does not yet appear in the Vedas.[14] The second piece of evidence excludes any doubt: Fire, you are the bile of the water (XVIII, 3, 5: *agne pittam apām asi*). This saying is repeated in the white and black *Yajurveda (Vājasaneyi-Saṃhitā* XVII,6; *Taittirīya-Saṃhitā* IV, 6, 1,).[15]

According to general linguistic usage, *pitta* means the bile and must still be held to this literal or far-ranging meaning. In the modern view, the bile is anatomically linked with its bladder. If, however, in the word *pittaśaya* of the section, *āśaya* = site, bed or location is a general reference to the gallbladder seems more than doubtful. For *āśaya,* as a technical term, is frankly a commonplace in the ancient anatomic, or better, physiologic topography. The first source of relevant knowledge from the sacrificial ritual can hardly be doubted. The liver, *yakan, yakṛt,* and perhaps also *taniman,* certainly belongs to the 18 parts of the sacrificial foods – even if it did not have the same meaning for the Indians as in Asia Minor – must be supposed to have been known. However, the monograph, *Ancient Indian Animal Sacrifice* by SCHWAB, records no details and the author can add no further synoptic material. Originally and practically, the designation *pitta* refers not only to its bladder content but also to the dark blood that flowed through the large vessels of the liver when this was removed from the abdominal cavity of the (regularly suffocated) sacrificial animal. Another pointer in this direc-

[14] The bile of the eagle *(suparṇa)* is contrasted here with the *āsurī,* which was given by WEBER *(Ind-Stud.* IV, 417/18) as the night opposed to the sun ⟨the sun as fire *(agni)* is given in the *Ṛgveda,* however, as the Lightener of Darkness *(doṣā-vastar)*⟩. Cf. Bloomfield, *Sacr. Books of the East* XLII, 268–9.

[15] Cf. Whitney-Lanmann, *Harvard Oriental Series* VIII, 850, note to 5.

tion generally is the close conceptual connexion of the bile and blood in disease depictions, and the occasionally surprisingly large amounts of blood which are ascribed to the human body.[16]

In contrast to the other groups, *Ca* introduces the *pitta* section in the *prameha* proportionately shortly in his established ideas. Precipitating causes stressed here are: hot, acid, salty, caustic and sharp foods *(nidāna-* 4,7: *uṣṇāmlalavaṇaksārakaṭuka-);* the other causes worth mentioning include an influence of warmth, probably corresponding to sunstroke, in which the property *tīkṣṇa* = scorching is mentioned. *Ca* groups the types of *pitta* as they are subsequently individually listed, and stresses that they correspond to the 6 types of the bile *(te ṣadbhiretaiḥ kṣāramlalavaṇakaṭuvisroṣṇaiḥ).* The principal description of the bile in *Ca* is found in *vimāna* 8,33: *pittamuṣṇatikṣṇam drutaṃ* (or *dravaṃ*) *visramamlaṃ kaṭukaṃca.* The word-form and its sequence there is therefore: hot *(uṣṇa),* scorching *(tīkṣṇa),* acid *(amla)* and sharp *(kaṭuka).* If the alterations in the individual designations are disregarded and the different arrangements observed according to the keywords, the following comparative list is obtained:

vimāna- 8,83	*nidāna-* 4,7	*nidāna-* 4,8 (with keyword)
1. *uṣṇa* (hot)	1. *kṣāra* (caustic)	1. *kṣārameha* (–)
2. *tīkṣṇa* (scorching)	2. *amla* (acid)	2. *kālameha (uṣṇa)*
3. *druta, drava* (flowing)	3. *lavaṇa* (salty)	3. *nīlameha (amla)*
4. *visra* (smelling of blood)	4. *kaṭu* (sharp)	4. *lohitameha (visra-lavaṇa-uṣṇa)*
5. *amla* (acid)	5. *visra* (smelling of blood)	5. *māñjiṣṭhameha (visra)*
6. *kaṭuka* (sharp)	6. *uṣṇa* (hot)	6. *haridrameha (kaṭuka)*

Even a fleeting glance at these lists shows the considerable derangements. For the arrangement here is not based on arbitrary or unimportant texts, but on a propaedeutics of the bile properties in *Ca* and a disease group determined by bile influence, in whose didactic exposition the announcement of the arrangement of the properties of the bile is placed directly beside

[16] In the statute-book of the *Yājnavalkya* (III, 105–6) the ratio of blood *(rakta)* to bile *(pitta)* = 8:5, at the conclusion of the *Garbha-Upanisad,* which belongs to the *Atharvaveda,* the heart *(hṛd)* is given as half the size of the gallbladder. Naturally, these measurements, even in the correlation selected here, cannot be regarded as absolute (cf. *Ca. śārīra-* 4,7)

the relevant and dependent special forms of the disease group. Such irregularities and exceptions, encountered not uncommonly in the old collections, we may note incidentally, can be brought about in later periods, perhaps by elaboration of the early portions through *Dṛdhabala,* which the last third of the *Ca* is known to have added to and collected. However, it is quite possible and, to a certain degree, probable that these types of inconsistencies already existed in the compilation of the texts of the *Agniveśa.*[17]

The actual names of the individual members of the *pitta* group are based on so-called color designations; this also involves the first member, *kṣārameha,* because in its description the reference to *varṇa* appears. The evaluation of the expressions which point to a coloring and its practical usefulness is difficult in the ancient Indian medical texts. The problems arising cannot be dealt with conclusively here; the attempt will only be made to clarify several points of contact with the pitta group. First, the designation *varṇa* (from *vṛ* = to conceal, etc.) does not quite correspond to the concept of the coloration, but is linked in the Vedic sphere with the types of fire as regards form and content. In all, *Ca* specifies seven different colors (*Indriya* 7,9: – *sarvā* – *saptavidhā*), namely *rakta* (red), *pīta* (yellow), *sita* (white – bright), *śyāva* (brown), *harita* (pale yellow – yellowish – green), *pāṇḍura* (white – yellow), *asita* (black). The bracketed translations correspond to the usual lexicographic identifications, but in large part do not apply here. For *Ca* says expressly that all these so-called colors have been formed out of fire *(taijasa),* and with this linguistic reference to heat *(tejas)* a bridge to the representation of *pitta* can generally be made according to precedent. In its group, ideas towards a combination of the red colors in 14 and 15 with fire in terms of content hardly arise; in 12, *maṣi* is specified as a fire color, already from the nature of its preparation from burnt bones, and if not through *ajasra,*[18] but defined closely in the given sense through *uṣṇa.*

---

[17] In noteworthy manner, JOLLY begins his assessment with the hint that the present status in *Ca* (as in *Su*) is certified only by the commentary of the *Cakrapāṇidatta,* whose temporal allocation to the 11th century is not even completely fixed. Nor is there any help over this time period from documents whose temporal relations are assured, like the Bower manuscript, so far as it has to do with the entire collections.

[18] In the *Ṛgveda, ajasra* occurs 19 times, referring to fire in I, 189, *4;* II, 35, *8;* III, 1, 2 21; 26,7; 54,I; VI, 16,*45;* 48,3; VII, 1.3,18; 5,*4;* VIII, 60,*4;* IX, 113,7, X, 6,2; 12,7; 45,I; 130,L; 185,3. The two other quotations (I, 100,*14;* IV,55,2) contain the relevant transfer to other gods.

Nīlameha can usefully be combined with the *kālameha* previously transcribed. This happens formally in *Vā* and *Mā* 12/13, where both these diseases are dealt with in one line of verse (cf. in *Garuḍapurāna* 159, *24*), whereas elsewhere each of the others has a special line devoted to it (18). As an interpolation is improbable, the assumption of a contextual connexion is not unjustified. This "blue" urine, hitherto taken invariably in the meaning of the word, may well be counted in the medical field as a blue miracle. It is constructed in *Ca* 13a with the reference to the bird *cāṣa.*[19] Now, the designation through "Tschaascha" quite probably has an onomatopoeic origin and therefore makes proof of a blue color difficult from the outset. Neither do the commentaries of the original text help further with their literal repetitions or occasional interrelation. If the principal elucidations in *Ca* are referred to, it seems remarkable that the previously listes socalled colors are characterized as *prabhā,* i.e., as radiations (*pra* = outward, *bhā* = to radiate). The concept taken into consideration here therefore strikingly resembles that of the Sehakt, as is recognizable in the *Ṛgveda,*[20] and as can also be demonstrated later.[21] However, *nīla* is expressly not named under *prabha,* but directly before under *chāyā* (*indriya-* 7,7); although *chāyā* is formed from *ci* = see, to seem, the meaning as shadow (or reflection or mirror-image) stands here in opposition to *prabha,* as is evident from the further exposition (*indriya-* 7,11). How far this opposition is consistent with the old fire texts may be left undiscussed. On the basis of the foregoing, *nīla* (or in agreed combination, also *kāla*) is difficult to classify under *asita,* but the shadow and light forms are presented in opposition. Among the not uncommon evidences for *nīla,* references occur at

---

[19] In *Ṛgveda* X, 97,*13,* case is mentioned alongside *kikivīdi,* and each of these two birds counts as the blue jay. In the commentary of the Rigveda translation (Vol. V, 559), with reference to *Taittīrīya-Saṃhitā* I, *1,* LUDWIG puts *casa* parallel with the great bird of prey *śyena,* which from its name should have a reddishwhitish color (GRASSMANN, Lexicon, *1417*); accordingly, the reference to the wings in *Ca* 13s alludes to *chāya* or the *sauparṇa,* in which the eagle steals the *soma,* the heavenly fire.

[20] Cf. *Asia Major* 1930, 336

[21] A pictorial presentation of the rays of sight, found by A. von LECOQ in a temple at Kutscha from the 2nd half of the 1st millennium, is published in the *Klinischen Monatsblättern für Augenheilkunde* 1928, 511–516.

times where *nīla* is included in a so-called color scale, but even then in acceptable opposition, as laid down above.[22]

The "yellow-root" urine may correspond to the coloration expressed. The descriptions in *Su* 12a and *Vā*, as in *Mā* 14c, through *dah* (to burn) establishes this – informally, it is true – in a taste property of the yellow root preparations, but then deviates significantly from the concept of the color.[23]

The short critical sketch about the colorations, which has been elaborated only for this topic, shows the dependence of the relevant attitudes on the old evaluation of fire. This state of affairs is also detectable in the other remaining properties of the *pitta* group.

The smell of blood or meat, described through *visra* in *Ca* 14a and *15*a as in *Vā* and *Mā* 16a, corresponds to the circumstances in the *Ṛgveda* I, 162, 10.

The smell *(gandha)* of "raw" *(āma)* blood or meat *(kravis)* is mentioned there fore the horse sacrifice. Its property equals that which "radiates" from the opened abdominal cavity *(yad ūvadhyam udarasyāpavāti)*; thereby the "rays" or, better translated, "flames" *(pū)* proves the awareness of a fire effect.[24]

The literal meaning of *kṣāramega* likewise contains "burning" *(kṣā)*.[25] *Kaṭuka* and *lavaṇa* stand chiefly in connexion with *kṣāra*.

---

[22] The colors are transformed at the body somewhat in the sense of degrees of brightness: shadow-dark, dusky, coppery, fiery and bright (glittering), *Ca indriya-* 1,5; *nīlaśyāmatāmraharitaśuklāśca varṇāh śarīre vaikārikā bhavanti.* In what way the meaning of *nīla* is to be defined is also shown by a passage of the *Atharvaveda,* where the discussion is of a raw vessel *(āma pātra)* with the properties *nīla* and *lohita* (IV, 17,*4*). The commentator (quoted by WHITNEY-LANMAN, *180*) explains *nīla* as smoke and *lohtia* as fire, and is therefore involved in the old-advanced attitudes which are further elucidated thereby, explaining the raw vessel of the text as an unbaked *(apakva)* earthen vessel *(mṛtpātra),* thus through the known connexion *āma – pakva.*

[23] The (actually proportionately late) term *haridrāmeha* misleads in inclining to the Aryan fire dogma, in the supposition that originally the disease name contained an inclusion of *haras* or corresponding derivative of the harmful flame; yet this close combination cannot be deduced with convincing validity from this passage alone.

[24] Cf. *Taittirīyasaṃhitā* IV, 6,*8k* and *Vājasaneyisaṃhitā* XXV, 33.

[25] In the general teaching on operations in *Su sūtra-* 7–14, to which *Ca* offers no equivalent, *kṣāra* with *agni* is designated as substitute for a sharper instrument (8,9: *anuśastrāni),* cf. 11, I. The attachment of *kṣāra* and *agni* in 7,II (mentioned here together also) to the blunt accessory instruments (*upayantra,* as opposed to the sharp instrument, i.e., *śastra,* the cutting) corresponds to a later general classification but not to the original conceptions, as emphasized by the previously listed sources in their textual dispositions.

This reference in *Ca sutra-* 26,14: *kąṭukalavaṇabhūyiṣṭha-* leads to the actual taste properties. Those of the *pitta* group, namely *amla, lavaṇa* and *kaṭuka,* are, in their primel combinations with earth, water and wind, each time set in relation with fire.[26] And in the special description, at least in *amla (Ca sūtra-* 26, *43)* and *kaṭuka (Ca sūtra-* 26, *47)* the fire *(agni)* is mentioned literally in first place; in *lavaṇa (Ca sūtra-* 26, *45)* that reference is paraphrased as "causing to cook" *(pācana).*

In the preliminary studies some essential material has been collected which provides information about the origin and – especially in *Ca* – the dominant views of the *pitta* group of the *prameha.* In the demonstration of the close connexion of this group with fire there appears the entering and precipitating impulse of older concepts of fire which calls for a general interpretation and enters paths which medical historical research hitherto may consider as strange or unusual. Abnormalities in the appearance of the urine probably elicited the reference to fire in practice, but would in no way have precipitated such an assessment first. For, in terms of cognition theory, the notion of fire is the superimposed concept which is only subsequently proportionately reduced to its components (gleam and glow). This is shown by the parts of the *pitta* group, whose properties are not assessed by appearance. Also, the visible properties of the fire action are not to be analysed in the sense of modern color criteria. Here an example seems noteworthy in which *pitta* is compared in its combination with *rakta* (blood), with *kṛṣṇa* (black) and finally with the rainbow *(Ca nidāna-* 2,*11: yat kṛṣṇamathavā nīlaṃ yadvā śakradhanuḥprabham).* However, there is no detectable finding here in any part – and this is especially relevant to the subject – which serves as any basis for the assumption of a urinary sugar flux.

On the other hand, the two other groups of the *prameha,* which are caused through *śleṣman* and *vāta,* exhibit in the context of the problem posed here a correlation which is occasioned by the mention of sugar or sweet. It will be shown that still other combinations exist in this context.

The following table provides an overview of the properties of the urine in the *śleṣman* group. The first column contains the properties ascribed to the *śleṣman* in *Ca vimāna-* 8,*83;* the second column lists the *śleṣman* properties contained in the essen-

[26] *Ca sūtra-* 26,*39: bhūmy (pṛthivy) agnibhūyiṣṭhatvādamlaḥ / toya(salilā)-agnibhūyiṣṭhatvāllavaṇaḥ / vāyvagnibhūyịṣthatvāt kaṭukaḥ.*

tially dependent places in the description of the *prameha* in *Ca nidāna-* 4,5;[27] and the third column compares the designations of the individual diseases 1–10, with the addition of their main qualities as there adduced (p. 24).

As in the *pitta* group the disorder of the sequence and the designations is striking in the following review. However, there is yet a further irregularity to be noticed here: that the *śleṣman*

1. *snigdha* (melting).	1. *śveta* (bright).	1. *udakameha*, *accha, bahu, sita, śīta, nirgandha. Su* 1: *śveta.*
2. *ślakṣṇa* (slippery).	2. śīta (cold).	2. *ikṣumeha*, *atyartha, madhura, sīta, picchila*, etc.
3. *mṛdu* (flexible).	3. *mūrta* (curdled).	3. *sāndrameha*, *sāndrī.*
4. *madhura* (sweet).	4. *picchila* (slimy).	4. *sāndraprasādameha*, *saṃhan, prasad.*
5. *sāra* (granular).	5. *accha* (transparent).	5. *śuklameha*, *śukla, piṣṭanibha*, etc.
6. *sāndra* (sticky).	6. *snigdha* (slippery).	6. *ṣukrameha*, *śukra* etc.
7. *manda* (sluggish).	7. *guru* (swollen).	7. *śītameha*, *atyartha, madhura, śīta, bhṛśa.*
8. *stimita* (hardly mobile).	8. *prasāda* (clarified).	8. *sikatāmeha*, *mūrta, doṣa, sikatā.*
9. *guru* (swollen).	9. *madhura* (sweet).	9. *śanairmeha*, *manda, avega, kṛccha, śanair.*
10. *śīta* (cold).	10. *sāndra* (sticky).	10. *ālālameha*, *tantubaddha, picchila.*
11. *vijjala* (greasy).	11. *manda* (sluggish).	11. –
12. *accha* (transparent).	12. –	12. –

[27] The text in the *Ca* edition, Lahore 1828/29 runs: *śvetaśitamūrtapicchilācchasnigdhaguruprasādamadhurasāndramandaiḥ;* it is doubtless preferable to the text of the large *Ca*-edition (Calcutta 1927 ff.): *śvetaśitamūrttapicchilācchasnigdhagurumadhurasāndraprasagandhaiḥ.*

of the *vimāna* has 12, that of the *nidāna* 11[28] and the disease designations only 10 constituents.

A glance at the first column, which describes the mucus, reveals descriptions like *snigdha, ślakṣṇa, mṛdu, sāndra, manda, stimita, guru, śīta, vijjala,* which supply clearly obvious properties of the mucus. To these can also be assigned *accha* = without shadow or reflection, comparable with the modern term "glassy". Under *sāra,* an allusion to a fruit-pip may be assumed, and therewith an expression which can be assimilated to the properties of the mucus. But *madhura* = sweet does not at all fit into the column; and if the last property of the mucus is provisionally omitted from the column of the *śleṣman* in the *nidāna,* all the other 10 attributes would be equally appropriate to the mucus.

Only in the 10 disease names and their descriptions do difficulties emerge, which cannot be directly removed if, except for the sweet substances, the signs are to be combined under the concept of mucus. For assessment of the group of the *śleṣman,* the parallel in *Ca cikitsā* 6, 7 (Lahore edn. 1929) must be brought in here with an editorial eye to the origin, younger for the entire section but old in its combined form at the relevant site. There the urine is depicted: like water or like sweet juice or sedimenting and above returned to rest, bright, with semen, cool or gradual, or like saliva or combined with san *(jalopamaṃ cekṣurasopamaṃ vā ghanaṃ copari viprasannam / śuklaṃ saśukraṃ śiśiraṃ śanairvā lāleva vā vālukayā yutaṃ vā //).* It can certainly not be denied that Vedic concepts are possibly alluded to at the beginning. *Su sūtra* gives the source of the water of heaven pride of place in a special chapter, and *Ca sūtra*- 26, *39* proceeds correspondingly, even if in other words. The water and the concepts linked with it do not therefore refer to the urine in a positive sense from the outset. If, with regard to the Vedas, the derivation of *prameha* from *mih* is observed, then the result is that of the 23 quotations from *mih* in the *Ṛgveda* a procedure on the earth in sacrifice can be assumed only three times,[29] but in the

[28] In the large *Ca* edition – cf. note 28 – only 10 parts are named here, because *gandha* is added for *manda*. That this text does not reliably appear with *gandha* has already been stated. Even if *gandha* is not intertreated as "smell of" but in the transferred meaning as "trace of", it yet remains noteworthy that the term *gandha* here appears conceptually vague from the modern scientific viewpoint and shows a similar lack of close definition within sense physiology as demonstrated previously for *varṇa*.

[29] *Ṛgveda* II, 3,*11 (ghṛta)*: IX, 107,6; X, 104, 2 *(soma)*

majority of 20 cases a reference to the macrocosmos, heaven or its representatives, the gods, and indeed very frequently to the distinct form of the Regent.[30] The god urinates on the earth;[31] this may sound strange to modern concepts but not to the old nomads of the *Ṛgveda.* And this urine possesses no pejorative valuation; the urine of the *Rudra* is healing *(jalāṣa, -bhesaja)* and highly esteemed.[32] The remedy is literally designated as urine through *mūtra.*[33] From these concepts, those of the strong rain, emerge the properties in *udakameha,* when the urine is here named *accha* (shadowless, therefore transparent),[34] *bahu* (abundant), *sita* (bright), *śīta* (cold), *nirgandha* (without sense perception).[35]

To these attitudes, for which previously only a few linkages were given to the underlying concepts, *ikṣumeha* is obviously added. When, in *Ca sūtra-* 26,39, that heavenly fluid *avyakta-rasa* (cf. note at p. 6) or in *Su sūtra-* 45,1 is named *anirdeśyarasa* (*anirdeśya* = indefinable), and translated in the sense of tasteless, as it happens, these sources must be considered as at least premature. For these waters are termed *saumyāḥ,* and shortly after it is taught that of these 6 rasa the sweet *rasa* has the predominance of the properties of the *soma (teṣāṃ ṣaṇṇām rasāñaṃ somagunātirekānmadhuro rasaḥ).* Even the oldest traditions offer no contrary criteria. It is a quite striking observation that, in the 23 examples quoted above from the *Ṛgveda* alone, *mih* is expressly linked with *madhu* 7 times.[36] This is evidence that originally the expression *madhu* was not used as a close definition in the sense of sugar disease. When, therefore, in *ikṣu-meha,* excessive *(atyartha),* sweet *(madhura),* probably in corre-

---

[30] E.g., *Agni (narāśaṅsa) Ṛgveda* I, 142,3; *Indra* VI, 29,3; 34,4; VIII, 4,10; *Marut* (the sons of the *Rudra)* I, 64, 6; 167,4; II, 34,13; *Aśvin* VIII, 10,2; *Dyāva-Pṛthivī* (heaven and earth) I, 22,13; *Uṣas* (dawn) I, 48,16. Note incidentally that in the Aryan concepts the rain is linked with those of fire and perhaps with the lightning of the thunderstorm, as in VII, 20,4; VIII, 61,18 *(vajra);* X. 96,3 *(rūpa haritā).*

[31] Thus in the war chant *Ṛgveda* X, 102,5, where the gods made the bull (of heaven, i.e., *Agni*) urinate in the middle of the fight (to the benefit of the family clan) *(amehayan vṛṣabham madhye ājeḥ).*

[32] *Ṛgveda* I, 43,4; II, 35,7; VII, 35,6; VIII, 29,5. *Atharvaveda* II, 27,6; VI, 57,2; XIX, 10,6.

[33] *Atharvaveda* VI, 44,3. The word *mūtra* does not occur in the *Ṛgveda.*

[34] *accha* = without shadow, reflection or mirror-image (cf. p. 20) and thereby material = transparent.

[35] Cf. p. 21 and note 1, p. 23.

[36] *Ṛgveda* 1, 22,3; 34,3; 47,4; 157,4; VI, 70,5; I, 142,3; IX, 107,6.

lation, and cold *(śīta)* are mentioned, these properties are assuredly related to old received attitudes; only with something slimy *(īṣat-picchila)* and sweetjuice-seeming *(kāṇḍekṣurasaṃkāśa)* is a reference to the preparation of the sugar from the cane credible, and that belatedly.[37]

However, the assumed reference to sugar-cane juice through the mucus is not guaranteed. For the one quotation from which the above proceeded says: Having the properties of the *soma,* surely the waters were formed between heaven and earth *(Ca sūtra-* 26,*39: saumyāḥ khalvāpo'ntarīkṣaprabhavāh),* and a connexion between *soma* and *śleṣman,* the special *doṣa* of the group, has already been demonstrated elsewhere previously (cf. p. 10). The intellectual linkage of the *soma* with the sweet substances in the Vedas, besides, can be taken as almost literal.[38] So it is probable that, here at least without real reference to the sugar disease, predominantly old views – especially of the *soma* – are received and released. Alluding to the keyword *mih,* the *Ṛgveda* IX,74,*4* also reports of the storm gods *Marut,* who abide between heaven and earth, that they "urinate *soma* down" *(ava mehanti)* as *hita* for the maker of the sacrifice (cf. note 2, p. 25). The allusions to the *soma* in the three following diseases rank with those to the *surā,* an intoxicating beverage which enjoyed great popularity in the profane life of the ancient Indians. Its designation in *Atharvaveda* II,26,*5* as *dhānya rasa* indicates a preparation from grain. The *surā* is usually considered as a brandy. However, insofar as it is doubtful whether distillation was known in earlier times, the references in the old medical texts provide no clues. In *Ca* 3–5 there are described three successive stages; in *sāndrameha* the viscous or turbid change (in the fermentation mixture), in *sāndraprasādameha* the settling, described particularly clearly in *Vā* and *Mā* 4, and in *śuklameha* the final result, which is transcribed with *súkla* or *sita* as a clear fluid, on which the Indians in the *surā* laid great value, like other peoples. The designation *piṣṭa* may depict the porridge-like nature of the deposit, but may also refer to the nature of the preparation as this emerges from the *Arthaśāstra* of the *Kauṭilya* (42), which also clarifies the confidence in the doctors with the

---

37 On types of cane-sugar, cf. U. CH. DUTT, Materia Medica, 266–268.

38 *Ṛgveda* IX, 107,*6*; *madhvā vajñam mimikṣa naḥ (soma):* sprinkle our fire-offering with sweet things.

surā preparation.[39] The abhīkṣṇam may also refer to the immediate downpouring of the *surā* after the conclusion of the process and *hṛṣṭa-roma* to the unleashing emotional state.

The sediment in the preparation of the *surā* might very well have further served for the representation of the seed, especially also outside medical circles as a valued sign that seed should sink in water.[40] At first glance in view of the close linguistic relationship of *r* and *l*, the arrangement of *śukra* and *śukla* in *Ca* may appear as a play on words; the originally contextual meaning of the brilliance and the indiscriminate use of both forms in the *Atharvaveda* elicit the assumption according to which a correlation of the old attitudes, embodied via fire through *soma, śukra,* etc., has been preserved.[41] However, it does not seem thereby legitimate to see these names as symbols or metaphors. Such ascriptions – be they ever so pleasing – are untenable even for the old epochs, and only correct in an acceptance of these fundamental views into the professional realism of medical science. Only one observation need be mentioned. The fire forms adduced here were originally favorable; but they appear in the earliest medical texts as unfavorable, i.e., as disease forms. This change in valuation can have occurred through the decisive large-scale changes in living conditions of the Aryans after their invasion of India; indicative signs are already to be found in the *Atharvaveda,* to be dealt with elsewhere. Hence, in a factual assessment *śukra* should probably be regarded as pus, arising from somewhere in the urinary tract. To clarify this assumption – not perhaps on reciprocal grounds – it may be recalled that in a not too remote period for ourselves, suppurative discharge from the urethra was considered as spermatorrhea.

---

[39] Edit. by SHAMA SASTRY, *120,*$_{8}$: *piṣṭasya; prasad* is frequently used in the descriptions, as also in letting the drink stand in a jug, which the King shall drink (*121,*$_{10}$: *kumbhīṃ rājapeyāṃ prasādayati).* Accordingly, *prasannā* is to be understood as the designation of an intoxicating drink, somewhat of the nature of a must; and similarly, *āsavā* is not to be conceived as a distillate, but as derived from pressus *(su).* The physician *(cikitsaka)* is mentioned at *120,*$_{12}$. Cf. J. J. MEYER, *Das altindische Buch vom Welt- und Staatsleben, 186,*$_{20}$. *188,*$_{10-22}$, *186,*$_{28}$.

[40] *Nāradasmṛti* 12,*10,* (quoted by JOLLY, *Medizin* 49). J. J. MEYER, l.c. *305,*$_{28-30}$, translates the passage as a note to his allusion on the part of *Kauṭilya* (Ed. *193,*$_{17}$), where however the discussion is of the undersinking *(majj)* of the excrement *(viṣṭhā).*

[41] Some references thereto in *Asia Major* 1930, *331–339.* Cf. also the comparison of *somapā* (drinking), *somasut* (pressing) and *śukrapūtapā* (clarified for drinking) in *Ṛgveda* VIII, 46,*26.*

No special process is detectable in the sparse description of the *śītameha*.

The three last diseases of the *sleṣman* group fall into an aspect which includes *prameha* with pain or difficulty in passing urine. Apart from the special texts, this combination is mentioned by *Ca sūtra-* 23,6: *mūtrakṛcchaṃ pramehaṃca.* The indirect foundation may be found in the fear of suppression of the excreta of the human body and its consequences; such a concern is manifested from all sides in illustrations from Indian life, reference to which is frequently made in the medical texts. *Ca* devotes a special chapter to the subject (*sūtra-* 7). A parallel to this combination can also be discovered in *Ca śarīra-* 8,16. There it is stated that a pregnant woman with the customary consumption of lizhard's flesh brings forth a child suffering from urinary gravel, bladder stone and urinary obstruction *(godhāmāṃsapriyā śārkariṇam śanarmehiṇam cā),* and – two clauses later – with constant consumption of sweets a child suffering from urinary flux, dumb or clumsy *(madhuranityā pramehiṇam mūkamatisthūlaṃ vā).*[42] In such a conceptual setting, the last three diseases should be attached to the *śleṣman* group. However, an actual, if uncommon, discharge of urinary concretions should not be unconditionally assumed in *sikatāmeha.* The basis of sensation sufficed for the nomenclature, as is obvious from the description, and as can have been caused by any kind of inflammatory changes in the urinary tract. The urinary oppression noted to occur from experience would especially justify the addition of the disease to the *prameha.* The same assessment fits the pains in *śanairmeha* and the indirect or direct passage of mucus in *ālālameha.*

In the last group of the *prameha,* which is evoked by the *vāta,* shortly before their description in verse, the remark is added that the special features of their naming stand in connexion with those of the properties of the wind *(Ca nidāna-* 4,9: *teṣāmapi vātaguṇaviśeṣenaiva nāmaviśeṣā bhavanti).* According to the main source in *Ca vimāna* – 8, 84, these properties of the winds are: drying *(rūksa),* fast *(laghu),* variable *(cala),* densely compact *(bahu),* speedy *(śīghra),* cold *(śita),* rough *(paruṣa),* clear *(viśada).*

42 In A. CH. KAVIRATNA, English Translation of *Charaka-Samhita, 830,* the actual translator, K. M. GANGULI, in *śārkarin,* deals with the designation of gravel or grit *(śarkara)* in the transferred meaning of ground brown sugar and obviously regards this first part of the disease as diabetes. If this concept also is not to be relied upon (even the textual commentaries offer no evidence for it), still perhaps the circumstances sketched above are an echo of the assumed connexion.

With the exception of a single verbal concordance in *Ca* 20c, and even there another meaning is probable, one will seek in vain for the concordance – announced in *Ca* – of the properties of the *vāta* with those of the four diseases ascribed to its influence. The discrepancy of the three groups of the *prameha* is here at its most blatant.

The ancient Indian physicians must probably also have been aware of this striking irregularity, probably even at the time of the composition or elaboration of the text, which were ascribed to the *Agniveśa*. For in the introduction to the special chapter of the *prameha*, besides the customary and usually exclusive classification according to *doṣa*, there appears a significant consideration of *dūṣya*.[43] This term *dūṣya* – not exactly uncommon in the medical nomenclature – refers to the substances which are (easily) exposed by decay, here to the disease matter: *vasā, majjan,*

---

[43] Similarly in the parallel in *Ca cikitsā-* 6,4. Also *Su nidāna-* 6,2 has the arrangement *doṣa-dūsya*, likewise *Vā nidāna-* 10,7 and *Mā prameha-* 4,6 repeated in the *Yogaratnākara*.
The heralded arrangement of doṣa and *dūṣya*, previously mentioned in *Ca* 6,4, is raised again in the general discussion of the *śleṣman* group. After some references to the causal role of immoderate lifestyles, *Ca nidāna-* 4,4 reports: *bahudravaḥ śleṣma doṣaviśeṣaḥ / bahubaddhaṃ medo māṃsam śarīrajakledaḥ śukraṃ śonitaṃ vasā majjā lasīkā rasaścauja iti samkhyātā dūṣyaviśesaḥ* / Here therefore the distinction *(viśeṣa)* between *doṣa* and *dūṣya* is made clear, and indeed through *drava* = running, flowing for *doṣa* and *baddha* = bound, stagnant for *dūṣya*. These two terms, which are also emphasized by their place in the text, are further reinforced by *bahu* (dense). Thus on the one hand there is *śleṣman* in fluid form, and on the other are the *dūṣya* listed as fat, flesh and, arising from the body, moistness, semen, blood, grease, marrow, *lasīkā*, juice, *ojas*, in a form which actually can be best described here as curdled. Further discussions follow on the combination of *śleṣman* and *dūṣya*, chiefly to fat (expressly mentioned six times) with the result of the passage of the last-named into the urine. This factual emphasis on the fat in the sense of *dūṣya* points to the *vāta* group. Hence, it is very probable that an original close definition of *dūṣya* according to this view existed, with an only later extension to all groups, as already evident in *Su nidāna-* 6,2. *Ca nidāna- 4,5* provides evidence for this observation; here, at the conclusion of the discussion of the influence of the *śleṣman*, it is said that its group is incurable *(asādhya)*. However, this assessment corresponds not only to the characteristics of the *vāta* group, but stands opposed to the correct evaluation of curability of the 10 *śleṣman* ailments a few sentences later *(te daśa pramehāḥ sādhyāh)*.
Actually, *dūṣya* refers more or less to the *dhātu* of the body: juice *(rasa)*, blood *(rakta)*, flesh *(māṃsa)*, fat *(medas)*, bones *(asthi)*, marrow *(majjā)*, semen *(śukra)* and also *ojas*. The designation (from *duṣ* = to become bad) cannot, however, be arranged conceptually under *dhātu*, but is a disease substance from the outset as has been shown for *doṣa* earlier.

lasīkā and *ojas*. According to the concepts about the course of the disease, and in consequence of an unsuitable mode of life of the patient, the *vāta* let his body-fat *(vasā)* sink down to the currents or canals leading to the urine *(mūtravahāṇi srotāṃsi pratipadyate)*, so that *vasāmeha* develops; similarly with the marrow and the two last constituents. The *lasīka*,[44] which belongs to the juice *(rasa)* according to its word-form, is depicted as dense or abundant *(bahu)*, and with it ascribed to the rut *(matta iva)* of the elephant, which passes urine indefatigably *(kṣaratyajastra)*. The stuff of the so-called life force *(ojas)*, which is itself sweet *(madhurasvabhāva)*, is concentrated *(kaṣāya)* by the drying influence *(raukṣya)* of the wind. Three *rasa* properties are named with the last references, which stand in stimulating reciprocal relationship to *vata*. If we exclude the loss of fat and marrow, an evaluation of whose presence in the urine appears uncertain and dependent on opinion, *hastimeha* approximates to the concept of diabetes mellitus, if in its assessment the amount and not the time is emphasized. Of course, this critical attitude cannot be confirmed textually.

The description of *madhumeha* seems to point to the sugary urinary flux with its linkage to *ojas*, because the sweet quality is emphasized in the latter. However, it may not be assumed without more ado that an experience of the sweet taste of the urine led retrospectively to its transference to the *ojas*. The arrangement of the concepts about *ojas* in those indicated above argues against this, for the explanations of *ojas* begin in *Su sūtra*- 15,*14* with comparison to *soma*.[45]

---

[44] Among the text sources which mention *dūṣya*, two are mentioned because they offer an explanation as to the meaning. In the special description of the *rasa* in *Ca sūtra*- 26,*49*, *tikta* is designated, which is moisture, fat, grease, *lasīkā*, discharge, sweat, urine, feces, bile and mucus, dried and drying, cold and light *(kledamedāvasā-lasīkā-pūyasveda-mūtrapurīṣa-pittaślesmopaśoṣaṇā rukṣaḥ śītā laghuśca)*. The quotation shows that *lasīkā* is placed between fats and badly smelling fluid discharges. In *Ca sārīra*- 7,*10*, which discusses the measure of the body fluid, it is stated that *lasīkā* have received their names from the efflux of a wound within the skin *(yat tvagantare vraṇagataṃ lasīkāśabdaṃ labhate)*. Hence, by *lasīkā* is actually to be understood a corresponding discharge from the skin; cf. the above reference to the elephant in rut.

[45] On the complicated views about *ojas*, treated very briefly by JOLLY in his *Medicine*, only a few remarks. A similar combination to that cited in *Su* above *(somātmakam)* occurs in *Ca* in the 10 disease states of the so-called breath of life *(daśaprānāyatāni)*, which term serves in *sūtra*-29 as an introductory text sentence and is referred to in *sārīra*- 7,7. In *Ca sūtra*- 17,*35*, *ojas* is referred to the blood in the heart *(hṛdi)*, it is yellow in color *(sapītakam)* and mucus *(63)*

The introductory causes for each of the three main groups of the *prameha,* which are based on the behavior and life-style of the patients,[46] exist in various combinations with views on general pathology and only in indirect connexion to the prameha, so that their discussion ceases here so as not to deviate into obscure territories and open questions. For similar reasons, the difficult unravelling of the relevant therapeutic measures is left alone here and touched on only briefly later.[47]

Prameha is less uncommonly associated with other diseases. *Ca nidāna-* 4,*5* contains only one reference, which, however, seem emphasized by its repetition *(12)* in this special statement on *prameha.* In both the disease names adduced here, *śarāvika* and *akachapikā,* the addition of *ādya* (= etc.) justifies the assumption that an allusion is being made to a generally recognized disease group, namely to that of the *piḍakā. Su nidāna-* 6,9–*13* treats of ten and *Ca sūtra-* 17,*39–65* of seven forms of this ailment. Also in the last special text, which is devoted to diseases of the head *(śiras),* the connexion of *prameha* with *piḍakā* is repeatedly emphasized. The meaning of *piḍakā* is lump, and its chief emergence in the skin as a painful and suppurative process suggests the corresponding inflammatory complications of diabetes mellitus. However, this modern critical attitude cannot be carried over to ancient Indian medicine. *Su nidāna-* 6,8 and 15 is hereby linked with fat and marrow, and *Ca sūtra-* 17,*53* clearly explains the basic concepts through the characteristics of the vāta group of the *prameha* by its reference to corrupt fat *(duṣṭamedas).*

Finally, there is some cardinal proof that the ancient Indians were acquainted with the sugar disease in the behavior of insects towards the urine being known to them. JOLLY says in his *Medicine, 84:* "Even how, diabetes is frequently discovered by the fact that files and whole trails of large black ants seek out

---

i.e., in the physiologic sense, not in that of the *doṣa. Ca śārīra-* 7,*10* assesses its amount at a halfhandful. *Ca sūtra-* 30,2 ff., takes an extended interest in *ojas,* including its importance for the embryo, which is taken up again in *śārīra-* 4,*11.* In *Ca sūtra-* 17,*38* there is also a reference to the combination of *vāta* and *ojas* and the severe form *(kṛcchra),* the *madhumeha,* dependent thereon.

[46] Apart from the chapter on *prameha, Ca Sūtra-* 28,*6* (in a short review of diseases of the fat) refers to the urinary flux in relation to the physical signs, which are especially treated at the start of *sūtra-* 21 and also mentioned elsewhere, e.g., *sūtra-* 28,9.

[47] The starting-point for an investigation of therapy may be provided by the recently confirmed Bower MS, whose revision by HOERNLE gives important help. Cf. the 6 recipes (II, 603–608) and the linked commentary.

the chamberpot." (CHEVERS: *Diseases of India*, p. 371 f.) This observation can be traced so far back into early times that the use of "chamberpot" is not to be taken[48] literally and the "even" is only demonstrative.

As the oldest evidence (in my opinion) for the process, *Ca nidāna-* shows a text at 4,*11* which concludes the ideas on *prameha:* the hastening of the flies and ants towards the body and urine of the patient *(ṣaṭpadapipilikābhiśca śarīramūtrābhisaraṇam).*[49] That the flies and ants are exceedingly inclined towards sweet things is stated by *Ca* in the discussion of the *madhura rasa (sūtra-* 26,*41: ṣaṭpadapipīlikānamiṣṭatamḥ).* The question was only whether, in the assessment expressed in *Ca,* the sweetness of the urine was to be reckoned precisely as the precipitating factor. However, such an express explanation, which in no uncertain manner excludes other possible causes, is strikingly lacking. And if the immediately adjacent part of *Ca* speaks of mistakes about the urine, and thereby actually emphasizez the smell of the flesh *(mūtre ca mūtradoṣān visraṃca śarīragandhaḥ),* it may be concluded therefrom that the previously described behavior of the insects in this last direction appears well-founded.[50]

The relatively late text section in the *Garuḍapurāṇa* 159,35 formall and factually separates the circumstance that the ants spread over the (ground with the) urine from: thirst, the sweetness of the micturition, the mucus efflux in the sugar disease, as well as the manifold types of disease (– *mutre 'pi dhāvantipipīlāśca (35) tṛṣṇā prameha prapicchan madhvāmaye syād vividho*

---

[48] Insofar as account-books and reports of popular packaging allow an assessment of the nature of urination, the use of such a utensil must be counted as at least extraordinary. The vessel *(bhājana)* in *Ca* 3 probably served for preparing must.

[49] The term *ṣaṭpada* (i.e., six-footed) is linked with the old classification of the Vedic Aryans into two-footed *(dvipad)* and four-footed *(catuṣpad).*

[50] *Su nidāna-* 6,7 speaks of the approach of flies or swarms of bees *(makṣikopasarpaṇamālasyaṃ)* and continues: *sāṃsopacayaḥ*; in the parallel position of the texts as provisional comparison of *māṃsa* (flesh) as dhātu and its *prameha* property in the stated increase may well have been in mind. *Ca cikitsa-* 6,*12* says no more in the repetition than before *(mūtre 'bhidāvanti pipīlikās).* The commentary, the *Carakatātparyatīkā,* goes no further into this passage. The commentator *Cakrapāṇi* adds no opinion to the main source, *Ca nidāna-* 4,*11* explaining any connexion. *Gaṅgādhara* goes no further: ṣaṭpateti maksika, śarure mūtre ca makṣikāpipīlikānām; only in the section which deals with *visra (mutre mutradosan kaphādisaṃ sargajamādhuryādidoṣān)* is the sweetness *(mādhurya)* mentioned. More on this later.

vikāraḥ). In what way the association of the aggregation of insects with urine – and body – is to be explained is shown, for instance, by a place in *Su sūtra-* 14, *13,* where the unpleasant sensations and smell of flesh *(visra)* of the decaying blood are associated with the observation that ants and flies arrive *(– visra-maniṣṭam pipīlikāmakṣikāṇāmaskandi ca).*[51] This text source is in the chapter which was used earlier (p. 10) for the main conclusions. And in this context there are also in *Ca* a few remarks which clarify the underlying attitudes.

Ca vimāna- 4,5, in the *rasa,* distinguishes the patient with a bad taste, characterized by the creeping of lice on to his body, and a sweet one with flies *(yūkopasarpaṇeṇa tvasya śarīravaira-syam makṣikopasarpaṇena śarīramādhuryam).* In *Ca indriya-* 2,9, two *rasa* are emphasized mainly among the patients, the bad-tasting *(vairasya or virasa)* and the good-tasting or sweet *(svādu),* in both cases in connexion with insects.[52] These intellectual associations flow from the earliest attitudes to disease concepts via the *rasa* (cf. note 2, p. 6).

Finally, the systematics of the *prameha* texts calls for a critical overview, which is restricted here from the viewpoint of the rasa doctrine. The six *rasa* break down into two groups, which behave antagonistically toward the two *doṣa* which dominate the 1. and 3. *prameha* groups, and also towards *śleṣman* and *vāta.* This correlation is described in *Ca vimāfna-* 1,*3: kaṭu – tikta – kaṣāya* stimulate *vāta, madhura – amla- lavaṇa* calm *vāta;* the influence on *śleṣman* is the opposite. It is noteworthy that in this text *pitta* and its *rasa* influences are not described at all. Cf. the following Table, A and B. Here, if the usual *rasa* references of the *pitta* are set down (Table, C) and compared with the relevant divisions in the so-called elements, as depicted in *Ca sūtra-* 26,*39,* there emerges the pertinent connexion between *pitta* and *agni* which has already been demonstrated at pp. 18–22. Cf. table, C and D3.

---

[51] The correct explanation of this passage is already to be credited to WECKERLING in *Die Tridoṣalehre in der indischen Medizin,* 36 and 48–49, where there is also a reference to the Indian commentary. U. CH. DUTT, HOERNLE and BHISAGRATNA all translate incorrectly.

[52] The specification of names for the adduced designation of insects – with the exception of ants – is very difficult for the early period. The relevant zoology in *Su kalpa* must constitute a later addition.

	madhura sweet	*amla* sour	*lavaṇa* salty	*kaṭu* sharp	*tikta* bitter	*kaṣāya* astringent
A. *vāta*	–	–	–	+	+	+
B. *śleṣman*	+	+	+	–	–	–
C. *pitta*	–	+	+	+	–	–
D. 1. *soma*	+					
2. *bhūmi* (earth)		+				+
3. *agni* (fire)		+	+	+		
4. *toya* (water)			+			
5. *vāyu* (wind)				+	+	+
6. *ākāśa*					+	

The relevance of rows A–C and D to the ancient Indian views is noteworthy in different ways. Particularly pertinent to the subject is the concordance between *vāta* and *vāyu* and that between *pitta* and *agni.* The *rasa* properties of the second or *pitta* group of the *prameha* in *Ca* are here established, also a clarification of the disturbances of membership of the group between *Ca* and *Su.*

The material about *prameha* is inadequate for a confirmed decision on the question whether the classification according to *doṣa* or to *rasa* is the older. The *doṣa* classification reveals a classification by content, yet the *rasa* taxonomy in general makes a more recent impression. For the development of the latter in the direction of taste appears, in the *Ca,* to be first completed. This observation corresponds, at least according to modern views, to a very clumsy use of terms designating sensory perceptions and their recording, for instance if *kṣāra* (caustic) is paraphrased with the aid of the later conventional expression for color *(varṇa),* when on the other hand it appears obviously oriented towards taste in *kṣaudrameha.*

In fact, the 20 specific diseases of the *prameha* appear more or less clearly arranged as derived from the constituent parts of the human body *(dhātu),* which are affected in sympathy. This is stated in *Ca cikitsa-* 6,6, according to which the three *doṣa* act on fat, blood, seminal fluid, grease, *lasīka,* marrow-juice, *ojas* and flesh and evoke the 20 *prameha* diseases, characterized through dūṣya, in those suffering from it *(kaphaḥ sapittaḥ pavanaśca doṣa medo 'sraśukrāmbuvasālasīkāḥ / majjārasaujaḥ piśitam ca dūṣyam pramehiṇām viṃśatireva mehāḥ).* This disease course is not thus mentioned elsewhere. But the atrophy *(kṣaya)* in the chapter on *piḍakā*, with its emphasized association with *prameha*, probably indicates this as the basis on which such concepts must have grown (*Ca sūtra*- *27,39* and correspondingly also *Ca sūtra*- 29,4). It is noteworthy in this connexion that in the "Key to Dreams" of the *Jagaddeva 2,31 (Svapnacintāmaṇi)* the two diseases *(prameha* and *kṣaya-roga)* are set out in parallel.[53] This textbook on dreams and their consequences for the well-being of men is only to be demarcated from Indian scientific medicine from the modern viewpoint.[54] Moreover, the author explains that he has borrowed from medical sources, and in the passages quoted attributes the cause of the urinary flux to fat consumption *(sneha)*. But he thereby attaches an etiology which emerges strikingly in the old medical texts, the precipitation of the disease through easily corruptible parts of the body, paraphrased as *dūṣya*. Even in the strictly medical texts this theory of fat emerged, which was originally limited to this and the constituent *vāta* group in *prameha*. *Ca* already shows the encroachment of the *dūṣya* evaluation on the *śleṣman* group, and *Su* also shows the same as regards the *pitta* group. This attention in *prameha* is subsequently maintained in an association with the *dosa*, as evidenced by the *Yogaratnākara*.

This short review justifies the conclusion that, not only is the urinary flux to be counted as a long-known disorder, on account of the external classification under the collective name of *prameha* and the early-established number of 20 specific diseases,[55] but the medical concepts of an internal origin for this disease extend beyond that time frontier which bounds the essentially professional traditions in the preserved texts. In the latter, *prameha* is found already dispersed among numerous associations with other disorders. In this sense, and according to the foregoing descriptions, an allusion through *anuṣaṅgin* (connected with) can probably be glimpsed in *Ca sūtra*- 25,22: *prameho 'nuṣaṅgaṇāṃ*. *Gaṅgādhara* comments, under properties, that it is a severe and obstinate disease *(prameho 'nuṣaṅgaṇām rogāṇāṃ nityasaṃlagnībhūtānāṃ śreṣṭhatamaḥ)*. The meaning of the uri-

[53] Published, translated and commented on by J. VON NEGELEIN, *Der Traumschlüssel des Jagaddeva, 288.*

[54] Established Indian medical science extends to the interpretation of dreams, as in *Ca indriya*- *5,15*.

[55] The Bower MS will serve as an example here; if we exclude the 6 special prescriptions in II, 603–608, the urinary flux is still mentioned 15 times, in groups with other diseases, as is usually the case in the MS: I, 41; II, 36, 70, 123, 230, 238, 243, 250, 359, 403, 632, 644, 942, 971, 1019; III, 69.

nary flux is also demonstrable in the lay literature. The *Artha-śāstra* of the *Kauṭiliya* is certainly not written from the viewpoint of medical science and introduces names of diseases relatively seldom; in its 177th *prakaraṇa,* however, we have *prameha.*

If, from the broad expansion of the disease concept of *prameha,* we extract those clues which argue for a knowledge of the sugar disease among the ancient Indian physicians, we may use only those proofs which use some sort of expression to designate the urine as sweet. For the other cardinal feature about the urine of diabetics (and also in diabetes insipidus), the increased amount of urine, is not to be inferred from the text with the necessary assurance, because here – apart from the increased taste sensation – the increase in the amount of urine is not sharply distinguished from the frequency of micturition. What is nowadays expressed as polyuria and pollakisuria appears actually obliterated. And the more or less subjective symptoms which can be extracted from the polymorphous descriptions in the text do not lend themselves to accurate assessment.

In early Aryan times, the urine was regarded as a remedy (cf. p. 26), and it was on this basis that it became part of the medicaments of Indian medical sciene. *Ca sūtra-* 1,*38* and *43* adds to the relevant 8 traditional types, but exclusively the urine of animals; only *Su* mentions in the penultimate *sūtra* chapter, briefly, of human urine, that it wards off poison *(ix,* 12: *mūtraṃ mānuṣaṃ tu viṣāpaham).*[56] On the other hand, in the introduction to the same chapter, Su warns against water which is unpurified, and here adduces urine and feces *(purisa)* together *(ix,4).*

There can naturally be no doubt that the urine in *prameha* was regarded as something bad and diseased. But the general attitude to its assessment remained divided and shows quite significantly favorable views. We give only one example: *Ca vimāna-*8,*115* places milk *(kṣūra)* next to urine in a therapeutic teaching paragraph of sweet things *(madhuraskandha).*

Among the possibilities of demonstrating sugar, the quickest is its establishment by tasting with the tongue *(rasanā).* On this precedent, such occasional observations doubtless cannot be

---

[56] *The Arthaśāstra of the Kauṭiliya* (ed. R. Shama Sastry, 412; trans. J. J. Meyer, *641*) cites a drink termed an intoxicant *(madanayoga)*; among its constituents, human urine *(naramūtra)* is listed.

excluded. But as a decisive measure here, such testing is in the highest degree improbable for the ancient tradition. For in the special chapters on prameha there is no mention of the taste test which ought to have been expected in such circumstances, and in the other old texts this author has found no clue arguing for confirmation of the presence of sugar in the urine with the tongue. On the contrary. *Ca vimāna-* 4,5 teaches that taste in (or at) the body of the patient – although it is the subject of a sensory perception – must be recognized as an inference, because the sense organ was not reached by immediate perception (appearance), therefore the patient shall be asked whether he experiences his own sensation (the taste in his mouth)[57] *(rasaṃtu khalvāturaśarīragatamindriyāvaiṣāikamapyanumānādavagacchet / na hyasya pratyakṣeṇa grahaṇamupapadyate / tasmādāturaparipraśnenaiva āturamukharasaṃ vidyāt).* Thereafter – as already shown at p. 35 – the distinctive feature is taught according to which the *yūka* (louse) seeks out what tastes badly or is tasteless *(vairasya)* in the body and the *makṣika* (fly or bee) what is sweet *(mādhurya).* The paragraph concludes with characteristics of blood-types from the behavior of the dog *(svan)* and crow *(kāka).*[58]

In contrast to the observations by means of hearing, sight, smell and taste, on which occasion they are required by the quotation in *Ca vimāna-* 4,5 in direct form, the indirect conclusion with taste occupies the foreground. That what is intended in this general textual instruction is the indirect assay of the urine by reference to the behavior of insects is shown by the practical explanation by *Dallana* in his *Nibandhasaṃgraha* in *Su sūtra-* 10,44, where, among others of the distinguishing features of the *rasa,* the discourse is of those which are perceptible in the var-

[57] This subjective symptom, that of sweetness in the mouth, is also mentioned in the summary to *Ca nidāna-* 4,11 *(mādhuryamāsyaya* or *mādhuryamāsye).*

[58] The mention of the dog and crow may be based on considerations of the early period; we need only refer to the importance of the dog in the Iranian tradition; that in the Indian is so far still unintelligible. That old attitudes are to be considered is shown by the form of the text: *svakākabhakṣanād dhārilohitam abhakṣaṇ ·āllohitapittamityanumātavyam* (if [the blood] of dog and crow are eaten, it will be recognized as *dharin* blood, if not, eaten as blood-bile). The last-named disease concept *(lohita-pitta* or *rakta-pitta),* which is only briefly explained by Cakrapani as *duṣṭa* (decayed, noxious) stands in opposition to *dhari-* (bearing, holding) though the object is missing. This is expanded by the commentators, apparently from the systematics of *Ca sūtra-* 1,16 *(śarīra-indriya*-sattava-ātman to dhārijīvita-nityaga-anubandha) and transcribed as *jīvana* (enlivening) and *jīvita* (life or lively); however, the correlation of the arrangement was not thereby observed.

ious types of *prameha (rasanendriyavijenyāḥ pramehādiṣu rasaviśeṣāḥ)*.[59]

If, then, it has been assumed, according to the earliest professional reports, that the ancient Indian physician may have diagnosed the sugar content of the urine in the sugary urinary flux for the first time in world medicine – and indeed the possibility of such an observation cannot be denied – an exact proof of such a medical realization has not yet been produced, and even the present study cannot supply one.

An essential contextual cause for this flawed conclusion lies in the difference between the development of medicine in India and in Europe; we may even speak of an opposition here. The discovery of the sweet taste of the urine by WILLIS in the middle of the 17h century did not, of course, yet mean the acutal demonstration of sugar and a complete explanation of the disease. However, his observation decisively excluded a long development of research into the urinary flux. On the contrary, the assessment of *prameha* from sweetness appeared even in the earliest professional reports, and was repeated and elaborated, and is indeed among evidence that this urinary property derived from spontaneous and favorable procedures of considerable breadth and frequeny in the life of the ancient Indians. It is not altogether clear through what circumstances the transition to a disease concept was induced. A reference to experiences in sacrificial revels[60] or to changes in life-style from other causes can therefore be only taken as suppositions, though as very approximate.

The difficulty in the development of the disease concept did not lie in the unexpected observation of a urine that was sweet or estimated as such, but in the fact that the original concept of things that were sweet, favorable or pleasant had been transplanted into a disease concept. The many-sided and many-membered disease picture of the *prameha* must be considered from

---

[59] Quoted from the Su translation by HOERNLE, *Bibliotheca indica N.S. No. 911,58*: "explains that this does not refer to the sense of taste of the physician, but of bees, ants and similar insects who are attracted by urine."

[60] Allusions are found here and there to the sacrificial revels, e.g., in *Ca nidāna-8,11: haviḥprāsāt pramehakuṣṭhānāṃ* where the excessive consumption of *havis*, i.e., of the sacrificial offering, therefore *soma*, milk, fat (designated as *madhu*) led to the diseases *prameha* and *kuṣṭha*. When it is mentioned in *Ca sūtra-* 25,*11 (ikṣumūtrajananānām)* that *ikṣu* generates much urine, we should not think exclusively of cane-sugar juice but also, from precedent, of an intoxicating drink (*surā* or suchlike) which was often sweetened.

the viewpoint in which sweetness diagnosis with the help of insects. On this basis, the Indian emphasis on the importance of the irregularity lay, not on the sweet taste, but on the nature of the disease. This is consistent with the lack of any reports that European doctors had heard something of the sugary urinary flux in their contact with Indians.[61] Accordingly, it must remain an open question whether the old Indian physicians recognized in the individual varieties of the *prameha* a pathologic sugary urine. Even the rejection of such an assumption cannot be positively disputed. Even empiric experiences are less probable in an affirmative conjecture, for otherwise honey or sugar would not have been emphasized as remedies for *prameha*.[62]

in: *Sudhoffs Archiv für Geschichte der Medizin 25 (1932), 1–42.*

[61] Salomon already mentions, in his monograph *(Geschichte der Glykosurie,* Dtsch. Archiv für klin. Medizin VIII, 1871, *520–521),* the qualified objection that JAMES BONTIUS (c. 1629), in his work on the diseases, natural history and remedies of East India, had not mentioned the sugary urinary flux at all. Even later, no corresponding affirmative reports had become known, although, from the documentary evidence, *prameha* was not a rare disease in medical teaching. Also CHRISTIE (1.c.,*287*) does not state that his sick doctor who came to him with a self-made diagnosis was particularly worthy of mention.

[62] *Su sūtra-* 45,*vi,6* and *9*, which treats of bee and plant honey. Sugar and honey are included in greater or lesser extent as remedies in the Bower MS (e.g., II, 493, 603, 604, 605, 607, 1019; III, 67).

Renaissance – 19th Century

Paracelsus and the Sugar Disease

by HANS SCHADEWALDT

In the collected edition of the works of Paracelsus by Karl Sudhoff (1853–1938) [17] there appears at four places the technical term 'Diabetes' and the adjective 'diabetic' or 'diabetica', sometimes in the linkage *'passio diabetica'*. Yet it emerges very much more often, and it is to be noted that at least one other place, in Volume 5, page 145, is still not included in the index volume to the 1960 edition of Sudhoff's *Collected Works of Paracelsus,* produced by Martin Müller (1878–1960) [13] (see also Meindl [12] and Schadewaldt [20]). Thus, Paracelsus (1493–1541) devoted rather much of his discussion to a disease still reckoned in his time as relatively rare. However, this is not be considered as something specific to his time, for diabetes had regularly also been as much discussed by the Byzantine authors and both by the medieval physicians, like Johannes Actuarius (d. 1283) and by the majority of Islamic physicians, such as Rhazes (c. 850–923) [18], Avicenna (980–1037) [3] and Avenzoar (c. 1092–1162) [2], to name only the most important, as by the physicians of the Renaissance period and the Humanist Era in which Paracelsus lived. Thus, one of the historians of the study of diabetes, Ernst Seckendorf [23], has quoted for the period from 1500 to 1670 alone 100 authors concerned with diabetes; and in the wide-ranging classical work on the history of diabetes by Max Salomon (1837–1912) a whole list of these Humanist authors are extensively quoted and their opinions discussed.

However, Paracelsus played a special part in the history of diabetes, for he was the first to depart from the Galenic scheme of things as regards the cause of diabetes and to advance what was, for his time, and undoubtedly original theory.

Like his predecessors in the East and West, he had adopted the name 'diabetes' from the ancient Greek terminology. A first authentic report of this concept of diabetes emerges from the work of the Greek physician Aretaios [1], who lived some decades before Galen (129–199 A.D.) and in whose medical writings we find:

"And hence also the disease has received the name Diabetes, as if it were a wine-pourer or siphon, precisely because the fluid does not remain in the body but uses the person as a tube through which it can flow out."

Yet, according to a treatise by the Byzantine physician, Caelius Aurelianus [5], of the 5th century A.D., well before Aretaios in the 3rd century B.C. Demetrios of Apamaia made a distinction between two types of dropsy, one of which he called 'diabetes' because of its inability to retain water,

"so that, whatever the patient drinks is immediately excreted as if passing through a tube"

derived from the Greek verb *diabainein*, which, tanslated, means 'to run through', in contrast to true hydrops. This actually corresponded to Galen's concept that this must be related to a form of atony of the kidneys in which whatever was drunk was got rid of by the body in equal amount and as fast as possible. Not only did Galen adopt the term 'diabetes', but he also used the expressions *dipsakos* (thirst disease) and *hyderos eis amida* (dropsy of the chamber-pot) or *diarrhoia eis oura* (urinary flux), thus underlining this completely mechanical concept, and emphasizing that as already mentioned the ancient authors regarded diabetes as a rare disease, so that Aretaios could remark, in the introduction to a brilliant clinical description of the disease:

"Diabetes is a puzzling illness and not very common in men."

Galen himself had seen only two diabetics, in whom he had been mainly impressed by the immoderate thirst. One drank whole jugs full of water without being able to slake his thirst in the least. He was also impressed that, in the other case, though he drank just as greedily, the entire amount of fluid was excreted in the urine after a short interval. But this explanation of diabetes as a pathologic change in the urine-forming organs had already been recorded by Cassius Felix [6], in his book on medicine in c.44 A.D., where he wrote:

"This disease is called 'Diabetes' by the Greeks because, no sooner has one drunk than the fluid, on account of the porosity of the internal organs, is emptied out through the urinary tract, as if passing through an empty space."

In fact, the well-known Greek *horror vacui* must have played an important part in elucidating the remarkable and clinically very accurately observed phenomenon of polydipsia and polyuria. Other authors of antiquity, like the Roman physician, Scribonius Largus [22], in his *Compositiones medicamentorum* (c. 17 A.D.), associated diabetes with a disease of the stomach in which the gastric juices were dried up, compelling the patients to empty jugfuls of water without being in the least able to slake their thirst, thus adding to the existing synonyms the term *dipsakos* (thirst disease), and this was transmitted in the Middle Ages by Galen, in his thesis that diabetes was a renal disorder, and then adopted without qualification by Paracelsus. But Galen, in his thesis, also advanced an ingenious but totally false analogy which was exposed only later. He opined that the remarkable illness, which he moreover termed *leiouria*, meaning no more than urinary flux, which was to be compared to the *lienteria* observed in atony of the stomach and bowel and just as in the gastrointestinal disease gave rise to ravenous hunger, could cause extraordinarily great feelings of thirst due to the renal disorder and likewise to the *horror vacui*, but which could not be sated because of the rapid passage of the fluid taken through the kidneys occasioned by excessive drinking.

Islamic medicine brought no new understandings, with the sole excription that Avicenna [3], in place of the term 'diabetes', relatively unused, even by the Greeks, for the branched siphon, originally derived from the warrior standing before the enemy with his legs apart and, in transmitted form, for the two-legged compass of the mathematician, introduced the technical term *Aldulab*, which more or less meant 'water-wheel', and also – I quote the Latin translation – distinguished between *lubricitas renum,* the specific diabetes of the Greeks, and a simple and, he said, harmless *multitudo urinae,* probably the first instance of the differential diagnosis between diabetes mellitus and diabetes insipidus.

It should not be forgotten that diabetes was considered by the physicians of antiquity as a severe disease that might even lead to premature death, as emphasized for instance by the Roman layman and encyclopedist, Aulus Cornelius Celsus (25 B.C. to 50 A.D.) [7]. Celsus did not actually use the Greek term 'diabetes' but spoke of *profusio urinae*, such that when the urine was passed in excessive amount and painlessly this was indicative of imminent wasting and danger. Similar views were expressed by Galen, whose concept was that not only what was drunk immediately was expelled from the body via the kidneys, but also, as firmly emphasized by Aretaios [1], that "flesh and bone melt together in the urine, moisture and cold are the prerequisite as in dropsy, but the fluid is expelled in the usual way via the kidneys and bladder. The patients never cease passing urine, but it runs without pause as if from wideopen channels. It takes some time for the origin and development if the disease, but once the symptoms are completely developed then that man will find himself near the end of his days, for then the wasting rapidly gains the upper hand and death soon follows after a wretched and painful life. The patients have an unquenchable thirst and drink and urinate to excess. However, the amount of urine passed exceeds that of the drink."

However, we find even in Aretaios [1] a hint of an etiologic impulse, which Paracelsus was to describe more thoroughly and precisely. Thus, it is stated in his brilliant clinical account:

"It is also not unlikely that a poisonous material exists in the bladder and the kidneys and stimulates them,"

before which the opinion was that the crisis of the disease might have been brought about by the unremarked accumulation of a dangerous substance in the body.

This substance Paracelsus now saw as one of his three *Principia*, the *Sal*. He expressed himself most exhaustively about the *diabetica passio* in his lectures of 1527–28 on the "tartaric diseases", to be found in Volume 5 of the collected works [17], Sudhoff's edition, page 103 ff. Here the opinion is expressed that a dry salt *(sal siccum)* could be the cause of the thirst of diabetics, which reached the kidneys as *sal urinae* and there gain "attachment" to a kindey vessel as cream of tartar (potassium bitartrate) and "creep into" the kindneys, "*et facit the renes* thirsty". It is expressly stated there under *Diabetica passio*, p. 104:

"inde est, quod spiritus salis renibus insidet and salts them"

and, at another place:

"*nam sitis semper venit ex sale, ita hoc sal* makes the *renes* become salted.

This new pathogenetic explanation of the origin of diabetes through "oversalting of the kidneys" also appears in Paracelsus's *Opus* or in the later written notes of his students at various other places, as in Volume 5, p. 75, 145 and 454, and Volume 3, p. 21.

However, it cannot be excluded that in another place Paracelsus briefly accepted the other version of antiquity, that the seat of the diabetic evil lay in the stomach. Thus, in Volume 2, p. 353, the opinion is expressed that obstruction of the gastric veins by salt could precipitate diabetes. Whether this passage is genuine is still disputed. In addition to Temkin (24) and Goldammer [9], Walter Pagel (b. 1898) and Heinrich Schipperges (b. 1918) [21] have yet again shown the difficulty in the exact definition of this *sal* of Paracelsus.

Paracelsus, apparently influenced by Neoplatonism, the Hermetics and the doctrine of the Christian Trinity, set up the three principles of sulfur, mercury and salt against the four elements of the ancients. If one proceeds from this, taking as a basis Paracelsus's conceptual model of the combustion of wood, as briefly discussed by Schipperges, then Sulfur, which is combustible, symbolized the active agent as flame; Mercury or Quicksilver would be the fumes created in the combustion process, and Sal, Salt, the incombustible, was left behind as the ash of the burnt wood. The emphasis on the analogy with the "Tartarus", the tartrate in the wine-barrel, makes it clear that *Sal* is not to be regarded here as elsewhere as the principle initiating decay, but as evidently a substance formed in the organism which, deposited in the kidneys, first produces the unaccustomed feeling of general thirst. It is interesting that, later, Paracelsus discovered in the urine of diabetics obvious crystals "with angles like saltpeter", and it may be assumed that this related to octahedral crystals. Paracelsus attributed the precipitation of this substance to the breakdown of a life-regulator, the socalled *Archaeus*; the deposition of the salt in the kidney would be an irreversible process, as residual salt is usually no longer soluble.

It is interesting that Paracelsus also spoke of a *dulcedo urinae*. This should not be interpreted as a presentiment of the sugar content of the urine in diabetics, but rather as compatible with the ideas of the alchemists of that time, in that the urine tasted neither sharp nor sour. However, it is still noteworthy that Paracelsus, who elsewhere in his writings gave the advice to taste the urine with the tongue, did not make use of this in his diabetic cases or at least made no mention of it. In no case, however, may one interpret the term *dulcedo* simply as "sweetness of the urine" and thereby claim Paracelsus as a precursor of Thomas Willis (1621–1675) [25], who expressly alluded in 1674 to the honey-sweet taste of diabetic urine: *Quasi melle aut saccharo imbutam*, thereby clearly defining the following word *dulcescere*, so that Willis must be regarded as the first to have recognized this third important symptom alongside polydipsia and polyuria. All the same, it is established that Paracelsus must have reported in detail on the fact that he had obtained eight "lots",* i.e., four ounces, of a salt from one urine-glass of diabetic urine, as in Volume 5, p. 179, in the Latin transcript of student:

Diabetica passio sitim provocat maximum urina eine Mass dat 8 Lot Salz urina destillata gibet zapfen wie sal petrae.

* A "lot" was an archaic German weight of about 10 grams (Trans.)

It follows from this that the urine flask of that period held between 750 and 1000 ml, and that four ounces must have been equivalent to some 120 g, so that this interesting fact may be taken as evidence of possible glycosuria, as asserted by the Greek diabetologist, Nikos S. Papaspyros [16] in 1952 in his *History of Diabetis Mellitus*. But the writings of Paracelsus himself give no clear evidence of this.

Among the symptoms of the disease that Paracelsus accorded pride of place, the most noteworthy were thirst, the excessive production of urine and tachycardia, with which were associated what were, for him, the noteworthy back pains and swelling of the feet, the latter immediately awakening the suspicion that Paracelsus, like so many of his predecessors, often did not clearly distinguish between "dropsy", an expression with he preferred to use in its German form of *Wassersucht*, and "diabetes" proper. In Volume 5, p. 103, he states for instance:

> *Diabetica passio est sal siccum resolutum. Signa: sitis cum chronico tempore* (alsewhere: *sitis abundans, sine requie), dolor spinae, tumores in pedibus aequales, urina multa, pulsus velox.*

and, mindful of the poor prognosis, he added in Volume 5, p. 145:

> *et in fine ad mortem.*

Moreover, that Paracelsus adhered to the "thirsty state of the kidneys" on the basis of the ancient theory of *horror vacui* we may conclude from his hint in Volume 5, p. 106:

> *Illa autem – per vim attractivam attrahunt humidi –*

Finally, it may be concluded that the new theory of Paracelsus quite significantly influenced further investigation and eliminated the kidneys as the site of origin of the disease, as against the other concept of a systemic metabolic disorder which only secondarily involved the kidneys. This new opinion, that diabetes was a systemic disorder, possibly of the blood, was energetically advocated by the Paracelsist, Johann Baptist van Helmont (1578–1644) [10] and the iatrochemist, Franciscus de le Boe Sylvius (1614–1672) [4]. Helmont assumed so-called *Sal volatile* from a discordance of composition of the body's juices. De le Boe expressed himself similarly, and so did Willis [25], to whom we owe the first clear indication of the sweet taste of the urine, and who discussed the theory whether the honey-like taste did not result from a precipitation of salt and sulfur in the blood, whereby this became corrupted and can no longer contain the amounts of fluid flowing within it. It may therefore be confidently maintained that the novel and original concept of Paracelsus, that a specific residue, the *Sal*, settled in the kidney, thereby producing functional impairment, and the shift in the debate from the anatomic lesion to a metabolic disturbance occurring in the entire organism, marked a real advance in the development of our understanding of diabetes; and it may be asserted that Paracelsus emerges as one of the first to concern himself with chemical investigations of diabetic urine, thereby discovering residues which he was unable to demonstrate in the urine of non-diabetics.

Unfortunately, because of the obscurity of the two concepts used by Paracelsus, relating to *Sal* and *Dulcedo*, it was impossible to obtain definite evidence as to the nature of the excretion substances involved, or, more exactly, to be able to show that Paracelsus, after the Sanskrit authors who had very probably already recognized the sweetness of diabetic urine, was the first Western author to have established this important diagnostic feature of glycosuria.

References

1. Aretaios: Opera omnia. In: C. Hude: Corpus medicorum graecorum, Bd. 2, 2. Auf., S. 65 ff. Berlin 1958.
2. Avenzoar: Opera, Lib. 2, Tract. 2, Cap. 6, fol. 25. Venedig 1490.
3. Avicenna: Liber canonis, Lib. 3, Fen. 19, Tract. 2, Cap. 17 f., fol. 684 ff. Basel 1556.
4. De le Boe-Sylvius, F.: Praxeos medica appendix. In: Opera medica, Cap. 5, S. 724 ff. Amsterdam 1680.
5. Caelius Aurelianus: On acute diseases and on chronic diseases (Latin and English). Hrsg. v. I. E. Drabkin, Chronic diseases: Book 3, Chapter 7, S. 776 f. Chicago 1950.
6. Cassius Felix: In: V. Rose: De Medicina ex Graecis Logicae Sectae Auctoribus Liber, § 46, S. 116. Leipzig 1879.
7. Celsus, A. C.: De medicina. In: F. Marx: Corpus medicorum latinorum. Bd. 1, Lib. 4, Cap. 20, 27, 2, S. 181 f. Leipzig 1915. German translation by F. Scheller, edited by W. Frieboes: Aulus Cornelius Celsus über die Arzneiwissenschaft, 2. Aufl., S. 204 f. Braunschweig 1906.
8. Galen: Opera. In: E. Littré: Corpus medicorum graecorum, Bd. 1, S. 781. Leipzig 1821; Bd. 3, S. 344. Leipzig 1822; S. 394. Leipzig 1824.
9. Goldammer, K.: Die Paracelsische Kosmologie und Materietheorie in ihrer wissenschaftsgeschichtlichen Stellung und Eigenart. Med.-hist. J. 6 (1971), 5–35.
10. Helmont, J. B. van: Opera omnia. S. 589. Frankfurt/Main 1682.

11. Johannes Actuarios: De utrinis libri VII. S. 125, 174 u. 236. Basel 1529.
12. Meindl, R.: Zur Geschichte der Zuckerharnruhr. Med. Diss., Göttingen 1948.
13. Müller, M.: Registerband zu Sudhoffs Paracelsusausgabe. Einsiedeln 1960 (Nova Acta Paracelsica Suppl. 1960).
14. Pagel, W.: An introduction to philosophical medicine in the era of the renaissance. New York 1958.
15. Pagel, W.: Das medizinische Weltbild des Paracelsus. Wiesbaden 1962.
16. Papaspyros, N. S.: The history of diabetes mellitus, 2nd. edn. Stuttgart 1964.
17. Paracelsus, B. T.: Sämtliche Werke, Bde. 1–14. Hrsg. v. K. Sudhoff, München–Berlin 1929–1933.
18. Rhazes: Opera, Lib. 9, Cap. 78, S. 263 f. Basel 1544.
19. Salomon, M.: Geschichte der Glycosurie von Hippokrates bis zum Anfange des 19. Jahrhunderts. Dtsch. Arch. klin. Med. 8 (1871), 489–582.
20. Schadewaldt, H.: Geschichte des Diabetes mellitus, S. 27 f. Berlin–Heidelberg–New York 1975.
21. Schipperges, H.: Paracelsus, S. 101. Stuttgart 1974.
22. Scribonius Largus: Compositiones medicamentorum. German translation, edited by F. Rinne: Das Rezeptbuch des Scribonius Largus. Hist. Stud. Pharmak. Inst., Dorpat 5 (1896), 1.
23. Seckendorf, E.: Kurze Geschichte des Diabetes mellitus. Med. Welt 5 (1931), 1443–1445.
24. Temkin, O.: The elusiveness of Paracelsus. Bull. Hist. Med. 26 (1952), 201–217.
25. Willis, T.: Therapeutice rationalis, Sect. 4, Cap. 3, S. 113 f. London 1674.

in: *Medizinische Klinik 72 (1977), S. 875–878.*

Lecture held on the Jubilee Congress of the International Paracelsus Society in Salzburg, October 10, 1976.

The First Description of the Symptoms of Experimental Pancreatic Diabetes by the Swiss Johann Conrad Brunner (1653–1727)[1]

by OLE CHRISTIAN ZIMMERMANN

Introduction

In 1889, by extirpating the pancreas in dogs, Mering and Minkowski produced conclusive evidence as to the role of the pancreas in diabetogenesis. But 200 years before them, Johann Conrad Brunner, a Swiss physician and research-worker, in the context of a quite different problem, had likewise removed the dog's pancreas. In describing the behavior of his experimental animals, he listed a series of important symptoms without suspecting what it was that he had discovered: namely, the clinical features of experimental diabetes; through his experiments, Brunner, even if unconsciously, was the true discoverer of this experimental form of pancreatic diabetes.

The relevant details are to be found in:[2]

1. Joh. Conrad Brunner, Experimenta nova circa Pancreas, accedit Diatribe de Lympha et genuino pancreatis usu, Amstelaedami, 1683.
2. Joh. Conrad Brunner, De Experimentis circa Pancreas novis confirmatis. Miscellanea curiosa sive Ephemeridum Medico – Physicarum Germanicarum Acad. Imp. Leopold. Natur. Curios. Dec. II Annus VII 1688, Norimbergae 1689. pag. 243/248.

---

[1] This work was carried out at the suggestion and under the guidance of Prof. Dr. med. et phil. G. Wolf-Heidegger.

[2] According to Brunner and v. Muralt (1919, p. 120), details of his pancreatic studies were also contained in some of Brunner's letters from the 80s of the 17th century. Unfortunately, however, these letters are not, to our knowledge, available at the present time.

Brunner's life and work[3]

Johann Conrad Brunner was born in 1653 in Diessenhofen, Canton Thurgau, son of the mayor, Erhard Brunner. His parents soon recognized the intellectual ability of the lad, and on the advice of the famous physician Johann Jakob Wepfer he attended the medical school at Strasbourg from 1669 to 1672. After zealous anatomical and surgical studies in Paris, London, Oxford, Leiden and Amsterdam he obtained his doctorate in Strasbourg in 1675 and returned to his home town of Diessenhofen, where he settled as physician and helper with the greatest conceivable success. It was here, in the quiet little Swiss town, that he initiated his highly interesting investigations of the pancreas and published some of his very important works, including *Experimenta nova circa Pancreas* (1683, Amsterdam) and *De Experimentis circa Pancreas novis confirmatis* (1689, Nuremberg). Also of inestimable value are his letters of this period, in which he devotes some attention to the experiments concerning the pancreas.

His profession as physician brought him in many countries. Emperors and kings, bishops and electors, counts and princes, all sought his counsel; in 1686 he was appointed to the Chair in Anatomy and Physiology at the University of Heidelberg.

His inaugural address at Heidelberg illuminates for us the theme of his life: "May Hippocrates and Aristotle be my friends, and Cartesius and any other; but may it ever be my truth, never to consent to swear by the sayings of any oracle whatever."

In 1711, he was ennobled as Baron of Brunn zu Hammerstein, and in 1720 he and his family were given the freedom of the city of Schaffhausen. On 2 October 1727 this greatest practitioner of his time concluded his indefatigable life.

"Brunner's research work was particularly concerned with problems of anatomy and physiology. In his paper, *De glandulis in duodeno intestino hominis detectis* of 1687, he reported the discovery of the duodenal glands, which, as Brunner's glands, have made his name immortal. Besides further anatomical and physiological treatises, he published works dealing with morbid anatomy and physics. He was also seen as an outstanding expert in botany and philosophy.

For Brunner as a doctor, reason and experience were the main supports of medical science. He believed that there was a speci-

---

[3] According to the older and more exhaustive reports of J. J. Scheuchzer (1733); M. Aepli (1787); C. Brunner (1888); C. Brunner und W. v. Muralt (1919); G. Wolf-Heidegger (1939).

fic remedy for every disease. Besides chemical and vegetable drugs, he valued venesection and dietary treatment. He was also one of the first to recognize the importance of cinchona bark in the treatment of fever.[4]" He has "done his country as much honor as ever a doctor did for his country.[5]"

Status of pancreatic research before Brunner's experimental studies

Before we study Brunner's researches into the pancreas and the phenomena following its extirpation, the status of pancreatic research before Brunner's experimental studies should be briefly clarified.

Historically regarded[6], the first use of the term 'pancreas'[7] is to be found in Hippocrates (460–377 BC). Even if both the anatomy and physiology of the pancreas were dubious for him and his pupils, science is still in his debt for the still-valid name of the organ.

It was not until five centuries later that the dominant medical figure of the Middle Ages, Galen (c. 130–200 AD), attributed to the pancreas particular importance for the human body. Galen regarded the pancreas as a mechanical protection for the nerves and vessels situated in the vicinity, as well as for the bile duct. Galen thought that it could achieve this purpose because it was "a soft, easily-yielding body" *(corpus molle et mediocriter cedens)*. Galen also spoke by way of intimation of a "viscous fluid, very similar to the saliva" *(lenta humiditas, salivae perquam similis)*. This did not come from the liver, like the bile, but from certain other glands *(ex glandulis item quibusdam aliis)*. Galen probably meant the pancreas when speaking of these glands.

At the threshold between the Middle Ages and the Modern Era stands the mighty figure of the founder of the new anatomy, Vesalius (1514–1564). He was acquainted with the precise anatomic position of the pancreas, for he says that it is "beneath

---

[4] From Wolf-Heidegger's account of J. C. Brunner, in "Große Schweizer Forscher", 1939, p. 84/85.

[5] Aepli, M. 1787.

[6] Here, we follow the interesting details in the inaugural dissertation of M. A. Schirmer "Beitrag zur Geschichte und Anatomie des Pankreas", Basel 1893.

[7] Originally, all glands were regarded as composed "entirely out of flesh" πᾶν κρέας. Then the term 'pancreas' remained for the 'Bauchspeicheldrüse'.

the stomach, firmly fused with the duodenum" and lies "retroperitoneally on the posterior wall of the posterior omentum" and with just the form and function of Galen's cushion. According to Vesalius, the pancreas did not function as a closure mechanism for the pylorus, as was asserted in his time.

In the following century, important investigators contributed to the more precise knowledge of pancreatic anatomy (we may particularly mention Wirsung, Vesling and Swalwe), but the actual function of the pancreas remained unclear.

Regner de Graaf of Schoonhoven, a contemporary of J. C. Brunner, was the first to refer to the great physiologic importance of the pancreas in the digestive process in his book, *Tractatus anatomico-medicus de succi pancreatici natura et usu.* However, his contemporaries somewhat over-valued the significance of the pancreatic juice as an essential factor in the course of digestive activity, as when we read, in the work of Theophil Bonet:[8] *"succus pancreatis plurimos morbos facit".*

J. C. Brunner found himself opposed to such a position on pancreatic research. He was not at all inclined to accept the existing findings as irrevocable. True to his motto: „May the Truth prevail for me", and inspired by an unrestrained enthusiasm for research, he undertook during 1673–1683 his studies on the extirpation of the pancreatic gland from the living dog, the first to do so.

From his accounts, especially from his work: *Experimenta nova circa Pancreas, accedit Diatribe de Lympha et genuino pancreatis usu,* of 1683, it emerges that Brunner started from the following formulation of the problem: Has the pancreas really got the vital significance that contemporaries attribute to it? Is the vitally necessary digestive process really linked with "the effervescence of the bile with the pancreatic juice", as his opponents repeatedly asserted? *(Effervescentia bilis cum succo pancreatis.)* Or can the animal organism not survive if the pancreas is lakking, whether this is due to artificial extirpation or to ligation of its excretory duct?

Is there not perhaps a functional substitute in the form of other glands which could take the place of failed pancreatic function?[9]

---

[8] Bonet, Theophile "Sepulchretum Sive anatomia practica", 1679, p. 626.

[9] A similar view was also reached by G. Martinotti, viz. that the functions of the pancreas could be replaced by an increased activity of Lieberkühn's glands, since after pancreatectomy a marked increase in nuclear mitotic figures could be demonstrated in the latter! (Sulla estirpazione del pancreas, Giornale della R. Academia di medicina di Torino, 1888. Suppl.)

In such a case, can some kind of changes of the nature of a functional adaptation take place, perhaps in those structures situated at and around the excretory duct of the pancreas and termed by Brunner the duodenal glands?

The experiments of the years 1673–1683, recorded in the abovementioned *Experimenta nova circa Pancreas,* gave the researcher himself the answer:

Deprived of their pancreas, his dogs continued to live. From this Brunner drew the conclusion that the pancreas could not have the vital importance that had hitherto been attributed to it. The pancreatic juice seemed to our researcher, not as absolutely specific but as approximately much the same kind as the juice of the other glands *(eiusdem fere cum aliarum glandularum liquore prosapiae);* otherwise his experimental animals would not have remained lively and agile after removal of the pancreas *(agiles atque veloces permansissent), they would not have fed as they used to do (nec ut antea comedissent)* or remained in possession of their strength and alertness *(vigore atque alacritate).*[10] On the basis of this knowledge, he further concluded that the pancreatic juice contained no acid and seemed to be replaced by the juice of other glands *(nature ipsa conglobatarum* – pancreatic glands! – *officium iis deficientibus, in conglomeratas* – other bowel glands! – *transferre videtur).*[11]

The elimination of the pancreatic juice was compensated by the fact that, through the overtime working of other filters (glands?) *(alia filtra)* latex accumulation was more abundant and fluid *(uberius ac fusius)* so that thereby the same important service for the food was made available from another source *(ut idem bonum ciborum massae aliunde resultet).*[12]

Here, Brunner refutes the view of his opponents (e.g., Franz de la Boe, known by the name of Sylvius) that the process of digestion is to be attributed to fermentation. According to Brunner, the breakdown of the food was organized by the gastric juice, which alone was acid.

However, we direct our attention – and this is the object of the present study – more to the *visible postoperative changes in the behavior of the dogs after removal of the pancreas* and summarize here the more important details from the experiments in the same work (*exp. nova circa P.* 1683).

---

[10] J. C. Brunner in Experimenta nova circa Pancreas, 1683, p. 119 f.

[11] ibid. p. 114.

[12] ibid. p. 119.

Thus we read in:

Experimentum VI (19 July 1679?)[13]

urinam reddidit durante et post experimentum . . . sitiit, ex rivulo per oppidum decurrente bibit impense . . . comedit adhine lac cum pulticula avanacea . . . dedi panis frustula aliquot quae avide devoravit . . . in prandio comedit panem, carnes aliaque edulia . . . noctu itidem ossa dentibus confregit ac devoravit	he urinated during the experiment and after the same . . . he was thirsty, so that he drank immoderately from the brook flowing through the town . . . later he ate milk with porridge . . . I gave him some bread scraps which he *greedily* devoured . . . at breakfast he ate bread, meat and other edibles . . . and also gnawed bones at night and devoured them

Experimentum VII (23. 3. 1683)[14]

... sitiit, bibitque oblatam lacte temperatam avide ...	... he was thirsty and *greedily* drank milk mixed with porridge

This reccurent and always repeated similar behavior of the experimental animals, in which we detect a quite specific symptom-complex, we can already establish as important for our theme. That Brunner did not see the polydipsia, polyuria and polyphagia as typical of the clinical picture of diabetes, but merely as the consequences of the operation, need not prevent us from recognizing Brunner as the true discoverer of experimental pancreatic diabetes.

It might be thought, after all these reported findings, that Brunner's contemporaries assented to his views about the pancreas, but they continued their opposition just as before his experimental physiologic observations. Brunner once remarks in a note: "About the drama afforded me by the dog minus his pancreas over three months, can you be surprised whereas others perhaps become annoyed?"[15]

And so Brunner saw himself as motivated, as we read in the preface to the relevant exposition – see the following text –, to confirm by further experiments the correctness of his findings portrayed above and the conclusions drawn from them:

---

[13] ibid. p. 37–40.
[14] ibid. p. 56.
[15] ibid. p. 12.

Observatio CXXXII. D. Joh. Conradi Brunneri[16]

Etsi experimentis luculentis negotium jam olim confecisse, et ingeniosam quorundam de usu Pancreatis sententiam satis superque refutasse, probabilemque aliam, eamque experientiae et veritati magis consentaneam inde elicuisse videri poteram; dantur tamen et qui de experimentorum meorum certitudine dubitant et qui decantatam bilis cum succo pancreatico effervescentiam subinde in suis scriptis crepant et a carie revocant. Multa laudabiliter inventa tempore interciderunt iterum, seu minus culta a posteris, seu studio et opera aliorum sepulta et oblivioni tradita, quae tamen nesse magni referret. Ne eadem fata experirentur, quae olim magno studio exantlavi circa pancreas experimenta neve veritas, quam eniti conabar, in ipso ortu iterum occideret, laboranti manus porrigere et dicta experimenta novis suffulcire mearum partium esse existimavi, ne penderent animis diutius alii, aut ego verba dedisse et publico imposuisse viderer; eoque magis, quod neminem novi, qui eadem et cum successu imitando me a falsitatis (quam impingere mihi conati fuerunt nonnulli) suspicione vindicarit, et rem extra omnem dubitationis aleam, etiam apud alios collocarit, quod tamen sequens experimentum haut obscure praestiturum confido

Though I could believe to have finished my duty and refused more than necessary the ingenious view of some people about the function of pancreas and to have developed an other view, more acceptable and consistent with truth and experiment, there are yet those who doubt the reliability of my experiments and preach again and again in their writings the outworn "effervescence of the bile with the pancreatic juice" and would commit it to oblivion (decay). Many a famed discovery perishes again with time, either because little attention is paid to it by posterity or buried by the scientific endeavors and exertions of others, and yet it would be highly important to know it. That the same fate should not befall the experiments on the pancreas which I once pursued with zealous efforts, and that the truth I sought to expound should not perish with its beginning, I thought it my duty to reach out my hand to it in its distress and to support the experiment mentioned with new ones so that others should not be left in doubt, and that I did not give the impression of having uttered only empty words, and the more so because I know no-one who, by imitating the same with success, could free me from suspicion of falsehood – which some have dared to me – and put the matter above all doubt and will, as I firmly believe, confirm the following experiment.

We take Brunner's description of this experiment as the basis and primary source of our study. This gives us the finest opportunity, by means of what is essentially important, to give our readers a glimpse of the work-place and humanly fascinating mode of creation of one of our greatest Swiss researchers.

---

[16] De Experimentis circa Pancreas novis confirmatis. Miscellanea curiosa sive Ephemeridum Medico-Physicarum German. Ann. VII, 1689, p. 243.

Brunner's experiment of 1685

Now we observe the investigator in his operative procedure, reminding ourselves that this master of his subject made the following experiment over 250 years ago. He says:[17]

Die VI. octobr. 1685 molossum apte ligavi et supra mensam ita composui, ut dextrum lypochondrium commode occurreret secanti. Resectis forfice pilis, cultrum iuxta limbum costarum notharum adegi fortiter, et vulnus congruae magnitudinis excitavi. E patefacto ita abdomine pancreas auspicato emicuit, quod dextre prehensum digitis per vulnus prolicui, et in apricum produxi floridum atque prolixum: quod dum praestiti diligenter cavi, aliorum ministẹrio, ne ventriculus aut intestina prorumperent, graviori utique patientis noxa. Partem inferiorem pancreatis omento undique annexam separavi, et arteriae ramum, ejus extremitatem subeuntum filo constrictum abscidi. In ductum eo loci, quo in intestinum penetrat inquisivi, et in superiorem ejus ramum primo incidi, mox utriusque conjunctionem assecutus, vulnusculum inflixi, et adaptato tubulo flatum immisi ita, ut partim in intestina mearit, partim remearit, et per ductum inferiorem evaserit eo loci, ubi arteria detruncata fuit; id quod ex bullis, quas excitavit et stridore perspicuum fuit. Quae quidem omnia notavi tanto diligentius, quanto magis omnem erroris suspicionem a me amoliri satagebam.

Abhinc ductum prope exitum arcte ligavi, superioremque primo ejus ramum detruncavi et ablata portione decurtavi studio, nec deinceps excusso, quod alias contigit, vinculo iterum coalescere posset: modo inferiorem quoque una cum substantia pancreatis (unde secundarius lateralis et exilis ductus ad meatum bilis ducit, vide Icon. lit. k.k.k.k.k.).

On 6 October 1685, I properly tied up a hound and so placed him on the table that the right hypochondrium lay convenient for incision. I cut off the hair with a scissors, inserted the knife forcibly at the margin of the false ribs and made a wound of the appropriate size. Fortunately, the pancreas at once glistened from the opened abdomen, I seized it cleverly with my fingers, drew it out through the wound and brought it to the light, fully developed and long and wide. While doing so, I took great care with the help of an assistant not to bring out the stomach or bowel to the greater harm of the patient.

The lower part of the pancreas, avery where attached to the omentum, I left free and ligated its arterial branch, which ran under its end, with a thread and cut it. I then sought the canal, where it enters the intestine, and first cut its branch in the upper part and then reached the place where the two join. I made a small wound, passed a cannula and blow into it so that the air partly entered the bowel, partly returned and escaped through the lower part of the canal where the artery was divided from the trunk. This was manifested by the produced bubbles and hissing.

I drew all this the more carefully because it was my endeavor to dispel any suspicion of error. – Then I firmly tied the canal at its exit and first divided the upper part of its branch from the trunk, removed a portion and shortened it considerably, so that it could not grow together again later after the repulsion of the ligature, as other-

[17] p. 243/244.

Partem superiorem pancreatis rescindere tum intestini cum eo coalitus, tum vasorum sanguiferorum frequentia, tum locus ibi reconditur remotior, quam ut cultro attingi queat, vetant; nec opus est. Ratus igitur omne pancreaticum intestinis commercium ademptum et commeatus viam interclusam esse partes saucias adipe porcino liquefacto calide perfusas unxi, et abdomini reddidi, quantum quidem potui delicatissime: vulnus rite consui, et eodem unguine perfudi: canem tandem vinculis solutum missum feci.

wise always happens. Then (I divided) also the lower part together with the substance of the pancreas, from which a secondary, lateral and insignificant duct leads to the bileduct (see figure, latters k.k.k.).
Removal of the upper part of the pancreas is made impossible by the internal connexions with the bowel, for the frequency of blood-containing vessels and the difficulty of access to the place where it is concealed are too remote to be reached with the knife. Nor is it necessary.
I could therefore assure myself that every connexion of the pancreas with the bowel was caught hold of and the junctional path interrupted; I now poured warm fluid lard over the wound area, rubbed it in and replaced it as carefully as possible in the abdomen. I sewed up the wound and poured the same ointment over it. Finally, I loosened the dog's bonds and set him free.

To make the nature and extent of Brunner's operation on the pancreas quite clear, we recapitulate it here briefly:

The caudal portion was freed from the omentum and removed. The duodenal portion was left because of the difficulties of extirpation. The inferior ramus of the pancreatic duct was removed together with the caudal portion. On the other hand, the superior ramus was left, but ligated near its end, sectioned and shortened by resection.

Thus, Brunner had attained his objective in this operation: namely, complete interruption of the junctional path of the pancreatic juice with the duodenum. He thus produced a complete elimination of the excretory portion of the pancreatic secretion. The resection of the upper branch of the excretory ducts assured him that the two duct-ends could; not reunite (as in previous experiments).

What reader of this detailed exposition can fail to consider Brunner's operative procedure astounding? How much more amazed must his assistants and surgeons have been as they watched their master operating, full of wonder. Brunner himself reports how "the surgeons, who willingly gave me a hand, looked on in wonderment as if absorbing the procedure with their eyes." *(intuentibus et rem quasi oculis usurpantibus, qui manus mihi commodarunt Chirurgis.)*

Brunner's Report[18]

As for the subsequent behavior of the dog released after his pancreatectomy, we read that he eagerly licked his wound and ran out into the open air. As an anatomist, Brunner meanwhile considered the extirpated part of the pancreas; it was "seven inches long and one and a half wide." When the dog was recaptured after two or three hours, having great exertion passed hard, lumpy and compact masses of excreta", he was still well for the whole day; but "in the evening he vomited blackish lumps, mixed with other stomach contents."

There now follow the reports that Brunner made in the form of a diary, constituting a regular case-history of the postoperative course:

Die VII. Octobris in aream domus procurrit, urinam redditurus, et insignem terrae tractum inundavit: redux lac aqua temperatum comedit: adipe porcino vulnus mane ac vesperi calide perfudi, et reliquam curam, de diaeta solicitus, cani commisi. Circa tertiam pomeridianam vomuit biliosa: noctu nihil comedit: nexus aliquot vulneris pro effluvio puris solvi.
Die VIII. Octobris vulnus curiose deligavi et nihil omisi eorum, quae ad experimenti successum facerent: nihil ciborum admisit, sed sitibundus bibit aquam: vomuit liquida flaventia; vesperi nonnihil jusculi sorbillavit.
Die IX. Octobris mane satis compositum inveni; scybala compacta durissima, muco tenaci incrustata magna vi et contentione excrevit: appetitus gliscebat, jusculum carnis frigidum (calida enim plerumque aversantur), abhinc pulticulam ex lacte et farina, quales tenellulis nostris in cunis offerimus, comedit; noctu esuriit et cibum sollicitavit; concessi viscerum vituli-

On 7 October, he ran into the courtyard to urinate and watered a considerable area of ground. Back again, he took in water mixed with milk. – I smeared the wound with warm lard morning and evening, leaving the rest of the nursing care to the dog, while I only looked after his diet. About 3 in the afternoon he vomited bile, in the night he ate nothing. I undid some of the stitches to let the pus out.
On 8 October I bandaged the wound carefully and neglected nothing that was important for the success of the experiment. He took no food at all, but drank water thirstily; he vomited yellow fluid, in the evening he lapped up some soup.
On 9 October, in the morning, I found him in fairly good condition; he passed compact, very hard excreta, covered with a very sticky layer of mucus, which he evacuated with much struggle and effort. His appetite improved; he ate cold meat-soup (he usually refused warm food) and then a mash of

[18] p. 245/246.

norum coctorum, et potus quantum sat erat; sic probe pastus quievit.
Die X. Oktobris perbelle sese habuit, famelicus cibum sollicitavit, vulnus elegans, et omnes secundi successus notas prae se tulit.
Die XI. Octobris sanus aufugit, et ad herum suum rediit: miratus is vulnus horrendum, pessime mihi imprecatus est: canem, cum per alium poposci, sese carnifici, si interfectum vellet, non medico traditurum respondit.
Per dimidium abhinc annum et quod excurrit domus custos fuit strenuus, fortis atque robustus, cursu saltuque velox, indem qui pridem, nec quicquam mutatus ab illo.

milk and flour as we give to infants in the cradle; he was hungry in the night and demanded to be fed, I allowed him cooked calve's tripe and drink until he was satisfied. So he slept well-fed.
On 10 October things went very well, he was hungry and wanted food, the wound was in good condition and showed every sign of a good outcome.
On 11 October he escaped healthily and went back to his master, who was amazed at the frightful wound and cursed me most evilly. As I had arranged for the dog to be supplied by a third party, he answered that if he ever had the dop destroyed, he would have it done by a slaughterer, not a doctor.
A half-year later and he was the watchdog of the house, brave, valiant and strong, as quick to run and jump as ever he was and completely unchanged.

In order not to spoil the connexion between Brunner's experiment and his exposition, we now add his report on the conduct of the necessary dissection in relation to the previous account.[19]

Tandem vero, ne experimenti jacturam facerem, et interiora perlustrandi voluptate privarer, omni arte et ingenio annixus fui, ut cane potirer; canicula proin cuius amore libidinosus incensus flagravit pellectum furtim mecum domum abduxi, philosophiae experimentali immolandum.

Finally, however, that I should not be cheated of my experiment, and not robbed of the pleasure of inspecting the interior, I sought with every art and guile to catch the dog in my hand. I enticed him thither with a bitch, towards which he was lasciviously inflamed, and so brought him secretely to my house in order to sacrifice him to experimental philosophy.

Canis pancreate spoliati anatome[20]

Perlustratis his oculos ad se rapuit, et rapuit merito *experimenti successus*, cuius gratia caetera acciderunt. Omentum cicatrici et hepar contiguo duodeno annexum fuit.

Anatomy of the pancreatectomized dog

. . . when I had surveyed this (namely, the situs viscerum) I turned my gaze, as may easily be understood, on the *result of the experiment*, through which cause the rest had happened.

[19] p. 246/248.

[20] We omit a paragraph from Brunner's original draft about some experiments to do with slaughter which is not of interest to our theme.

The omentum was attached to the scar and the liver to the duodenum.

Pars inferior pancreatis, quam caudam eius appellare liceat, plane *defuit*, vide lit. c.c.c.c., quippe resectus olim: *superior* autem *emarcuit et exaruit*, nonnisi (quod mirum) medium digitum longa, vix minimum seu auricularem *lata*, et calamum meum, quo hac exaro crassa; lit. d.d.d.d., caeterum *indurata* et *grandinosa* ceu olim quoque in experimentorum meorum tertio annotavi. Osculum ductus pancreatici stylum ex intestino ad transversi digiti distantiam admisit, lit. f. (scilicet ante ligaturam in experimento olim factam *ubi sani nonnihil nucis juglandis magnitudine* superfuit: lit. e.e.e.) ulterius nec stylum nec flatum adigere potui. *Ductum* investigavi in arido, seu potius pancreatis cadavere; *caecum* autem inveni, induratum, *solito crassiorem et impervium*, lit. g.g.g.g. praesertim eo in loco, ubi ligatura olim facta fuit; callus etenim firmissimus ibidem ferrum pene elusit, lit. h. Singula haec quum monstrari melius quam describi queant, rem emnem icone ante oculos posuisse juvabit.[21]

The *lower part of the pancreas*, which one may call its tail, *was entirely absent* (see letters c.c.c.), as it had at one time been amputated. The *upper part* however was *wasted and withered*, curiously only the length of the middle finger, barely the with of the little (ear-) finger, and as thick as the penholder with which I write this (letters d.d.d.), and otherwise *hardened and granular*, as I had noted earlier in the third of my experiments. –
The orifice of the pancreatic duct admitted a probe from the intestine to a distance of a fingerbreadth (letter f.), namely, from the ligature made at the earlier experiment to the place where *something healthy the size of a walnut* was present (letters e.e.e.) and I could not introduce either probe or air-bubble further. I sought to trace the *Ductus pancreatis* in the dried-up piece or better in the cadaver of the pancreas, and found it however blind and hardened, unusually thick and impenetrable (letters g.g.g.) especially at the place where the ligature was formerly made. A very firm callus almost split the knife (letter h.). As, however, these details can be better shown in picture than described, it is useful to present the whole subject pictorially.

... Vesica turgida fuit et lotio distenta, etsi paulo ante obitum hanc exonerarit, rutilabat quoque impense. In hepate nihil vitii apparuit, neque in liene; vesicula fellis naturalis fuit.

. . . The bladder was distended and tense with urine, although the dog had relieved itself shortly before his end. There was nothing amiss in the liver, nor in the spleen. The gallbladder was normal . . . (See our comments regarding the extent of the operation on pages 116/117).

[21] We omit some parts of the dissection report which are not relevant to our study.

Brunner as unconscious discoverer of the more important symptoms of diabetes.

From the viewpoint of the clinical phenomena of diabetes, we now group the symptoms described by Brunner into three main groups of diabetic symptoms, viz. polydipsia, polyuria and polyphagia, thus providing, with unexceptionable and compulsive clarity, a consistent picture of the typical symptom-complex of diabetes.

As the patient, in most cases, is particularly alarmed by the increased thirst at the beginning of his illness, and the doctor is at once inclined to suspect diabetes, we were struck by the immoderate thirst and the resultant polyuria shown in the behavior of all Brunner's experimental animals. There also emerged in the pancreatectomized dogs (as in diabetics) increased hunger, and with this polyphagia, in the closest connexion with the elimination of pancreatic function.

For the sake of thoroughness, we cite again in this context all those places in Brunner's writings[22] which argue most plainly for these three main symptoms:

1. Polydipsie	
1. sitiit, ex rivulo per oppidum decurrente bibit *impense.*[23]	he was thirsty and drank *immoderately* from the brook flowing through the town
2. sitiit, bibitque oblatam lacte temperatam *avide.*	he was thirsty and *eagerly* drank porridge made with milk.[23]
3. *sitibundus* bibit aquam.	*Thirsty*, he drank water.
2. Polyurie	
4. urinam reddidit durante et post experimentum.	he urinated during the experiment and after the same
5. in aream domus procurrit, urinam redditurus, et *insignem* terrae tractum inundavit.	he ran into the courtyard to urinate and watered a *considerable* area of ground.
6. vesica *turgida* fuit et lotio distenta, etsi paulo ante obitum hanc exonerarit.	The bladder was *distended* and tense with urine, although the dog had relieved itself shortly before his end.
3. Polyphagie	
7. panem, carnes aliaque edulia *devoravit avide.*	he *avidly devoured* bread, meat and other edibles.

[22] From: Experimenta nova Pancreas, 1683: 1. p. 38 experimentum VI. 2. p. 56 experimentum VII. 4. p. 37 experimentum VI. 7. and 8. p. 24 experimentum IV. 9. and 10. p. 38 experimentum VI. 11. and 12. p. 39 experimentum VI. 13. p. 41 experimentum VI. From: De Experimentis novis confirmatis, 1689: 3. 5. 14. p. 245. 6. p. 248.

[23] Italics ours, also italic passages in No. 2–14.

8. oblata *quaevis avide devoravit*, pultes, panem, carnes, ossa aliaque.	*He ate greedily whatever he was thrown*, thick porridge, bread, meat, bones and other things
9. comedit lac cum pulticula avenacea . . . vesperi *iterum* comedit.	he ate milk with oatmeal porridge . . . in the evening he ate *again*
10. dedi panis frustula aliquot, quae *avide devoravit*.	I gave the dog some breadcrusts which he *devoured avidly*
11. in prandio comedit panem, carnes aliaque edulia.	at breakfast he ate bread, meat and other edibles
12. . . . *noctu itidem* ossa dentibus confregit ac devoravit.	. . . he likewise gnawed bones in the night and *devoured* them
13. . . . *magis famelicus* exstitit atque *vorax*, gallinas venatus, earum *aliquot* praeda captas *devoravit*.	. . . he became *hungrier* and *greedier* and chased hens, of which he *devoured* several as his booty
14. nihil ciborum admisit, sed *sitibundus bibit* aquam . . . vesperi nonnihil jusculi sorbillavit . . . *appetitus gliscebat*, jusculum carnis frigidum, abhinc pulticulum ex lacte et farina . . . comedit; noctu *esuriit* et cibum sollicitavit; concessi viscerum vitulinorum coctorum, et potus quantum sat erat; . . .	at first he took no food at all, but drank water *thirstily* . . . in the evening he lapped up some soup . . . his *appetite improved;* he ate cold meat-soup, and then a mash of milk and flour, in the night he was *hungry again* and demanded food, II allowed him cooked calf's tripe and drink until he was satisfied.

The reader of this protocol, which could be very easily supplemented by many similar reports to the same effect, now comes unhesitatingly to the same perception as Wolf-Heidegger in 1939 on the occasion of a thorough revision of Brunner's writings for biographic purposes, namely, that Brunner, even if unconsciously, was the true discoverer of the pathologic-physiologic connexion in which these symptoms form the bridge between diabetes and the pancreas.

A critical assessment of Brunner's investigations

It thus emerges from his earlier and later studies that Brunner had described important symptoms of diabetes.

Why then, we ask, having compiled all these important symptoms, did not Brunner think of the diagnosis of 'diabetes'? Diabetes was certainly known in antiquity, and Brunner, as a learned researcher and physician, knew this. Galen and his school had already seen the existence of this disease as an emerging cachexia caused by enormous amounts of urine.[24]

---

[24] E. Grafe 'Diabetes mellitus' in 'Neue Deutsche Klinik', 1928, Vol. II. p. 640 and 'Lehrbuch der Inneren Medizin', 1936, Vol. II. p. 134.

In his pancreatectomized dogs, Brunner had of course been unable to demonstrate a cachexia, although he did observe the polyuria; but, remarkably, this in itself had not led him to postulate a diabetes. And yet, in that very century, new evidence on diabetes had become known thanks to the researches of Thomas Willis (1674) (establishment of two categories of diabetic phenomena: diabetes mellitus and diabetes insipidus).[25]

In Brunner's justification it must be stressed that he represented the symptom-complex[26] he had discovered only in the time-span of his operation. He must have regarded the polydipsia, polyuria and polyphagia as temporary consequences of the operation, as they disappeared; and as his experimental animals recovered after a certain period the clinical picture faded until no visible symptoms at all were any longer present. Thus, the dogs made a complete recovery.

What, then, became of his experimental animals? He himself reports in many places that after the lapse of a certain period they returned to their normal conditions of life, just as before the operation. We extract some passages from earlier reports, which state:[27]

1. . . . *ut antea*, comedit, bibit, excrementa rite constituta dejecit, urinam reddidit: reliqua vitae munia vegete obiit; excurrit alacris, et ut verbo dicam *nihil novi nec immutati* animadvertere locuit.	. . . *as before,* he ate, drank, passed normally formed stools and passed urine; he pursued his other habits briskly and, in a word, *nothing new or in any way changed* could be observed.
2. Interea sensim convaluit canis, . . . comedit, bibit, alvi faeces et urinam, *ut antea* excrevit, reliquas caeterum vitae functiones *uti prior* rite obiit.	In the meantime the dog became completely well again . . . he ate, drank and passed stools and urine *just as before,* for the rest he pursued his former habits *just as usual.*
3. Postridie appetitus melior et ipse canis fuit vegetior, tandem vorax, mordax, cursu ac saltu velox, alios canes adortus plerumque victor recessit. *ὅλως ίε εἰπεῖν*, vitae functiones *ut antea obiit.*	The next day his appetite was better again and the dog himself livelier; at last he became greedy and snappish, quick to run and jump, attacked other dogs and usually returned the victor. To put it briefly, he resumed his habits as *before.*

[25] In 'Handwörterbuch der gesamten Medizin', 1891, Vol. II, p. 1012.

[26] Which did not include cachexia!

[27] From: Experimenta nova circa Pancreas, 1683. 1. p. 12/13 exper. I. 2. p. 14/15 exper II. 3. p. 18 exper III. 4. Aus: Experimentis circa Pancreas novis Confirmatis, p. 246, 1689.

Or we may recall the postoperative behavior of the pancreatectomized dog in the reported experiment of 1685, thoroughly reported above, in which we read:

4. . . . on the 6th day "he escaped healthily and went back to his master . . . A half-year later and he was the watchdog of the house, brave, valiant and strong, as quick to run and jump *as ever he was and completely unchanged*".

The question now arises: why did Brunner's pancreatectomized animals recover and remain alive, and why, on the other hand, did those of later experimental physiologists mostly perish? To anticipate briefly: In Brunner's experimental animals there occurred a regeneration of the residual pancreas left behind at operation, especially as regards its internal secretory portions, which was not the case with the experimental animals of the later physiologists in which the pancreas was totally extirpated (we return to this in detail later).

Apart from amazement at the fact that a 17th century physician found it all possible to undertake a major operation of this kind with what must now strike us strangely primitive instruments, yet without subsequent signs of peritonitis that would more or less herald a fatal outcome, it is obvious that the cause of death did not arise from possible external operative complications, as briefly mentioned, but was essentially unrelated to operative considerations.

Brunner was aware that the certain elimination of all pancreatic functions (obviously he was acquainted only with the excretory component of the pancreas) could only be obtained by total extirpation. Though he did not achieve this total extirpation, he nevertheless succeeded in completely interrupting the entry of the pancreatic juice into the duodenum (see Brunner's operative procedure, pp. 116/117).

Brunner therefore did only a partial extirpation, as the above report with his own drawings makes clear. This type of operative procedure leads us to two different conclusions: on the one hand, the fact of the appearance of diabetic symptoms as a consequence of the *extirpation;* on the other hand, the possibility of regeneration as a consequence of *only partial* extirpation.

The diabetic symptoms in the dogs must primarily have arisen after extirpation of the pancreas, as Brunner in his studies and we ourselves in the experiment reproduced above concluded (cf.

---

[28] See G. Wolf-Heidegger 'Zur Genese der Langerhansschen Inseln des Pankreas'. 1936.

p. 6, where that part of the pancreas arising from the dorsal *Anlage* material was totally extirpated, whereas a residual organ remained from the derivative of the ventral rudiment).

According to embryologic studies[28], the caudal part derived from the dorsal *Anlage* contains a profusion of islet cells, whereas the duodenal portion arising from the ventral *Anlage* is relatively poor in endocrine tissue. If, then, in Brunner's extirpations of the tail portion with its rich content of islet tissue, its function as a distributor of insulin comes to a halt, while the residual head portion has only few islet cells, primary diabetic phenomena must next appear. In fact, we know, from the experimental literature[29] about the course and extent of experimental pancreatic tissue suffice to render the developing diabetes mild and abortive. Even fragments of a tenth to a twentieth of the pancreas suffice to bring about such a "Sandmeyer diabetes", which exhibits a rapid tendency to recovery.

However, the small number of islet cells in the residual portion means that complete regulation of carbohydrate metabolism is not obtained, so that symptoms of diabetes must develop, if only at first.

We must further ask how it is that the dog which has initially developed a diabetic disorder can later completely lose these symptoms. How is its complete recovery at all possible when the very part of the pancreas that regulates carbohydrate metabolism is lacking? From our knowledge of the *regenerative capacity of the pancreatic tissue*[30], we may adduce the following:

The small amount of islet tissue in that small healthy portion[31],

---

[29] Especially E. Grafe 'Diabetes mellitus' in 'Neue deutsche Klinik'. 1928. Vol. II. p. 637.

[30] As we now know, regeneration of the endocrine part of the pancreas is quite possible, postulating a certain period (see *inter alia* the work of Martinotti 1888, Ukai 1926, Grauer 1926, Shaw and Latimer 1926, Cameron 1926, Tschassownikow 1928, Canger 1938).

According to Kyrle (1908) and Weichselbaum (1909), even both types of tissue, *parenchyma and islets, may regenerate.* Initially, a new and similar tissue develops from its own current cellstock, but if this source is inadequate, the small excretory ducts are called on to collaborate in the formation of new tissue. Also, according to Laguesse (1927), who speaks of a *balancement* of both types of tissue and hence the possibility of a reciprocal conversion of acini into islets and conversely, a new-formation of islets from the epithelium of the small excretory ducts can take place.

[31] See p. 121 of our study

which was found to be of walnut size on dissection, must have hypertrophied and taken the place of the exocrine parenchyma[32] that perished as a result of the tying of the duct. After duct ligature, islet hypertrophy is even reinforced, as shown by the classical ligature experiment of Banting and Best[33], to whose experimental pattern Brunner's procedure strictly conforms as regards the portion of pancreas left behind.

Finally, we would like to establish: In the dogs pancreatectomized by Brunner, diabetic phenomena developed initially despite an only partial extirpation. Because fragments of pancreatic tissue were left behind at operation, regeneration of islet cells was possible, and because of this the initially developing diabetic symptoms later disappeared. Hence, in our opinion this type of diabetes, first produced by Brunner, is most suitably designated as *temporary experimental diabetes.*

Although Brunner, because of the reasons and circumstances given above, did not and even could not arrive at a diagnosis of diabetes, it is our desire that this great anatomist and physician – to whom we owe so much valuable knowledge in the field of anatomy and physiology – should be accorded the glorious place in diabetic research that he deserves.

With due regard for the efforts and achievements of his predecessors, Brunner introduced his work, *Experimenta nova circa Pancreas,* with Seneca's words: *Multum egerunt, qui ante nos fuerunt.* We would end our discussion of the first description of the symptoms of experimental pancreatic diabetes with the samewords and thereby remember the exemplary researcher and human being, Johann Conrad Brunner: *Multum egerunt, qui ante nos fuerunt.*

Summary

By means of reports by the Swiss, Johann Conrad Brunner (1653–1727) on his experimental extirpation of the pancreas in

[32] A compensatory enlargement and increase of the Langerhans' islets can also occur in man. We refer here to a case observed by Christlieb (1933); in a 69-year-old woman the absence of the pancreatic tail and one of the sections appended to the body was established. In the existing part of the pancreas I found considerable multiplication and enlargement of the islets, which must be interpreted as a hypertrophy.

[33] (Toronto, 1921).

dogs, it is shown that, some 200 years before v. Mering and Minkowski, Brunner had described the most important clinical features of experimental pancreatic diabetes in his experimental animals in a clear and objective fashion.

References[34]

Aepli, J. M.: Dr. Johann Conrad Brunner, Arch. gemeinnützig. phys. und med. Kenntn. I, 2, Zürich 1787.

Banting, F. G. and Best, C. H.: Journal of labor, and clin. med. 7, 1922.

Biest, C. H.: Die innere Sekretion des Pankreas, in: Die Drüsen mit innerer Sekretion. Wien–Leipzig 1937. (Übersetzung von Glandular Physiology and Therapy).

Bonet, Th.: Sepulchretum sive anatomia practica. S. 626, 1679.

Brunner, C.: Dr. Johannes Conrad Brunner, in Virchow und v. Holtzendorff. Gemeinverst. Vorträge, N.F. Ser. 3, 62, Hamburg 1888.

Brunner, C. und v. Muralt, W.: Aus den Briefen hervorragender Schweizer Ärzte des 17. Jhdts., Schwabe, Basel 1919.

Brunner, J. C.: Experimenta circa Pancreas, accedit Diatribe de Lympha et genuino pancreatis usu, Amstelodaemi 1683.

– De Experimentis circa Pancreas novis confirmatis.Miscellanea curiosa sive Ephemeridum Medico – Physicarum German. Acad. imp. Leopold Natur. Curios. Dec. II. Annus VI 1688, S.243–248. Norimbergae 1689.

– Glandulae duodeni seu pancreas secundarium, Frankfurt–Heidelberg 1715.

Cameron, G. R.: Journal of Pathol. and Bacteriol. 29, 1926, ibid. 30, 1927.

Canger, G.: Arch. ital. Chir. 51, S. 41–53, 1938.

Christlieb: Virchows Arch. f. path. Anat. Bd. 289, S. 244–246, 1933.

Galen: zitiert in Schirmer, M. A. und Grafe, E.

Graaf, Regner de: zitiert in Schirmer, M. A.

Grafe, E.: Pankreasdiabetes in Handbuch der inneren Medizin, Bd. II, S. 134. J. Springer Berlin, 1936/37.

– Diabetes mellitus, in Neue Deutsche Klinik, Bd. II, S. 631 u. 640, Urban und Schwarzenberg, Berlin und Wien, 1928.

Grauer, Th.: Amer. Journal of Anat., 38, S.233–253, 1926.

Hippokrates: zitiert in Schirmer, M. A.

Kyrle, J.: Zentralbl. f. Physiologie Bd. 21, 1907.

– Archiv f. mikr. Anat. und Entwicklungsgesch. Bd. 72, S. 141, 1908.

Kyrle, J. und Weichselbaum, A.: Archiv f. mikr. Anat. Bd. 74, S. 223, 1908.

[34] After the preparation of the present study, we obtained from a review of the literature in *Gesnerus* (Bd. 1, Heft 2, 1944) knowledge from an american study on Brunner's experiments on the pancreas (R. H. Major: Johann Conrad Brunner and his experiments on the pancreas. Annals of Medical History 3, 91–100, 1941). Unfortunately, despite every endeavor, it was impossible to obtain this article.

Laguesse, E.: Journal physiol. et pathol. gén. 1. Jan. 1911. Bull. d'histol. appliquée 4, 1927.
ferner zitiert in Biedl. A. Handwörterbuch der Nat.-Wissenschaften, 2. Aufl. Bd VIII, S. 1237. Fischer Jean, 1933.
ferner zitiert in Herxheimer, G. und Carpentier, E. Beitr. path. Anat. Bd. 76, 1927.
Latiner, E. O.: siehe Shaw, J. W. und Latimer, E. O.
Martinotti, G.: Giornale della R. Academia di Medicina di Torino Anno LI, Vol. 36, S. 348 ff. 1888. Ibidem S. 383 ff.
v. Mering, J. und Minkowski, O.: Arch. f. exp. Pathol. und Pharmakol. Br. 26, S. 371, 1889.
Minkowski, O.: Berliner klin. Wchschr. No. 54, 1924. Arch. f. exp. Pathol. und Pharmakol. Bd. 31, 1893.
Scheuchzer, J. J.: Bibliotheca Helvetica, Zürich, 1733.
Schirmer, M. A.: Beitrag zur Geschichte und Anatomie des Pankreas, Inauguraldissertation Basel, 1893.
Shaw, J. W. und Latimer, E. O.: Amer. Journ. of physiology, Bd. 76, S. 49–53, 1926.
Swalwe: zitiert in Schirmer, M. A.
Sylvius: zitiert in Brunner, C.
Tschassownikow, N.: Anat. Anz. 65, S. 17–27, 1928.
Ukai, S.: Morphologie und Biologie des Pankreas.
I. Mttlg. allg. Pathol., pathol. Anat. Japan, 3, S. 1–25, 1926
II.ibidem S. 27–64, 1926
III. ibidem S. 65–87, 1926
IV. ibidem S. 89–170, 1926
V. ibidem S. 173–188, 1926.
Vesalius: zitiert in Schirmer, M. A.
Vesling: zitiert in Schirmer, M. A.
Weichselbaum, A.: siehe Kyrle, J. und Weichselbaum, A.
Willis, Th.: zitiert in Villaret, A. Handwörterbuch der ges. Med. Bd. II, S. 1012. Stuttgart, 1891.
Wirsung: zitiert in Schirmer, M. A.
Wolf-Heidegger, G.: Zur Genese der Langerhans'schen Inseln des Pankreas, Med. Diss. Bonn 1936.
– Johann Conrad Brunner, in: Große Schweizer Forscher, S. 84/85, Atlantis-Verlag Zürich, 1939.

in: *Gesnerus 2 (1945) 109–130.*

John Rollo

by Alexander Marble

In 1797 there was published in England a book entitled in part, *An Account of Two Cases of the Diabetes Mellitus.* In it John Rollo, M.D., a surgeon of the Royal Artillery, recorded in detail his observations regarding the course of diabetes in two patients treated by means of a special diet. As a result, his methods of treatment and ideas regarding the origin of diabetes were widely discussed in England and on the Continent with acceptance by some and rejection by others. Rollo has become known as the first, or certainly one of the first, to plan definite diets for diabetic patients.

Rollo was born in Scotland and received his medical education at Edinburgh. He became a surgeon in the English army in 1776 and served in the West Indies, being stationed on the island of St. Lucia in 1778 and 1779 and on Barbados in 1791. He appears to have been a man of inquiring mind with both talent and energy. As a military physician, his interest in disease was general. His account entitled *Observations on the Diseases in the Army on St. Lucia* was published in 1781. This was followed in 1785 by *Remarks on the Disease lately described by Dr. Hendy* (that form of elephantiasis so common as to be known as "Barbados leg") and in 1786 by *Observations on the Acute Dysentery.* He was advanced to the grade of Surgeon-General in 1794. In 1801 there appeared his *Short Account of the Royal Artillery Hospital at Woolwich* and in 1804 a *Medical Report on Cases of Inoculation* in which he supported the views of Jenner. Rollo died in 1809 at Woolwich, the seat of the Royal Artillery Academy and now a borough of London [1].

A second edition of the book on diabetes was published in 1798 and a third in 1806. Rollo was frequently consulted regarding cases of diabetes and his book carried notes and communications regarding patients seen by other physicians who had applied his method of treatment and had written to him regarding the results. In his work Rollo had the cooperation of William

Cruickshank, artillery surgeon, chemist and apothecary, who carried out studies on the quantity and nature of the suger in urine.

Rollo's account of the circumcances under which he became interested in the treatment of diabetes reads in part as follows: [2]

"In the year 1777 . . . I saw a case of the Diabetes Mellitus in a weaver at Edinburgh. He had been at least four months in the Royal Infirmary without having derived any advantage, and was chiedy under the care of the late Dr. Hope, Professor of Botany. When the patient was discharged, a Mr. Johnstone, then a Student of Physic, and myself, detained him a few days, and paid his expenses, in order to bleed him, and obtain some of his urine, so as to ascertain the appearances and spontaneous changes. I well remember that the blood and urine exhibited the appearances discribed by Dr. Dobson; but the papers, and a portion of the saccharine extract which I carried with me abroad, were lost in the hurricane at Barbados in 1789."

"From that period I had not met with a case of Diabetes, although I had observed an extensive range of disease in America, the West Indies, and in England, until 1796."

"Captain Meredith, of the Royal Artillery, being an acquaintance. I had seen him very frequently, previous to his going on camp duty in 1794, but then he had no disease; however, he always had impressed me, from his being a large corpulent person, with the idea that he was not unlikely to fall into disease. (*Editor: Another instance of Rollo's clinical acuteness.*)"

"On the 12th of June, 1796, he visited me, and though I was at once struck with the diminution of his size, yet, at the same time, the colour of his face being ruddy, I received no impression, otherwise than of his being in health: a moment's conversation, however, convinced me of the contrary . . . . "

"He complained of great thirst and a keenness of appetite; his skin was hot, dry and parched; and his pulse small and quick. He told me his complaints had been attributed to an old disease, and a liver affection. The thirst, dry skin, and quick pulse, marking a febrile state, depending probably on some local circumstance, and connecting these with the keenness of appetite, Diabetes immediately suggested itself to me. I enquired into the state of his urine, which I found in quantity and colour to be characteristic of the disease; and was at the same time much surprised, that for the two or three months he had been under the care of a Physician and Surgeon, the circumstance of the increased urine had not been known to them. The patient told me, as he drank so much, the quantity of urine had appeared to him a necessary consequence; and of course never having been asked about it, he gave no information. I directed him to keep the urine he next passed, and, on examination, it was found to be sweet; in consequence of which the disease became sufficiently ascertained."

At another point in the case history, Rollo states that Captain Meredith was 34 years of age and was 71 3/4 inches tall. At the time of beginning of the special treatment, the symptoms of diabetes had been present seven months or more and his weight had fallen from 232 to 162 pounds.

A view held by some at that time was that diabetes was a primary affection of the kidneys. However, Rollo developed the idea that the disease was "a primary and peculiar affection" of the stomach in which, due to some morbid changes in "the natural powers of digestion and assimilation," sugar or saccharine material was formed in that organ, chiefly from vegetable matter. It was on this basis that he advocated the use of an animal diet together with certain medication designed to quiet the overactive stomach and to diminish the appetite. Following initial bloodlettings, Rollo's treatment of Captain Meredith was as follows:

"1st. The diet to consist of animal food principally, and to be thus regulated:

Breakfast. One and a half pint of milk and half a pint of lime-water, mixed together; and bread and butter.

Noon. Plain blood-puddings, made of blood and suet only.

Dinner. Game, or old meats, which have been long kept; and as far as the stomach may bear, fat and rancid old meats, as pork. To eat in moderation.

Supper. The same as breakfast."

"2dly. A drachm of kali sulphuratum to be dissolved in four quarts of water which has been boiled, and to be used for daily drink.

No other article whatever, either eatable or drinkable, to be allowed, than what has been stated."

"3dly. The skin to be annointed with hog's lard every morning. Flannel to be worn next the skin. The gentlest exercise to be only permitted; but confinement to be preferred."

"4thly. A draught at bed-time of twenty drops of tartarized antimonial wine and twenty-five of tincture of opium; and the quantities to be gradually increased. In reserve, as substances diminishing action, tobacco and foxglove."

"5thly. An ulceration, about the size of half a crown, to be produced and maintained externally, and immediately opposite to each kidney. And,

"6thly. A pill of equal parts aloes and soap, to keep the bowels regularly open."

Captain Meredith began the above treatment on Oct. 19, 1796. Two days later the quantity of urine passed in twenty-four hours had fallen from seven or eight quarts to six quarts. By November 1 the quantity did not exceed four quarts and on November 4 "he drank only three pints of water, and made only two quarts of urine, which to him and his servants (who had been in the habit of tasting his urine from curiosity) was not sweet." As time went on, the opium at bedtime was discontinued and the rubbing with hog's lard was left off. The latter was found to be a "troublesome and disagreeable" part of the treatment. Rollo decided to simplify therapy to include those features which were considered really essential: animal food, confinement with limitation of activity, and hepatized ammonia. The hepatized ammonia (ammonium sulphide) was used in place of "kali sulphuratum," originally prescribed, with the thought that it might be "a more certain and active medicine than the other on the stomach, in diminishing its action."

Captain Meredith was directed to keep notes regarding his symptoms, diet, medication and progress of his illness. He did this quite faithfully, recording his transgressions as well as his attempts at cooperation. When at times he indulged in apples, bread and beer, Rollo found it necessary "to point out in stronger language the impropriety of such deviations." By December 30 the patient was free from abnormal thirst and polyuria, was regaining some of his lost weight and felt well. Continuation of treatment with a somewhat more liberal allowance of bread in the diet was prescribed.

Rollo's second case was an unnamed "General Officer," aged 57, with symptoms of diabetes dating back at least three years. His primary disease was complicated by other conditions and he was not nearly as cooperative as Captain Meredith. He died nineteen months after first being seen, having been under Rollo's direct observation for less than two months. During the last three months of his life he had returned to an unrestricted diet including apple-pudding, tea with suger, and wine.

Rollo, with the aid of Cruickshank, carried out laboratory studies with his patients to ascertain the results of treatment and to elucidate the nature of diabetes. The fluid intake, urine output and the body weight were determined. The urine was tasted to indicate the presence of sugar and subjected to experiments before and after evaporation to determine its chemical composition and content of sugar. At the beginning of treatment when Captain Meredith was passing up to twelve quarts of urine in twenty-four hours, the following notes were made:

> "Mr. Cruickshank took 36 ounces troy weight of urine voided today, and it yielded by evaporation three ounces and one drachm of saccharine extract, of the appearance of molasses, but thicker, having nearly the consistence of wax, and somewhat tenacious. If, therefore, the whole of the day's urine had been evaporated it would have yielded about 29 ounces troy weight, an astonishing quantity to be formed and seperated form the system. By standig in the air it became moist, and of nearly the consistence, smell and appearance of treacle."
>
> "Treating some of this extract with the nitrous acid, he procured the saccarine or oxalic acid; and with a smaller proportion of the acid it produced a substance, which in resemblance, and smell, could not be distinguished from honey."

From studies on blood, Rollo and Cruickshank concluded that sugar might be present without being detectable by taste and that if two or three ounces of serum from the blood of a diabetic patient were taken at a proper time after eating, it was probable that saccharine matter might be obtained. From such studies and from the finding of normal-appearing kidneys at autopsies on diabetic individuals, Rollo argued against the idea that diabetes was primarily a renal disease. Instead, he conceived of the process as follows:

> "The serum of blood apparently containing less saccharine matter than the urine, may depend on the power of the kidneys in separating it in common with the other saline matters of the blood; but proving a new and peculiar stimulus, their action is increased, and the saccharine matter consequently separated speedily and in proportion to its formation in the stomach."

In summing up and evaluating Rollo's contributions, we find among his erroneous ideas and bizarre treatment much that was good. He conceived of diabetes as being a disease of the stomach with overactivity of that organ with the secretion of an abnormal gastric juice and the formation of sugar in the stomach chierly from foods of vegetable, as opposed to animal, origin. Hence the source of sugar formed in the stomach was to be reduced by using a diet liberal in protein and fat and restricted in carbohydrate (though milk was included provisionally under animal food). In order to quiet the stomach and reduce the appetite, drugs were given to produce anorexia and nausea. These included potassium sulphate (later ammonium sulphide), antimony, opium, tobacco and digitalis. "Fat and rancid old meats" likewise tended to discourage appetite. The end-result of Rollo's plan of treatment was an over-all restriction in calories, particularly those derived from carbohydrate. In this connection it is instructive to note that when Captain Meridith had improved and glycosuria was thought to have disappeared, Rollo in liberalizing the diet directed him to begin with the "use of cabbage, or greens of a similar nature, boiled onions, or salad without acid sauce; also mustard, horseradish, and common radish when in season."

Although Rollo's method of treatment was widely used and often enthusiastically endorsed, at least in part, by many physicians, it never gained general adoption in any country, except perhaps in England. Even there, a decline in popularity gradually took place which may be "attributed to the crudeness and imperfections in the method itself, the careless and faulty application of it by most physicians, the rebellion of patients – who generally, sooner or later, secretly or openly broke the intolerable dietary restrictions and relapsed – the failure of the method to check the severest cases, and the frequent bad results . . . . of changing diabetic patients suddenly from a mixed diet to a strict protein-fat regimen [3]." Nevertheless, Rollo's contribution to the development of knowledge regarding diabetes and its treatment was significant and has won for him lasting recognition.

References

1. Moore, N.: Sketch of John Rollo in Dictionary of National Biography, New York, Macmillan Co., 17:169–70, 1909.
2. Rollo, John: Cases of the Diabetes Mellitus, with the Results of the Trials of Certain Acids, and other Substances, in the Cure of the Lues Venerea, 2nd ed., London, T. Giller for C. Dilly, 1798.
3. Allen, Frederick M., Stillman, Edgar, and Fitz, Reginald: Total Dietary Regulation in the Treatment of Diabetes. New York, The Rockefeller Institute for Medical Research, Monograph No. 11, 1919. pages 14–20.

in: *Diabetes (1956) 325–327.*

Matthew Dobson (1735–1784). Clinical Investigator of Diabetes Mellitus

anonymous

Matthew Dobson, born in Yorkshire, was the son of a nonconformist minister and had planned at one time to follow his father's professional path [1]. When he decided upon medicine, he became a student at the University of Edinburgh; there he graduated in 1756 upon presentation of a dissertation on menstruation. Dobson commenced practice in Liverpool, served on the staff of the Liverpool Infirmary, and, in 1770, was advanced to physician, a position held for a decade until ill health forced him to retire to Bath where he died.

The uncertainty regarding Dobson's birth date is consistent with the lack of information concerning many details of his personal and public life. He has been described as a natural philosopher, an experimental physiologist, and a skilled clinical observer. *A Medical Commentary on Fixed Air* (carbon dioxide), dedicated to William Cullen, was the only subject that received monographic treatment. His experiments on physiological stress experienced by humans at critical high temperature and observations on the petrifying properties of water at Matlock were communicated through Dr. Fothergill to the Royal Society of London, of which each was a member, and were published in their *Philosophical Transactions*. Dobson's clinical studies, which included the treatment of internal hydrocephalus with large doses of mercury salts, appeared in *Medical Observations and Inquiries*, the organ of Society of Physicians in London. Dobson's most important work was his observations and experiments on patients with diabetes mellitus. He described the extraction of a sweet substance from the urine an serum of one patient, a 33-year-old male, who was afflicted with clinical diabetes mellitus. The symptoms currently recognized as characteristic included polydipsia, polyphagia, polyuria, weight loss, dry skin, and paroxysmal fever. He described five experiments and concluded with eight observations and queries. In these, he sensed the metabolic defect in discussing etiology and suggested an enhanced assimilation of nutrients by the body in treatment. The report was communicated by Dr. Fothergill; excerpts are as follows [2].

Experiment II.

Eight ounces of blood taken from the arm of this patient, exhibited, after standig a proper time, the following appearances . . . The *serum* was opaque, and much resembled common cheese whey; it was sweetish, but I thought not so sweet as the urine.

Experiment V.

Two quarts of this urine were, by a gentle heat, evaporated to dryness, under the inspection of Mr. Poole, apothecary to the hospital, and Mr. Walthall, one of the house apprentices. There remained, after the evaporation, a white cake which . . . was granulated, and broke easily between the fingers; it smelled sweet like brown sugar, neither could it, by the taste, be distinguished from sugar, except that the sweetness left a slight sense of coolness on the palate.

These experiments suggest the following:

Observations and Queries.

1. That the fluid which was separated by the kidneys of this patient, had very little of the nature or sensible qualities of urine, but contained a substance which readily passed through the vinous, acetous, and putrefactive fermentations.

3. It appears from Experiment V. that a considerable quantity of saccharine matter passed off by the kidneys, in this case of diabetes, and probably does so in every instance of this disease, where the urine has a sweet taste. From Experiment II. it further appears, that this saccharine matter was not formed in the secretory organ, but previously existed in the serum of the blood.

5. This idea of the disease, also, well explains its emaciating effects, from so large a proportion of the alimentary matter being drawn off by the kidneys, before it is perfectly assimilated, and applied to the purposes of nutrition. The *diabetes* proves, in some cases, a very rapid consumption: I have known it terminate fatally in less than five weeks. In others, it becomes a chronic complaint.

8. This idea of the nature of the *diabetes*, suggests more clearly and explicitly the method of cure. For if it is a disease of the system in general, if it is to be considered as a species of imperfect digestion and assimilation, the obvious indications of cure are, to strengthen the digestive powers, to promote a due sanguification, and establish a perfect assimilation througth the whole oeconomy.

References

[1] Williams, O. T.: Matthew Dobson, Physician to the Liverpool Infirmary, 1770–1780: One Who Extended the Confines of Knowledge, Liverpool Medicochir J 32:245–254, 1912.
[2] Dobson, M.: Experiments and Observations on the Urine in a Diabetes, Med. Obs. Inq. 5:298–316, 1776

in: *Jama 205 (1968) 108.*

Then and Now: 100 Years of Diabetes Mellitus

by HORST and JOSEPH SCHUMACHER

Summary

The authors point out that diabetes mellitus is still not much more than the glittering shell of a notion without precise and established content. As an immense number of works have been published concerning this subject, the authors attempt to make a general extensive survey of the development of present concepts of this disease. Various theories on causal mechanisms based on endocrine, humoral and central nervous processes are discussed as they were developed by scientific research during the last century.

Chapter 1 reports on the four fields which contributed to knowledge before the discovery of insulin. These fields are: physiological chemistry, physiological pathology based on experiment, pathological anatomy and endocrinology.

Chapter 2 describes the insulin era (including old insulin, Hagedorn and Best).

Chapter 3 reports on the development of newer conceptions. The aim of this work is to enable the non-specialist doctor to understand the results of modern research, including special fields such as intermediate metabolism and endocrinology, and also to help him understand the latest publications (such as discussion of the newer remedies based on the sulfonamides, pathogenesis, prophylaxis and treatment of the much-feared diabetic angiopathies, etc.).

I

"Diabetes mellitus" (DM), even today, is not much more than a glittering shell of a concept lacking precise established content. We use the name for the sake of understanding. A pretension beyond its competence makes it inevitable that the name of the disease gains a power over and beyond its task as a schematic aid, and finally leads to its schematic application to the patient himself. Especially exposed to this danger is the doctor desirous of informing himself about the treatment of "diabetes" from a "concise manual", for he will not find there the problem as actually posed by each individual case. On the other hand, the overall literature is so extensive – the last decade saw tens of thousands of publications – and therefore so contradictory that even specialists fail to assess the true worth of new paths and opinions. We are not in a position, even today, to know which of the many single discoveries will be accepted in the history of the nosology of DM as milestones on the way to the objective. Precisely because of this, a short historical survey of the development of the ambiguity of DM may be the best way of seeing this in its specificity.

The beginning of systematic research into DM may be taken as the middle of the last century with reasonable accuracy. The systematic application of biologic experiments and methods of quantitative analysis to the new "zoochemistry" had brought about an unexpected abundance of new insights into the chemical synthesis of plant and animal substances, the process of their breakdown, absorption and assimilation and their function in the living organism, which might now be fruitful in the investigation of the "enigma of mellituria". From this time on at least four parallel lines of development were followed, which, by countercriticism and suggestions, have shaped the changing picture of diabetic theory and therapy up to the arrival of the insulin era.

The following data from a larger work by the present authors aid a historic understanding of the new developments. Around 1800, DM was still rated as a disorder very seldom seen. There are reasons for assuming that most diabetics suffered intercurrent illnesses without the underlying disease being diagnosed. The description of the clinical symptoms listed, as we do today, the characteristic pruritus, the gingivitis, the loosening of the teeth, the 'malum perforans', the furunculosis, intense feelings of hunger and thirst, increasing exhaustion, disturbed potency, etc. Further, we can also register certain changes in the voice, psychological changes and numerous other symptoms, evident to the fine observation of the physicians of the time. It was known that a "sugar-like substance" could be qualitatively demonstrated in the urine. Dobson, Cullen, Rollo, Frank and Zipp inferred the presence of sugar also in the blood from the sweet taste of the saliva, sweat and even the blood itself. But attempts to demonstrate the blood-sugar chemically failed initially, for lack of appropriate methods.

Autopsies showed changes in the liver, spleen, kidneys and a particular flaccidity of the muscles, heart, etc. (Summary by A. W. v. Stosch: *Versuch einer Pathologie und Therapie des Diabetes mellitus,* Berlin 1828); the variability of the morbid anatomic findings, especially the fact that they may be completely absent even though there is urinary flux, even then gave rise to the idea that these were not to be considered as the cause but as more or less random effects of the diabetic diathesis.

As regards etiology, a distinction was made according to the custom of that time between "predisposing" and "precipitating" causes (cold, gout, scrofula, psychologic upsets, mode of life, pregnancy, etc.). According to the preferred views of the disease, the predisposition lay in the "structure", the "combination of humors" or in particular chemical or physical states of the organism.

A hereditary disposition was accepted by Rondolet, Thomas, Brisbane, Prout and Peter Frank, but not conceded by other authors as not proven. One of the most important causes was taken to be the over-acidification of the entire organism, which was therefore placed at the beginning and not the end of the disease. Haase and others, based on the physiological chemical views of the outgoing 18th century, saw the fundamental cause as a "hyperoxidation of the gastric and intestinal juices". The excess of acid produced the development of "an excessive amount of sugary matter from the vegetable nutrients", analogous to the known chemical process of the production of sugar from starch in the retort. Hufeland assigned this process to the kidneys, where sugar was produced through the action of the urine on the chyle (Journ. d. prakt. Heilk., Bd. 65, I, p. 39).

The theory of v. Stosch was also a pregnant one. He distinguished a positive and a negative factor in the autonomic nervous system. The consequences of paralysis of the negative factor, which produced "chylification" of the nutriment, would be incomplete animalization and hyperperoxidation of the chyle, which would now be excreted as "crude excremental material" by the kidneys and therefore also the occurrence in the urine of sugar that had not been transformed in the blood, as shown by subsequent wasting and cachexia. Hence the classical overproduction theory of v. Noorden and the non-utilization theory of Seegen, Minkowski and Fr. v. Müller.

The theories of a therapy for diabetes are of especial interest to the historian even, who sees in them the transformation of the hitherto valid general system of therapeutics and can observe how so many of the "external" and "naturopathic" measures applied even today go back to old concepts of a century and a half ago.

The keynote of all treatment was based on the old Hippocratic axiom that the disease was healed by its "opposite" or "contrary". The number of "enantioses" (opposites) increased during the first fifty years of the last century to correspond to the growing number of disease theories and became limitless. The older concepts preferably related to the qualitative changes and sought, for example, to compensate for the loss of "sweetness" (= the most valuable part of the nutrients) by the most nitrogen-rich nutrients and so restore the "right combination". John Rollo – who also gave diabetes mellitus its name – attributed to the diabetic a "predominantly vegetable character" on the grounds of his inability in "chylification", "sanguification" and "animalization" of the nutriment (*An account of two cases of the diabetes mellitus . . .* London 1797, p. 387 ff.) and therefore prescribed an animal diet. Aqua calcaria, charcoal and all kinds of alkalis were given to combat the "acidification". Far more important was a second therapeutic system which sought "scientifically" to correct the quantitative changes and, in one variation or another, remained in use until the insulin era. The principle was the reduction of secretions and excretions by drugs acting neurally, chemically or mechanically; the limitation of the excretion of digestive juices was intended to reduce both the need for nourishment and its conversion into sugar, while the damping-down of renal function would hinder the increased excretion of sugar. The "sedative method" – developed especially in France – made use of various narcotics for this purpose, especially opium with allegedly the best results. The chemical method employed the most varied styptics and astringents to produce local contraction of the vessels and thereby reduce secretion. Besides astringents, medicines were popular that, according to Schönlein, "produce an intense vascular irritation and a state bordering on inflammation, and so likewise limit secretion", e.g., cantharides in increasing doses, "until the patients exhibit the first signs of nephritis". The *Lehrbuch der speziellen Heilmittellehre* of the Freiburger, J. A. Werber, gives hundred of drugs meant to prevent the excretion of sugar in one way or another. A third method made use of the "derivantia" for the same purpose: excretion of the digestive juices by salivation ("aversion therapy"), vomiting, diarrhea, "diversion through the skin"by external application of turpentine, copaiba balsam, cantharides, hot baths, etc.

As the concept of the "renal threshold" for sugar was still unknown, belief in the healing outcome of the medications mentioned persisted until the exact demonstration of the blood-sugar disclosed the illusion and guided research into new paths.

The physiologic-chemical orientation

The inauguration of the new epoch in diabetic research stood first and most impressively under the sign of "animal chemistry" or "physiologic chemistry", as it was soon called. Above all, German physiology, after the conquest of the "romantic interlude", with its all-biological speculations, turned to thoroughly mechanistic or chemical concepts, whose steady development up to then had been given a great impulse by French research. It adopted from Marcelin Berthelot the fixed aim "to banish life from all explanations involving organic chemistry".

In Otto Funke, the Freiburg physiologist, we can learn (1) how the "animal matter" was no longer really reckoned as "living", but rather only "lives" through the "continuing physical and chemical changes and movements which proceed according to certain laws, and which, in their turn, are conditioned "by the supply of certain substances" taken in with the food. Even Rudolf Virchow saw chemistry as the true foundation of physiologic and pathologic processes. This theoretic scientific – not to say ideologic – anchorage in physiologic chemistry explains the particular path taken by the theory and therapy of diabetes up to the fundamental discoveries of v. Mering and Minkowski. The publications of Liebig on the possible applications of chemistry to agriculture, physiology and pathology in 1840 and 1842 contributed decisively to the shaping of this direction of research. Particularly significant were his analyses of the expired air and the residual substances in the excreta and the important establishment that the nutriment must contain certain minimal quantities of protein (as "plastic" material for synthesis), fat and carbohydrate (as "respiratory substances"). Frerichs, Lehmann, Bidder, Carl Schmidt, Limpert, Falck, Voit, Pettenkofer and others perfected Liebig's methods and corrected many initial errors. Thus,

Frerichs found as early as 1849, by feeding dogs on a purely meat diet, that protein, too, could act as a "respiratory" substance; still more important was the finding that protein, given in excess, is likewise burned (Carl Schmidt, Lehmann, Bidder) and that the organism falls back on its own body protein when hungry and in severe diabetes. The therapeutic application of the meat diet in diabetes thus gained an entirely new theoretic basis.

The special interest of diabetic research now turned to the question of the enzymes active in digestion by the application of precise chemical and physical techniques, continuing French studies and adopted also in Germany. The physical and chemical properties of the saliva were investigated – its diastatic capacity had been demonstrated by Erhard Fr. Leuchs as far back as 1831 –, the individual components were analysed, their changes under different physiologic and pathologic states observed, the action on the different starches in the raw and the cooked state tested, also in acid and alkaline settings and in the presence of the most varied ingredients. This led to the observation that, under certain circumstances, the enzymes designated as "sugar-forming" in the saliva, pancreatic and small intestinal juices could lose their diastatic capacity. It now seemed possible to approach the solution of the problem of diabetes, at least from one aspect, a problem formulated for researchers of all orientations around the middle of the 18th century, according to E. F. v. Gorup-Besanez, as follows: either sugar production in the diabetic organism is so increased that the conditions for its further conversions no longer suffice, or the organism is unable to utilize physiologically the sugar supplied in normal amounts (2). Therefore, "antienzymal" agents were given, e.g., carbolic acid, sodium salicylate, iodoform, and especially sodium carbonate in large doses in order to decrease the remarkably increased or accelerated conversion of starchy materials into sugar. However, these theories were very soon deprived of their basis, if only through clinical observation that even with complete removal of all amylases a glycemia could develop and, secondly, because Trommer and others demonstrated precisely that even in the healthy organism ingested starch is converted into sugar without residue.

Historically important in this context is a sentence from the textbook Funke already mentioned: "Since the rapid oxidation of sugar in alkaline solutions had been discovered, one was at once ready with the hypothesis (Mialke, 1839) that the accumulation of the blood-sugar . . . in diabetes is based on a reduction of blood alkalis." This sentence is evidence of the critical attitude of the "exact scientific thought" that usually rapidly overcame errors. Lehmann, Uhle, Poggiale, Jeannel and Pavy injected "large amounts of caustic or carbonate alkalis and found that they reduced neither the sugar nor the acid content of the diabetic urine.

This critique extended even to fundamentals. Liebig and others in the 1840s had assumed with Lavoisier that, in the synthesis of the "respiratory substances", a simple oxidation process in the lungs was concerned (hence the basis of the view that a sojourn in oxygen-rich air with physical exertion was advantageous for diabetics). In 1867, E. F. v. Gorup-Besanez called attention to the danger that physiological chemistry might become "chemical physiology". Although an opponent of vitalism, he nevertheless presented the view that the organism, "in its structure and development has no analog in inanimate nature and that its singularity calls for a specific method of investigation". The historical outcome of this view, advanced by him and many other German workers, was that the results of other lines of research were incorporated into the mode of thought of physiological chemistry, as will be seen later.

The most important advance, and the most significant for diabetic research, in the physiological chemistry of these years lay in the understanding that the mere assertion of the balance between substance intake and output might give much valuable information about the end-results of the metabolic process, but that it had nothing to say about the processes of the so-called intermediate metabolism. The concept, dating back to Lavoisier, of the synthesis of the ingested nutrients as a combustion process is certainly retained for the process as a whole; but, first, this synthesis was displaced into the blood and then into the tissues (Hoppe-Seyler, J. J. Müller, Schönbein, etc.) and, second, it was valid for an increasing number of researchers that it is "obvious that the carbon dioxide . . . is not an immediate combustion product of the blood constituents, but only the end-phase of a series of intermediate oxidation and chemical processes". In his "chemical biostatics" of 1867, Gorup-Besanez postulated series of theoretically possible intermediate products which "illustrate the breakdown of the organic constituents of the animal body from the most complex to the simplest forms" (3), e.g., olein, oleic acid, capronic acid, butyric acid, acetic acid, formic acid, sugar, succinic acid, lactic acid, oxalic acid. Just as theoretic was the next assumption that some intermediate products, such as succinic and oxalic acids, derived their chemical structure both from the albuminates and from the fats and carbohydrates. We now know more precisely that these theories, though fundamentally correct, were erroneous in detail; at the time, however, they entered unremarked into a new epoch of diabetic research, both in the field of therapy and especially on the prevalence of intermediate metabolism. The sometimes supposed, sometimes actual confirmation of these hypotheses through increasingly refined and ingenous metabolic studies, led immediately to a series of consequences: first, if certain products of glucose synthesis could also be formed from protein, then the strict protein-fat therapy with exclusion of all vegetables lost its rationale; further, nutritional studies suggested that in particular the glycogen formed from protein was chemically identical with that derived from carbohydrates; all this confirmed the clinical observation that in severe diabetes the withdrawal of carbohydrates did not prevent mellituria.

A second consequence led to the (provisional) solution of the problem of the source of the ketone bodies. The new concepts of intermediate metabolism suggested the concept that, in severe diabetes, particularly in its end-stages, the observed intoxication was to be attributed, either to the arrest of synthesis at a certain stage, or to the formation of newer and pathogenetically more active intermediate products. In 1857, Wilhelm Anton succeeded in demonstrating acetone in the expired air and urine of a woman in diabetic coma, and thought he had found the sought toxin. In 1860, Joseph Kaulich made an exact analysis of the acetone and described its effects on the organism. In 1874, A. Kussmaul, who was occupied with the "terminal symptom complex of the sugar disease (Kussmaul's breathing – diabetic coma) based on a number of cases, confirmed the fact of the acetonemia but found that doses of 6 g produced no disease phenomena in man and only symptoms of intoxication in dogs. Similar findings were made by Buhl, Tappeiner, Albertoni and Frerichs, who increased the dose to 12 g without harm, so denying acetone a pathologic significance.

The explanation was provided by the Old Master of diabetic research, Bernhard Naunyn, and his pupils. Back in 1865, Gerhardt had found that diabetic urine contained not only acetone but also ethyl-diacetate ("acetic ether"), giving rise to the acid treatment but with separate individual additions of bread, potatoes, etc., and with constant monitoring of the blood and urinary sugar. Most authors took the view that it was better to put up with a minor excretion of sugar than to force through a cessation of the mellituria at the expense of the overall physical state, especially as Külz and Troje had found that increased administration of carbohydrates did not give rise to a parallel rise in urinary sugar.

The development of special *"carbohydrate regimes"* goes back to v. Düring and Rudolf E. Külz. Düring prescribed, besides 250 g of meat daily, 80–120 g of rice, semolina or buckwheat grits with an unlimited intake of old-baked white bread, and claimed to have obtained amazing results of treatment thereby. In his *Beiträgen zur Pathologie und Therapie des Diabetes mellitus* (Marburg 1874 and 1875), Külz published his observations on harmful and harmless carbohydrates and assigned to the latter class levulose, inulin, inositol, mannitol, quercitol and, with its specifically different action, lactose. The outcome was that the diabetic menu now contained vegetables and tubers previously forbidden: Jerusalem artichokes, comfrey, celery, peas, etc. Winternitz based his milk cure on these findings, Donkin his recommendation of asses milk. Even alcohol in small amounts was advised (C. A. Ewald and others). But only the "oats cure" of Carl v. Noorden and the "porridge-fruit cure" of his pupil, Wilhelm Falta, found general acceptance and remained in use for particular gastrointestinal disorders in diabetics even after the discovery of insulin. Another type of diet is associated with the names of Newburgh-Marsh and Petrén. The designation of this diet as "especially rich in fat" is only correct in relation to Allen's "hunger cure". In the 1880s and 90s, many authors advised that fat should be given "in as large a quantity as could be digested to combat the decrease in carbohydrates and the increased breakdown of proteins, as may be noted in Munck and Uffelmann's *Ernährung des gesunden und kranken Menschen* (Vienna and Leipzig 1895 [3], p. 549 f.). Only the oats cure of v. Noorden could tolerate, at least initially, administration of fat in the amounts equivalent to those of the Petrén diet. The special feature of the latter lay rather in the extreme restriction of both carbohydrates and protein. In Germany, despite allegedly good results, it found no acceptance.

The third special form of diet was marked by reduction of all three basic substances to a minimum. It was also related to the diet in which v. Düring employed methods related to naturopathy. It was Naunyn who established this "strict diet" as a remedial diet – with the interpolation of separate "hunger days" – on a scientific basis. Guglielmo Guelpa, who attributed diabetes to an auto-intoxication, intensified the deprivation of nutrients by purgative cures (1910 and 1917); Allen practiced it in an even stricter form in America. The significance of the "hunger diet" explains why Joslin divides the period before the discovery of insulin into a "Naunyn era" (1898–1914) and an "Allen era" (1914–1922). One may, if one wishes, consider the Naunyn and Allen deprivation cures as successful. The general life-expectation rose and deaths in coma fell allegedly to 40%; but instead, as E. Grafe rightly points out, the patients, wasted to a skeleton, died the frightful "death of inanition".

II Physiologic Experiment

This is in the foreground of the second main line of development. The best characterization of this orientation for his time was given by the oft-mentioned Gorup-Besanez, who defines the goal-setting of physiologic experiment in his *Textbook* of 1867 as follows: "It serves to ascertain the importance of individual parts of the organism for the whole, partly through establishing their behavior towards specific stimuli and effects, partly from the effect which their removal, damage or pathologic change has on the entire organism or on particular organs."

Its prototype is Claude Bernard, the pupil, collaborator and successor of Francois Magendie, the "spokesman and inaugurator of modern experimental trends in physiology and medicine", as Rothschuh has rightly called him.

Bernard linked the findings of exact physical and chemical research with those of morphologic-biologic answers to increasingly new and fruitful problems. The principle that the function of the blood and tissues was, as it were, effected only from outside and according to general physical and chemical laws was amplified by him as the concept of the *milieu intérieur* with its own biologic conformity to law, a concept whose full fruitfulness has been recognized only in recent years.

Therefore, as regards the problem of the sugar disease, the most important problem lay with the organ responsible for blood-sugar formation, and the next with the regulatory mechanism whose disturbance must be responsible for the overproduction of sugar in the diabetic's blood. He injected sugar solutions into the veins of rabbits in 1843 and found that this reappeared unaltered in the urine. By catherizing the most varied trunk veins in dogs – on 9 January 1855 and regularly during a lecture demonstration of "cardiac catheterization" – he sought to demonstrate that under certain conditions sugar could always be found in the circulating blood "between liver and lungs". The difference between the (small or absent) sugar content in the portal vein and the (rich) content in the hepatic veins, and the demonstration of sugar in the liver itself, led him to the discovery confirmed by Lehmann, that the liver was the site of constant sugar formation (contrary to Figuer, Colin, Longet, Bérard, etc., whose views were refuted by the careful studies of Lehmann and Meissner). He also showed that the sugar content of the blood in the hepatic veins was largely independent of the nature of the nutriment, whether animal or vegetable. In the search for the substance from which the liver produced sugar, he found an odorless and tasteless nitrogen-free material which stained blue with iodine and which he could convert into sugar by means of the salivary or pancreatic enzymes or mineral acids. Soon afterwards, Hensen found this same substance with the properties attributed to it by Bernard (8). In 1857, Pelouze estimated it (falsely) as $C_{12}H_{12}O_{12}$. In 1859, Bernard and the physiologist Moritz Schiff (also a pupil of Magendie) managed to demonstrate it microscopically (9). Because of its similarity to vegetable starch, Bernard termed it "animal starch" *(amidon animale)* and, on the basis of its function, as a sugar-forming agent *(substance glycogène)*. Bernard and Henses succeeded in demonstrating also, in the liver and to some extent in the portal blood, an enzyme capable of splitting glycogen with release of energy. The question whether this related to diastatic enzymes of the saliva or pancreatic juice entering the liver with the current of portal blood or whether it was a specific and as yet unknown enzyme remained unsolved, as it could not be separated with the means then available. The discovery that sugar formation was not completely suppressed even in hungry animals (Poggiale) and during winter hibernation (Valentin), whereas there is an accumulation of liver glycogen in frogs in winter (Schiff), was taken as evidence for the thesis that the mother-substance of glycogen was not to be sought immediately in the ingested nutrients, but rather in the "blood elements" which underwent "natural breakdown" in the liver and from one part of which glycogen – and possibly fat – was synthesized, while the other part was excreted as bile.

Thus the organ responsible for the development of diabetes seemed to have been found: and also founded was the weighty view of Bernard and his school, long prominent in therapy, that limitation of carbohydrate in the intake of diabetics is an unnecessary and cruel deprivation.

However, the further development along this particular line shows, here again, an interesting fact in scientific theory: how even so-called methods of exact science in problem-setting and solution or in the interpretation of "objective" experimental findings are dependent on current historical conditioning factors and dominant theories. This is shown very clearly by Bernard's next step, the *piqûre* that was to become famous, especially from its derived concept of the "neuropathic sugar-urinary flux".

In 1840, the surgeon and anatomist Benedikt Stilling, also a pupil of Magendie and Bernard, had introduced the concept of "vasomotor nerves" with his sensational *Physiologisch-pathologische Untersuchungen über die Spinal-Irritation* (Leipzig). In 1851, Bernard began his investigation into the conditions of vascular innervation. On cutting the cervical sympathetic, he regularly found dilatation, increased circulation and higher temperature of the homolateral ear in the rabbit. With the intention of demonstrating the consequences of transection, injury or irritation of the vasomotor nerves on the circulatory conditions in the liver vessels, he arrived by anatomic and experimental procedures at the ala cinerea, which he supposed to be the site of origin of the vagi; when he finally injured certain sites in the lower part of the rhomboid groove in the floor in the fourth ventricle, between the cerebellum and medulla oblongata, in the living animal, the animal after a short interval began to excrete an abundant, acid-reacting, sugar-containing urine (10). On opening the abdomen, he found the liver in a state of marked congestion and still very hyperemic even at autopsy.

Uhle (1852), Schrader (1852), v. Becker, W. Kühne (1858) and especially Moritz Schiff then confirmed Bernard's findings in only slightly modified experiments. The epoch had begun of attempts to induce glycosuria artificially by destruction or stimulation of the various nerve-tracts (Schiff, Pavy, Eckard, Klebs, Munck, Hensen, Grafe), by the action of various poisons (curare, chloroform, ether, amyl nitrite, carbon disulphide) or by psychic insults (e.g. simple tying-up in cats and rabbits).

Medical history tends to record the *piqûre* as "a unique success of exact scientific thought". Yet this is correct neither for the uniqueness nor for the unfortunate effects on theory and on the practical diagnosis and treatment of diabetes mellitus. We now know that the "results" of the various types of *piqûre* were due to be attributed increased adrenalin output – as every surgeon knows – or to stimulation of the centripetal and centrifugal pathways of the "sugar center" actually situated in the gray matter of the third ventricle. Moreover, it was found even then that the 6 to at most 24 hours of artificial glycosuria had little in common with true diabetes mellitus. Much more decisive for the whole orientation was the decreased reaction, either of the liver glycogen or of the liver itself, after the blocking of certain nerves. In 1856, Schiff observed that the glycosuria persisted if he tied the liver vessels in frogs before the *piqûre*. Bernard found the same results after transection of the vagi or the spinal cord at particular sites, and drew from the rapidly ensuing death of the experimental animals the very important conclusion – still disputed by Abeles in 1875 and by Cohnheim in 1880 – that the source of the physiologic blood-sugar could be assumed to be the liver and its glycogen content (12). The glycosuria failed to appear if the liver had become glycogen-free due to protracted hunger, fever, strenuous muscular activity, convulsions or high-grade fatty degeneration due to phosphorus or arsenical poisoning. Especially impressive was the complete disappearance of the physiologic blood-sugar after extirpation of the liver – according to Bock and Hoffmann within 45 minutes (13) – or after its "switching" by simple or reversed "Eck's fistula" (1877).

This seemed to have proved the thesis of "angioneurotic diabetes", postulated by Bernard, Schiff, Landois and others and briefly propounded as follows: the liver forms glycogen from materials in the nutrients (and the body itself), which is converted under the influence of an enzyme into blood-sugar and supplied to the blood in physiologically necessary amounts. For their part, the liver vessels remain under the influence of the vasomotor nerves, which produce in them such a "moderate tonus" as is just necessary and adequate for the formation of the physiologic amount of blood-sugar. If they are paralyzed by certain toxic, nosologic, traumatic or psychich effects – or if the vasodilator nerves are stimulate – the liver vessels are widened, the enzyme formed from destroyed blood corpuscles acts more intensively on the glycogen and thus produces hyperglycaemia; there follow glycosuria and the other wellknown features of the sugar disease.

Despite many counter-arguments over details, into which we shall not go further here, this view of diabetes can explain how it is that it does stand out uniquely in the history of nosology. Morbid anatomy and histochemistry sought zealously for tumors, scleroses and every other possible tissue change in the liver, on the one hand, and in the medulla oblongata, cerebellum and afferent nerves on the other. The clinician saw in numerous neurologic phenomena – disturbances of sensation and motility, reflex anomalies, occipital and trigeminal neuralgias, physical and mental fatigue, frequent depression, etc. – genuine manifestations of a disorder of the nervous system in line with the theory. Even diabetic coma was designated as "the most important phenomenon of a neurologic nature" by Strümpell in 1897 (14), to adduce a particularly descriptive example, and this in 1897, after the important findings of Kussmaul, Naunyn, v. Jaksch, Stadelmann, Minkowski and others.

Just as drug treatment had been subject to change in the latter half of the 18th century, so now it changed with the numerous differing views on the existance of nervous disorders. Many clinicians who, with Griesinger (1844), saw these as the effects of cerebral irritation or, with Beard, of spinal irritation, prescribed "tranquillizing" agents, especially opium in high doses; others, who interpreted the nerve weakness as congenital or as an acquired disorder (due, for instance, to inadequate or inappropriate nutrition or to excesses of all kinds), discarded all narcotics and hypnotica (with the exception of bromides), especially opium and its derivatives. They recommended, on the other hand, iron, arsenic, copper, phosphorus and quinine in the most various formulations. At the same time, great value was attached to psychic treatment, relaxation from vocational duties, spa cures and – since Trousseau, Zimmer, Bouchardot and Külz had emphasized the favorable influence of well-spaced muscular exertion – appropriate physical activity.

The theory of "angioneurotic diabetes" becam historically fateful in a double aspect. The concept of the importance of the liver in the origin of diabetes lessened interest in Minkowski's studies of the pancreas and is, as we must now retrospectively accept, certainly partly responsible for the remarkable fact that this discovery had to battle on until well into the 1930s to gain general recognition. The view of the role of nervous regulation of the blood-sugar level has its own history. In 1892, Thiroloix in Paris established his own theory of *diabète nerveuse,* further elaborated by Pflüger, in support of resistance to the pancreatic theory (15). He attributed the artificial diabetes produced by Minkowski, not to the extirpation of the pancreas, but to the lesioning of an "antidiabetic nervous central organ situated in the duodenum" (16), irritation of which was responsible for the development of diabetes.

To what extent the theory of angioneurotic diabetes may have obstructed the path to insulin cannot, naturally, now be certain. However, it is very obvious, even today, how many current concepts in diabetes therapy are attributable to its influence, e.g., the ideas, commoner of course at the beginning of the insulin era than now, about the insulin "cure", fasting or vegetarian days, etc., and "calming the irritated pancreatic system".

Moreover, the further development of the general orientation took place partly on the basis of specific studies, partly through the initiative of renowned clinicians who assessed the value of all the lines of research and often made their own contributions. Yet Claude Bernard himself had been able to postulate that, in true diabetes, the capacity of the liver to polymerize glucose to glycogen and to store it as such was reduced. Külz and others found in numerous precise studies in minor and severe cases of diabetes that the overproduction of sugar by the liver was not of such great importance, that rather the diabetic might synthesize less blood-sugar as an end-process. Thus the path of physiologic experiment led increasingly to the originally still hypothetical concept, that the blood of the diabetic lacked an enzyme which under physiologic conditions guaranteed the breakdown or utilization of the blood glucose.

Orientations in morbid anatomy

The third line of development in diabetes research is characterized by the unceasing endeavor to call into play the findings of pathologic anatomy, especially the anatomy and histology of the pancreas, to elucidate the puzzling features of the sugar disease. At autopsy, the spleen was usually found grossly normal, seldom atrophic, the gastrointestinal tract without significant changes, the kidneys were often strikingly large, even oftener there was the glycogenous degeneration of Henle's loops described by Ehrlich, with glycogen in the form of flakes or pellets in the epithelium. Under the influence of Bernard's theory and that of his pupils, particular attention was paid to the liver and the nervous system, but only occasionally were tumors or scleroses found in the cerebellum or medulla. The so-called Lindau's tumors in the cerebellum were found remarkably often in combination with associated angiomatoses of the retina and cyst formation in the pancreas. Frerichs found microscopic capillary hemorrhages and myelitic changes in the medulla. In the liver, the single but often recurring finding was the small number of "glycogen corpuscles". Proportionally often there was found atrophy of the pancreas, especially in older age-groups and in marasmus, usually without demonstrable structural changes, occasionally anemia, hyperemia and hemorrhage, rarely calculus formation, occasionally cysts, lipomatosis, hyalinosis, amyloidosis, tissue necroses and neoformations, especially cirrhosis. But these findings were also seen in non-diabetics, whereas nothing striking was to be established in known diabetics.

The first account of the glandular cells of the pancreas stems from Claude Bernard, who saw them as a counterpart to the submandibular and sublingual glands. In 1869, the 22-year-old Paul Langerhans, then the pupil of Virchow, in his *Beiträge zur mikroskopischen Anatomie der Bauchspeicheldrüse* (Berlin thesis 1869), described the islet-shaped cell clumps in the pancreatic tissue which Gustave Édouard Laguesse named the "islets of Langerhans" in 1893 in honour of their discoverer. The discovery aroused no particular interest in the field of pathology; and from the standpoint of cellular pathology the pancreas was hardly included in the group of affections because none of the characteristic cellular lesions were found there. Of course, Opie (1900), Weichselbaum and Stangel (1901), Herzog (1902) and Heiberg (1906) frequently found hydropic or hyaline degeneration or atrophy of the islets in diabetics, but these changes were nonspecific and also occurred in non-diabetics.

This knowledge of the proportionately rare changes in the morbid anatomy, as also in the cellular pathology, proved of little value in therapy. Theoretically, it was assumed that the diabetes – like fatty degenerayion and gout – was based on a degeneration of the body cells (loss of the "oxidative" power of the cells with consequent arteriosclerotic changes), hence the ban on alcohol and other noxa which were assumed to promote cell degeneration, the use of potassium iodide preparations and the prescription of physical measures (especially baths, massage, exercises) to which was attributed a favorable effect on the cells.

It was not until the turn of the century that major refinements in histologic methods allowed postulates about the role of the pancreas in diabetes. E. L. Opie found that individual cell-nuclei of the Langerhans' islets were different from the others in their size (1900) (17).

Lane (1907) and Bensley (1911) rendered the alpha-cells (so-called by them) visible by staining with gentian-violet orange. After fixation with potassium bichromate sublimate, the beta-cells then showed violet nuclei, while the alpha-cells were stained a diffuse yellow. Lane concluded from this staining behavior that there are chemically different substances with different functions. Bensley saw besides the regularly predominant number of "clear cells".

These findings too were almost completely ignored for decades. The fourth line of development was determined by knowledge of:

The Endocrinology of the Pancreas

The history of diabetes contains numerous names of those – such as Chopart, Bright, Bouchardat, Griesinger, von Recklinghausen, Lancereaux, etc. – who have linked this disease with the pancreas. However, closer study makes it repeatedly clear that these authors referred to changes in the chemistry of the neurovascular system or of the cells, and that in general they gave no thought to the fourth possibility of the regulation of the *consensus partuum.*[1] As these studies form the subject of a special article, only the most important are dealt with here, to some extent in tabular form.

The history of the discovery of pancreatic diabetes in 1869 was thoroughly discussed by Minkowski himself in this journal (76 [1929], 8, pp. 311–315). To the debate about priority between him and Lepine about the introduction of the concept of "internal secretion", it must now be added that the term had already been used by Claude Bernard, even if in a some-

---

[1] Also J. v. Mering and Minkowski, both then at Strassburg, hit by chance, as it were, on the knowledge of the consequences of pancreatectomy. However, Mering had long been occupied with the problems of carbohydrate metabolism and in 1886 was able to produce long-term glycosuria by giving phloridzin.

what different sense, and that it was first used in its modern significance in 1905 by Ernest Henry Starling in a lecture on *Chemical Correlation of the Functions of the Body*, in connexion with the introduction of the hormonal concept.

Decivise for the experimental results of Minkowski was, first, his successful total extirpation of the pancreas without residue, something the skilled operator Bernard had taken as impossible; second, the production of a diabetes which approached the nosologic in many aspects; and third, the demonstration by Minkowski and Hédon that the diabetes could be prevented or regression induced by the subcutaneous implantation of fragments of the pancreas.

The experiment to prepare the pure active enzyme and to study its action on carbohydrate metabolism foundered on the then unknown fact that, as proteo-hormone of pancreatic trypsin, it was rapidly destroyed. It was not until the turn of the century that Diamare could identify the organ already found in cartilaginous fish in 1846 and termed "blood-gland" as corresponding to the Langerhans' islets separated from the pancreas, and then without anyone drawing the corresponding conclusions.

The following dates may be listed in detail:

1893 Minkowski (18) injected dogs made diabetic with pancreatic juice extracted with physiological saline. Severe necroses.

1893 Battistini reported success in 2 cases.

1894 Goldscheider and Fürbringer did the same experiment with a glycerine extract. No success (19).

1898 Blumenthal treated pancreatic juice with alcohol, thereby unintentionally inactivating the trypsin. The injection caused necrosis formation. His experiment had no imitators (20).

1903–1906 Cohnheim undertook numerous experiments; he heated expressed pancreatic juice, treated it with alcohol, and often saw 100% glycolysis in the expressed muscle juice. His technique was patented but not followed up (21).

1908 Zuelzer at al. processed calf's pancreas, treated the extract with alcohol, and markedly improved artificial diabetes in a dog (22). Forschbach at Minkowski's clinic, to whom he sent the preparation for assay, confirmed the reversal of glycosuria and ketone excretion, but given to patients it caused rigors, fever, bounding pulse and sweating.

Others authors, who obtained favorable results with extracts obtained by modified techniques, include Gley (1905), Rennie and Fraser (1907), E. Acott (1910–11), Murlin and Kramer (1913–16), Kleiner and Meltzer (1915), Paulesco (1921). Especially noteworthy also are the findings of Camille Reuter, a colleague of Abderhalden, to whom probably the production of a really very pure preparation should be credited. Zuelzer, who reported on this in 1923 (23), opines, probably rightly, that the convulsions produced by Reuter's preparation must be attributed to the high dosage and the resultant hypoglycemia, which was not unknown at that time. Thus, the preparation discovered foundered on its own good quality in a tragic accident.

After the failure – and possibly also because of the important attitude of Pflüger – had led to a certain resignation, Frederick Grant Banting and Charles Herbert Best under MacLeod in Toronto took the decisive step. Through a publication by O. M. Barring (1920) their attention had been drawn to the investigations of W. Schulze (1900) (24) and especially of L. W. Sobolew (1902) (25); these had established that after tying of the excretory duct of the pancreas the enzyme-forming gland parenchyma atrophied, but that the animal did not become diabetic as long as the islets remained intact. This, as Sobolew himself had already hinted, offered a way of obtaining the active glycolytic agent in pure form. Moreover, Ibrahim had established (1909) that in calf embryos in the fourth month the islets, but not the acini, were already functional. Banting and Best took both paths. They succeeded in obtaining from both the expressed juice of the normal pancreas and from the separated islet system a preparation which was capable of reducing both the glycosuria and the ketonuria in diabetic dogs. They called this, after the precedent of J. de Meyer, "insulin".

III The Insulin Era

In 1921, C. von Noorden, at a convention of the German Society for Internal Medicine, had, in a "Review of the present state of diabetes research", characterized the attempts hitherto at a drug or organotherapeutic treatment of the sugar disease as ineffectual.

A little later, at the beginning of 1922, Banting and Best were able to report the first therapeutic successes of their "insulin" (26). The first results concerned the finding that, after administration of the material obtained by them into pancreatectomized dogs, a reduction of the blood-sugar dependent on the dosage could be obtained which reverted to the previous state after some hours. Moreover, there was an increase in the liver glycogen with a simultaneous regression of its fat content and the lipemia, disappearance of the ketone bodies with a marked improvement in the general condition, and in increase in the body-weight and capacity for exertion. In further studies, performed additionally by MacLeod, Collip and Noble, it was learned that the state of coma was different from the "hypoglycemic reaction" and that the latter could be eliminated by administration of glucose and adrenalin.

The hypoglycemic effect of insulin served for the establishment of the "Toronto unit", and in practice of exact dosage. At first, the introduction of insulin by no means constituted the "mighty revolution" in the treatment of diabetes mellitus that is occasionally depicted. More nearly, one may speak of such in America at the time of the so-called "wild insulin era", in which the treatment was carried out according to the simplified principle: "as much carbohydrate that no ketonuria develops, as much insulin so long as there is no glycosuria." A better view of the state of therapy during the period termed by Joslin "the first insulin era" (1922–1925) is given by a small pamphlet by C. von Noorden and S. Isaak (Berlin 1925) with the indicative title "Family doctor and the insulin treatment of the sugar disease". Von Noorden and numerous other authors repeatedly emphasized that treatment had now become, not simpler, but much more complicated, and that assessment and treatment must be modified for each individual case. Insulin treatment of the "slight" and largely also of the "moderately severe" cases was rejected. This rejection was based, first, on the risk of complications (resulting from "impurity" of the preparation, initially obtained mostly from the pig's pancreas), then on the fear of hypoglycemic shock and also on the need for several injections daily because of the short duration of action of the insulin then available. A necessary prerequisite for the best possible treatment was the establishment of the individual carbohydrate tolerance, i.e., the quantity of carbohydrate at which the urine remained just sugar free. One began either with a hunger day or a completely carbohydrate-free diet, and then nutrition was built up again but with a diet poor in all the basic substances. Additions of 2 to 2 days, interruption of the regime twice weekly by a carbohydrate-free or vegetarian day. If sugar appeared, an insulin injection beginning with doses of 5–15 units, the injections given at least twice daily, before the main meals, and 6–7 times daily in insulin-refractory cases. If acetonuria persisted, 1–3 days on oats (von Noorden) or Falta's porridge days were inserted. Up to 6 months in hospital was required for the "period of adjustment".

The normal diabetic diet should be as near as possible to the nutritional minimum according to Bouchardat's repeatedly adduced principle: *manger le moins possible*. Most clinicians in the first years of the insulin era advocated the greatest limitation of carbohydrate intake. In compensation, fat was given (Petrén and Newburgh-Marsh) in quantities up to 300 g or protein. Others preferred the "double nutrient system" or inserted – at short intervals – vegetable days, oats days, porridge or fruit days, on the principle of sparing and relaxing the islet system. Others (e.g., the clinicians Porges and Adlersburg in Vienna, Sansum and Geyelin in America), conversely required the most carbohydrate-rich diet possible with abundant fat (Adlersburg–Porges) or protein supplement. The guiding principle was to whip up intrinsic insulin production and at the same time prevent acidosis. Thereby Sansum aimed at thorough removal of the hyperglycemia, if necessary by extremely high dosage of insulin.

Bertram, Katsch, Himsworth and others gave a diet as rich in carbohydrate as possible – without going to extremes – with moderate amounts of protein and marked fat restriction and thereby obtained, after eliminating any ketonuria with insulin, sugar values of 0.16–0.18% and glycosuria of 10–30 g, because in this way the patients had subjective well-being and the objectively greatest exertion capacity ("new school"). This was in sharp opposition to the "old school", represented in Germany especially by Grafe, in America by Joslin and his school, who endeavored to keep carbohydrate values to a minimum.

Insulin treatment celebrated its greatest triumph with the overcoming of the coma that had previously almost always been fatal. In addition to the alcohol used earlier, insulin was given in "very high doses" as von Noorden, Brugsch and others write, i.e., 120–300 units divided into 8–15 doses. Simultaneously, most administered 10 g of levulose or oxanthin (a triose) and often also up to 100 g of sodium bicarbonate.

An important relief for doctor and patient was the introduction of insulin preparations with depôt action, achieved after great endeavor by Hagedorn et al. by the addition of protamine from the sperm of *Salmo irideus.* We should also here mention Bertram, who devoted much of his energy to this field.

Newer Concepts

There have been great changes in the evaluation of the sugar disease in the last 30 years. In the *Handbuch der Inneren Medizin,* Vol. VII, 2, 1954, 99, J. Kühnhau states, as the certain outcome of research and as a starting-point for all diagnostic and therapeutic considerations, that diabetes mellitus does not exist as a disease *sui generis.* "The same clinical picture, comprising longstanding hyperglycemia and glycosuria, disturbances of fat and protein synthesis, nitrogen-loss and a tendency to the accumulation of ketone bodies, can develop on the basis of quite different endocrine, humoral and central venous causal mechanisms, in which insulin deficiency is only one, if a specially important, factor." Even the advocates of the theory of the absolutely central position of the pancreas in intermediate metabolism realize the fact that diabetes can no longer be regarded as a mere disturbance of carbohydrate metabolism produced by lack of insulin, but as a complex general disorder of metabolism determined by an immense number of factors, not all of which are yet known to us.

They way to a better concept is mainly outlined by the development of general endocrinology.

One endocrine organ after another has been linked with intermediate metabolism and hence with diabetes mellitus. In 1930, Houssay and Biasotti discovered what they called the diabetogenic principle of the hypophysis. The diabetes of the Minkowski dog could be considerably improved by elimination of the anterior lobe of the pituitary. The injection of anterior lobe extracts produced in normal experimental animals (Houssay, Biasotti, Riltei) and in man (Lassen, Hansen) a temporary diabetes ("idiohypophysical diabetes" of F. G. Young, *Lancet* 1936, 2, 297). In 1937, for the first time since the discovery of pancreatectomy-induced diabetes, Young succeeded in producing a permanent diabetes by the protracted daily injection of anterior lobe extracts ("metahypophysical diabetes", *Lancet* 1937, 2, 372), which proved strinkingly insulin-sensitive, as opposed to the "idiophysical" diabetes which was almost entirely insulin-resistant. The phenomena (polyuria, polydipsia, glycosuria and hyperglycemia) persisted even if no further anterior lobe extract was given (the "Young" dog). This provided an extremely interesting analogy to the already clinically familiar "asthenic" insulin-sensitive diabetes and the "sthenic", relatively insulin-resistant, diabetes of later life. Histologically, H. Ferner found involution of the alpha-cells and Dohan-Fish-Lukens, Young and Richardson a degeneration of the betal-cells with vacuole formation.

A significant advance in the study of the diabetogenic effect of the anterior pituitary lobe was the production of the "pure" somatropic hormone (STH) by Li, Evans and Simpson in 1945. Known as chondrotropin or growth hormone since 1924, it had prompted an enormous number of experiments with increasingly contradictory results. Probably, the "pure" preparations of this protein substance of molecular weight 45,000 were still crude substances. STH produces accelerated growth in young dogs and cats and, but only when they are grown, a permanent diabetes; in rats – which, to a certain extent, are always growing – and in pregnancy and lactation it has no diabetogenic effect. It is certainly involved in the development of acromegaly, though not yet to a measurable extent. 40% of all acromegalies are associated with glycosuria, sometimes with and sometimes without other diabetic symptoms. There is often enlargement of the sella turcica, and nearly always overaction of the eosinophil cells of the anterior lobe.

The experimental results of the Young animal and clinical considerations in acromegaly, rare as this is, prompted the question if and how the pituitary hormone, especially the STH, was involved in the development of ordinary diabetes. A causal connexion with the diabetes of children and adolescents seemed excluded, for these were almost always cases of true pancreatic diabetes based on an inherited islet inefficiency. White and Pincus (31) pointed out that the manifestation of the diabetes was usually preceded by symptoms of over-function of the anterior lobe, since 86% of diabetic children were significantly taller and heavier than their metabolically normal counterparts at the onset of the disease. But the further course showed, not the expected symptoms of hypophyseal diabetes, but the classical picture of insulin-deficiency disease.

H. Ferner (32) claimed to have given an impressive explanation of this fact. He assumed that the "alpha-cytotropic factor of the hypophysis", which was probably identical with the growth hormone, produced an increase of the alpha-cells and secondarily a predominance of the glucagon system over the insulin system. Even in childhood diabetes, in which pathologic changes in the pancreas of the nature of the cellular pathology of Weichselbaum (1910) are nearly always absent, the shift in the alpha-beta relationship is strongly expressed, the alpha-cells often constituting 75% as against 20% in healthy individuals.

Ferner based his ideas on the fact that hypophysectomy leads to atrophy and numerical reduction of the alpha-cells after some months, but which is rapidly restimulated by STH-induced growth. Kracht et al. confirmed this result, but found no stimulatory action of STH on the alpha-cells of the normal animal (33). Other authors therefore rejected a diabetogenic action of STH, or sought it in the peripheral effects of the growth hormone. STH compensates for the growth inhibition of the thymus, has a "myoglycostatic" effect (Russell–Wilhelmi) and a muscle glycogen preserving effect in the starved animal, and furthers protein formation from fat. It is probable that certain effects on the different stages of the synthesis and breakdown of carbohydrate and protein, direct or indirect, must be taken into consideration; but for all these functions the presence of insulin was necessary, without which hyperglycemia and acetone-body formation developed (Bennett–Kreiss, Li–Evans, Simpson–Bennett–Laundrie). We thereby arrive at a clinical picture – in congenital insufficiency of the islet system or due to a "whipped-up" effect – which is now perceived as a true pancreatic diabetes, even though it has arisen through "counter-regulation" (Bertram).

ACTH or corticotropin, the adrenocorticotropic hormone of the hypophysis, works both with and against STH. ACTH alone hardly leads to diabetes (Bookman 1953). However, Reich found in animal experiments that it heightened the diabetogenic action of STH.

It controls the adrenal cortex and exerts its effects via this cortex; bilateral adrenalectomy leads to atrophy of the basophil cells of the anterior pituitary lobe, while, conversely, lack of ACTH produces atrophy of the adrenal cortex. In particular, ACTH controls the synthesis and release of corticosterone (Kendall's compound B), 11-desoxycorticosterone (electrolyte exchange hormone, Reichstein's compound Q), 17-oxycorticosterone (Reichstein's compound S) and 11-dehydrocorticosterone (Kendall's compound A). These hormones act to inhibit fat breakdown and glycogenolysis, and favor fat formation and glycogenesis. In this way a deficiency produces deficiency of the phosphorylation processes in carbohydrate economy, with a decline in the glycogen reserve in the liver and muscles (adynamy), and fat resynthesis is disturbed, as is phosphorylation of the lactoflavines; hence there is a decrease in the yellow respiratory enzyme, a reduction in basic turnover and of body heat, with simultaneous increase of the residual nitrogen, cholesterol and K- and Mg-values. The administration of desoxycorticosterone promotes regression of these phenomena, whereas the other adrenal cortical hormones are much less effective. However, ACTH also influences carbohydrate economy via the adrenal cortex in quite another way, and is probably responsible, via highly complicated processes, for the various forms of diabetes mellitus.

If the production of ergotropic ACTH exceeds the norm, the glucocorticoids are also increased. As these work against glucagon, not only are the beta-cells stressed as described above but also the alpha-cells. Their exhaustion produces all the symptoms associated with maturity-onset diabetes: disturbances of lipid metabolism, fatty degeneration of the liver and vessels, obesity. As a "regulatory diabetes", this steroid diabetes is very insulin-resistant, but often responds promptly to administration of testosterone (as a "pituitary restraint") and almost always to desoxycorticosterone, often given for quite other purposes.

But other paths also lead from the same ACTH to explain the insulin-sensitive juvenile diabetes, expressed quite otherwise in many symptoms and regularly associated with ketone-body formation, also the Mauriac syndrome (diabetes, hepatomegaly, infantilism), but above all also the disturbance of phosphatide synthesis in the liver, of the phosphatide content of the peripheral nerves in severe diabetes, and the arteriosclerosis and dreaded diabetic angiopathies, now described by Max Bürger as specific (*Angiopathia diabetica,* Stuttgart 1854). Here, we touch on parts of the territories of physiology and pathology (absorption of nutrients, regulation of metabolism, hormonal and nervous correlations, significance of minerals, vitamins, enzymes, etc.), each of which has its own history, method of working and problems. The "now" of diabetes research can only be ascertained by a knowledge of the state of the study of each of these branches. If authors adopt an attitude on the basis of individual chapters, they are well aware of the difficulties. Publications of new findings appear every day which make old-fashioned what was regarded as newest yesterday, which often contradict each other, and which – and this is the worst – as partial results of partial disciplines, are seen neither in direct correlation with the clinical aspect of the diabetes problem, nor without any distinction other than "important" or "unimportant".

And yet, a cognisance of the "Now" of the state of the partial discipline appears necessary for every doctor who has to adopt an attitude to the individual case based on his own physiologic view of the pressing problems of diabetes theory (e.g., prophylaxis and treatment of the dreaded complications of DM, diet, etc.), who – in other words – wishes to avoid a standardized "program". For what Theodor Brugsch (30) said at the time of the first triumph of the insulin era is still valid: "Diabetes is a personal disease and successful treatment depends on the right approach to the personal factor even if, to all appearances, organistically the site of the lesion is the pancreas."

References

1. Lehrbuch der Physiol. Bd. 1, Leipz. (1860), S. 1.
2. Gorup-Besanez, E. F. v., Lehrbuch d. physiol. Chemie, 2. Aufl., Braunschweig (1867), S. 201 f.
3. Gorup-Besanez a. a. O. 42 f.
4. Knoop, F., Hofmeisters Beitr., 6 (1905), S. 150.
5. Embden, G. u. Marx, A., Hofmeisters Beitr., 11 (1908), S. 318.
6. Embden, G. u. Salomon, H. u. Schmidt, F., Hofmeisters Beitr. 8 (1906), S. 129.
7. Ringer, A. J. u. Lusk, G., ebd. 66 (1910), S. 106.
8. Verh. d. Würzb. phys.-med. Ges., 7 (1856), S. 219.
9. Compt. rend. T XLVIII 18 (1859), S. 880.
10. Gaz. med. Paris 5 (1852), S. 72.
11. Eckhard, E., Beitr. Anat., 4 (1867), 6 (1872), 8 (1977).
12. Bernard, Cl., Leç. de la phys. et path. du syst. nerv. T. I, S. 432.
13. Experimentalstudien über Diabetes, Berlin (1874).
14. Strümpell, A., Lehrbuch d. spez. Path. u. Ther. d. inneren Krankh. II, 11. Aufl., Leipz. (1897), S. 575 f.
15. Pflüger, E., Über die Natur d. Kräfte, durch welche das Duodenum den Kohlehydratstoffwechsel beeinflußt, Pflügers Arch. Physiol., 110 (1907), S. 227.
16. This journ., 76 (1929), S. 313.
17. Opie, E. L., On the histology of the islands of Langerhans of the pancreas. Bull. Hopkins, 11 (1900), S. 205–209.
18. Arch. f. exper. Path. u. Pharmac., Leipz., 31 (1893), S. 85.

19. Dtsch. med. Wschr., 20 (1894), S. 293, 376.
20. Zschr. diät.-phys. Therap., 1 (1898), S. 250.
21. Zschr. physiol. Chem., 39 (1903), S. 336; 42 (1904), S. 401; 43 (1905), S. 547; 47 (1906), S. 253.
22. Dtsch. med. Wschr., 34 (1908), S. 1880.
23. Ebd., 19 (1923), S. 1551.
24. Arch. mikrosk. Anat., 56 (1900), S. 491.
25. Ebd. 168 (1902), S. 91.
26. J. laborat. clin. Med., 7 (1922), S. 251, S. 464; Canad. Med. Ass. J., 12 (1922), S. 141.
27. in: Joslin, E. P. u. Mitarb., The Treatment of diabetes m., 8. Aufl., Philadelphia (1946), S. 56.
28. Klin. Wschr. (1951), S. 397; vgl. ebd. (1950), S. 388 u. Ferner, H., Das Inselsystem d. Pankreas, Stuttgart (1952).
29. Naturwissenschaften, 40 (1953), S. 607.
30. Zschr. ärztl. Fortbild., 19 (1924), S. 586.

Summary: The author points out that diabetes mellitus is still not much more than the glittering shell of a notion without precisely established content. As an immense number of works have been published concerning this subject, the author attempts to give a general extensive survey on the development of the present conception of this disease. Various theories on causal mechanisms based on endocrine humoral and central-nervous processes are discussed, as they were developed by scientific research during the last century.

Chapter 1 reports on the four fields which contributed to knowledge until the discovery of insulin. These fields are: physiological chemistry, physiological pathology based on experiment, pathological anatomy, and endocrinology.

Chapter 2 describes the era of insulin (including old-insulin, Hagedorn, and Best).

Chapter 3 reports on the development of newer conceptions. The aim of this work is to make it possible for the non specialised doctor to understand the results of modern research, including special fields such as intermediary metabolism and endocrinology, and to help him also, to comprehend the latest publications (for instance discussion of the new remedies based on sulphonamides, pathogenesis, prophylaxis, and therapy of the dreaded diabetic angiopathias etc.).

Résumé: A l'heure actuelle on peut considérer encore le diabète sucré comme la coque brillante d'un concept sans contenu parfaitement bien définissable. D'autre part la quantité des publications parues sur le diabète s'est multipliée à foison. Le présent travail a pour but de donner une vue d'ensemble sur l'évolution de l'image pathologique en se basant sur les différents mécanismes hormonaux, humoraux et nerveux centraux. On décrit ainsi les différentes conceptions qu'on s'est fait sur cette maladie durant la dernière centaine d'années d'une façon critique historique et en rapport avec les théories actuellement en cours.

Dans le premier chapitre on montre les quatre grandes directions qu'ont prises nos connaissances sur le diabète: la voie chimico-physiologique, la voie physio-pathologique expérimentale, la voie anatomo-pathologique et la voie endocrinologique, jusqu'à la découverte de l'insuline. Le chapitre suivant donne une description de l'époque de l'insuline (les périodes de l'ancienne insuline, de Hagedorn et de Best). Dans le troisième chapitre on décrit le développement des nouveaux points de vue.

En écrivant cet article on a eu pour but de permettre également aux médecins non spécialisés dans les domaines de plus en plus nombreux et touffus du métabolisme intermédiaire et de l'endocrinologie de se faire une idée synoptique résumée des résultats des recherches modernes dans ce domaine et de comprendre plus ou moins les principes exposés dans les publications récentes (par exemple la discussion sur le mode d'action et du point d'attaque des médicaments appartenant au groupe des sulfamides utilisés actuellement ou encore, sur la pathogénie, la prophylaxie et le traitement des angiopathies diabétiques tellement redoutées, etc.).

Aus: *Münchener Medizinische Wochenschrift 98 (1956) 517–521, 581–585, 601–604*

On the Development of Anatomical Research on the Pancreas from Vesalius to Bichat

Part I: from Vesalius to Kerckring

by HANS-MICHAEL DITTRICH and HERWIG HAHN von DORSCHE

As scientific knowledge requires a historical analysis of each problem as it arises for any prognostic study, it is also necessary to analyse the process of research into the pancreas.

In the scientific field, as in others, the 15th century saw the development of an orientation towards the application of the results of natural studies and the revival of classical Greco-Roman culture. With the ousting of the metaphysical view of life, man moved to the apex of the hierarchy of Being. This tendency received a special impetus through Platonism as a reaction to the Aristotelism that had hitherto been emphasized. Thus arose Renaissance Humanism, which attributed the dignity, freedom and independence of Man to his own reason and learning.

1. The position of anatomy in the Renaissance

In Renaissance medicine, anatomy was still inextricable linked with physiology. Medical science as a whole saw its task as the transmission of the ancient concepts of HIPPOCRATES (460–377 BC) and GALEN (129–199 AD). All contemporary physicians were prejudiced in favor of these authorities and under the influence of numerous speculative late scholastic theories. The type of the so-called "philological doctor" played a great part in this tradition of ancient knowledge. Such doctors naturally overvalued the inductive method and were totally alien and opposed to experiment, so that no practical results were to be expected from this source.

The new type of man also changed the tasks of medical research. With the orientation of art to the depiction of the human body, there was a growing necessity for the acquisition of more accurate anatomical knowledge. Towards the end of the 15th century the schematic illustrations that had prevailed in the anatomy texts for almost a thousand years were replaced by new and realistic figures. The discovery of printing by means of movable metal type by JOHANN GUTENBERG (1400–1468) introduced a new epoch of storage of information which had a revolutionary effect in all fields of scholarship, based on the technique of the woodcut for purposed of illustration.

It is no accident that the practical instruction in anatomy at Salerno, which had begun with animal dissection, progressed to the study of human cadavers (Bologna c.1300), and that this led to the separate development of anatomy as the basis of medicine. Already in the 14th and 15th centuries, the findings of the dissections carried out meant that new facts became known about the structure of the human body. The most important advances took place in Italy, then highly developed economically. Thus, among others, ALLESSANDRO ACHILLINI (1463–1512) successfully studied the anatomy of the cranial bones, worked on the auditory ossicles in this context, and discovered the opening of the common bile-duct into the duodenum.

On the basis of over 100 dissections, BERENGARIO DA CARPI (1470–1550) published good descriptions of the laryngeal cartilages, the lacrimal apparatus and the heart and also provided a graphic picture of the cecum and the hepatic circulation. ALESSANDRO BENEDITTI (d. 1512) discovered the excretory ducts of the glands at the entrance to the female genitalia later to be named after PARTHOLIN. The Vidian canal in the bony base of the skull was named after GUIDO GUIDI (d. 1569). However, the leading textbook of anatomy of this period originated from MONDINO DEI LUZZI (d. 1326) and was used as a primary source until VESALIUS brought out his *Fabrica.*

This period of the emergence of anatomy as a separate discipline also saw the beginnings of pathological anatomy. JEAN FERNEL (1506–1558) esteemed the knowledge of anatomy as important for the doctor as a knowledge of the seat of war for the historian. VOLCHER KOYTER (1534–1590) was already performing autopsies in cases where the cause of death was unclear.

In terms of the nature of the times, anatomy prior to VESALIUS was oriented rather to the discovery of anatomic detail, often delighting in discovering curiosities, but was unable to trace the main connexions in the human body. It was only with ANDREAS VESALIUS (1514–1564) that modern anatomy was founded.

2. Pancreatic research from Vesalius to Wirsung

The uncritical handing down of Galenic teaching was interrupted by ANDREAS VESALIUS (1514–1564). He himself carried out numerous dissections on human cadavers and so arrived inductively at conclusions which demonstrated the essential inadequacy of teleogically based Galenic anatomy. In his work, *De humani corporis fabrica libri septem* (1543) he dealt predominantly with the pancreas in the chapter on the stomach, duodenum and omentum (Lib. V, Cap. 3; Lib. V, Cap. 5 and Lib. V, Cap. 4) and depicted it as two independent glandular parts, corresponding to the head on the one hand and the body and tail on the other. On p. 497 he describes it as follows:

"Apart from the fat, which is common with the membranes of the omentum, the deeper membrane which is interposed at the hinder part of the stomach is required for a quite large glandular body. Because the same is reddish in dogs and has the color of ordinary muscle, it was called by the Greeks *καλλίκρεας* and *πάγκρεας*. In men this body is more white than red and extends to the portal vein and the branches of the arteries and nerves found there, so that in its full extent it supports only the deep membrane of the omentum, that this should be more secure, and also provides the stomach with a support on which it rests. Thus is constituted the organ and the substance which lies under the duodenum, of which it has been previously falsely believed that it closes the under opening of the stomach (so that nothing undigested can flow out)" (Rev. SCHIRMER, 1893, p. 8/9).

The Greifswald medical historian HEINRICH HAESER (1881) assessed VESALIUS's work as follows:

"The 'pancreas' on the other hand, by which is to be understood not our *Bauchspeicheldrüse* (abdominal salivary gland) which was only discovered later but a convolution of glands lying in the midst of the mesentery, is likewise only to be accorded the importance of serving as a support for the vessels."

To this judgment one can give only a qualified assent. It must be borne in mind that VESALIUS studied the pancreas of the dog rather than of man, himself saying that it was very large and easy to recognize because of its flesh color. For this reason, according to N. BROCKSTEDT (1968), the described structure and function differ in many ways from the actual anatomic conditions in man. Thus, as regards pancreatic research, VESALIUS remained with the results of his zoologic studies, and his information about the pancreas is contradictory:

- On the one hand, he does not adhere to the opinion of GALEN and his supporters, that the pylorus possesses a specific "glandular muscle" *(glandosa carnis)* which has contractile properties, because he could find no muscle fibers as in the bladder.

- On the other hand, he advanced the concept that, as well as the supporting function of the pancreas, this organ had the additional task of impregnating the lumen of the entire bowel so as to prevent it from drying up.

Thus VESALIUS did not break with tradition, as also when he clearly emphasized the fusion of the pancreas with the duodenum. He still did not recognize the secretory capacity of the gland. His intellectual experiments – as BROCKSTEDT (1968) emphasizes – had the outcome that he designated the pancreatic juice as a "lentus humor", although the secretion is extremely thin and watery. Vesalius's contemporaries scarcely differed from him. CHARLES ESTIENNE (1504–1564), born in Paris, likewise in his work, *La dissection des parties du corps humain* (Paris 1564) advocated the view that the pancreas had a protective function for the vessels and bile-ducts and served as a *fulcimentum* (support) or *pulvinarium* (cushion) for the stomach against the hard vertebral column. A similar idea occurs with REALDO COLOMBO (1516–1559), who worked in Padua as a disciple of VESALIUS. In his *De re anatomica* of 1559 he writes, of the basic function of the pancreas:

". . . and its chief office consists in this, that it restrains the intestines so that they should not become entangled and complicated, or fall downwards." (Rev. SCHENK, 1609).

Besides its supporting function, COLOMBO saw the task of preventing a volvulus and incarceration of the bowel. GABRIELE FALLOPPIO (1523–1562), an admirer of VESALIUS, also interested himself in the pancreas. He was the first to question the concept, almost rigidly established as dogma, of the mechanical protective function of the pancreas as his observations in animals showed this to be meaningless in the horizontally placed bodies of quadripeds. In his *Observationes anatomices* (1562) he states:

"The anatomists add something no less uncertain when they assert that the said gland (pancreas) is made to support the stomach. If that were true, this structure would be found to be completely useless in animals which proceed sloping forward, for in these the pancreas lies above the stomach and not beneath it. However, the true use of the same is that is has an incised canal which is surely conducted along that prominent vein which leads from the liver hilum to the spleen. It spreads over this as if it were a cushion and protects it from all compressing influences."

By the *insculptum canalem,* he means the groove through which the splenic vein reaches the portal vein.

In this period of morphologic pancreatic research, not only AMBROISE PARE (1510–1590) but also the Swiss, FELIX PLATTER (1563–1633), as an adherent of VESALIUS, defended the concept of the supportive function of the pancreas. In his work, *De corporis humani structura et usu tabulis methodice explicati, iconibus acute illustrati* (Basel 1583), he adduced:

"A gland-like body, situated at the underside of the stomach and duodenum, called the pancreas, has important branches there attached to the head for strengthening and supports the stomach so that there is no pressure on the vessels; this is rather its true definition than that it is merely a support for the stomach."

In his *Anatomicae praelectiones* of 1586, ARCHANGELO PICCOLOMINI (1526–1609), a younger contemporary of VESALIUS, proposed a correction of the concept "pancreas" in the form of *"pandenon"*. Because of its white color and soft structure, some anatomists – like JACOB DE BACK, for example – called the pancreas *"Lastes"*. However, these terms did not prevail.

The fleshy glandular character was also emphasized by the anatomist GEORGI BERTINI in his Campani medicina of 1587, where he wrote:

"Pancreas vero et caro glandulosa, plurimis glandulis scatens, vasorum divisionem solidiorem ac securiorem efficiens, simulque fulciens."

The anatomist and botanist CASPAR BAUHIN (1560–1624) based himself almost exclusively on VESALIUS, even adopting a poor reproduction of his illustrations, and described the pancreas in his *De corporis humani fabrica* (Basel 1590) as follows:

"It is a gland-like body interposed in the stomach bed and attached to the duodenum, whitish in men and reddish in dogs. Its function is 1. as GALEN maintained, to preserve undamaged and uninjured the veins, arteries and nerves which are distributed in delicate branches; 2. so that the stomach should not be damaged by contact with the spine; 3. so that the artery is not excessively compressed by the stomach; and finally that it fills the empty space between the stomach and the liver." (Rev. Schirmer 1893, p. 11)

BAUHIN developed the *fulcimentum* theory further in that he conceived the pancreas as *vesica fellea lienis* (gallbladder of the spleen) and regarded it as a kind of storage organ for the black splenic humor (melancholia). Here the old humoral pathology is revived in pancreatic research. He further believed that from this gland *infiniti vapores humidi et calidi* were emitted to surround the stomach as a sort of water-bath. He still advanced this concept 19 years later in his *Institutiones anatomicae virilis et muliebris* of 1609.

If we survey previous investigations and publications on the pancreas, we can note that the Galenic dogma of the supportive function of the pancreas was onyl gradually ousted. The anatomists concentrated exclusively on description of its fleshy substance, without detecting the connexion between the pancreas and the duodenum, not to mention its actual glandular function. It already marked a great step forward that the pancreas should be seen in connexion with the alimentary tract by Vesalius in his pancreas-stomach relationship, and as a storage organ by BAUHIN. The direction of anatomic research was predominantly governed by morphologic structural considerations.

When SCHIRMER asserted in 1893 that "up to the year 1641, nothing of any consequence was to be found in the entire literature" (p. 11), this is incorrect. The discoverer of the chyliferous vessels, GASPARRE ASELLI of Cremona (c. 1581–1626) also designated as "pancreas" certain mesenteric gland conglomerates in 1627. As he ascribed a lymph-node function to his "pancreas", a similar function was also ascribed to the true pancreas. He regarded the pancreas as a sponge for sucking up the chyle, which was passed on to the liver and spleen. This error nevertheless proved no mean stimulus to the investigation of pancreatic function, an investigation that was reserved for the iatrochemists. But of course, before this there had to come the discovery of the connexion between the pancreas and the duodenum.

The first concrete evidence that the pancreatic duct constituted a connexion between the pancreas and the duodenum came from the anatomist and botanist MORITZ HOF(F)MANN (1621 or 1622–1698). He discovered this in 1642 in a turkey-cock, in Padua, and he attached such importance to this discovery that he specified in his will that the current professor of anatomy should receive a guilder annually to commemorate his name by demonstrating the pancreatic duct. He was constrained to this singular step by the discovery of the pancreatic duct in man by JOHANN GEORG WIRSUNG (or Wirsüng) (1600–1643). HOFFMANN, delighted with his discovery, had informed WIRSUNG. Soon after this, the latter, in the presence of the young THOMAS BARTHOLINUS (1616–1680), in March 1642, demonstrated the excretory duct in man also by extremely skilled dissection, and had his discovery engraved on a copper plate. According to L. CHOULANT (1858), only two examples were known, in Basel and Padua, and only after unearthing the original block in Padua could further prints be made. The news of the discovery of the pancreatic duct rapidly spread throughout Europe. According to ALBRECHT VON HALLER, a banquet was held annually in Altdorf to celebrate this event.

The most important achievments of Wirsung are:

- the discovery of the pancreatic duct in man
- the first determination of a double excretory duct (though he did not recognize this as a constant component)
- the first description of the pancreatic juice.

WIRSUNG was nevertheless so influenced by the old Galenical opinions that he himself could not assess the importance of the great discovery and its consequences. With great modesty, he therefore turned in a letter of 7 July 1643 to his former teacher, JOHANNES RIOLAN (1580–1657) with a request to check these exciting findings. WIRSUNG also enclosed a copper plate and wrote:

"Though at a distance, the memory of respectful friendship is renewed: so it is with me, famous and high-ranking man, formerly also my teacher, always held in honor by me; although I have been deprived of your presence for 23 years, and you were the first to introduce me to anatomy, so can I indeed be no other than respectful and mindful, and especially of that time when I was your pupil and was instructed and inaugurated by your very clear lectures, and am also mindful of the many kindnesses you have shown me and express my infinite thanks; and at the same time renew the memory of your fidelity, which is impressed on my mind. This will be confirmed to you by that famous man who was formerly my teacher, CASPAR HOFFMANN, Professor at Altdorf. On his advice, I venture to trouble you with these few words, as I used to do. Likewise the famous PAUL MARQUARD SLEGEL, professor in Jena, my friend, who came from your Paris school to our discussions, the bearer of these lines, will witness. I have requested the famous HOFMANN for his views on the use and function of a newly discovered duct in the pancreas and have asked him also to refer to you; however, as I have received nothing from him or from you, I write this because of the great distance and the difficulty in sending letters. And because I now have a very favorable opportunity, I humbly repeat my request through the bearer and have recourse, now as formerly, to the true source, my first teacher, my refuge. As for the duct mentioned, of which an illustration is enclosed, the case is thus: the opening or beginning, if one may consider it the beginning, where the larger trunk is found, lies as may be noted in the duodenum beside the bile-duct. The probe can be inserted from the bowel towards the pancreas only with difficulty, but from the latter to the bowel quite easily, and goes through the middle of the entire pancreas along its length towards the spleen, has innumerable ramifications, and finally quite small twiglets as far as the wall above, below and underneath the splenic vessels, and itself sends out winding branches through the pancreas but does not enter the spleen. At times I have found in both men and animals a double form, a short one at the most usual place and a longer one more deeply. Likewise, I found this not only in human bodies of adults, newborn and unborn, but also in apes, dogs, cats, pigs, hens, mice and frogs, and short in all I have thoroughly investigated. Shall I call it an artery or vein? I found no blood in the same, but a turbid fluid which acted like a corrosive fluid on the silver probe. These are the facts: but, as I do not know what it is or what use and function it has, I submit it humbly for your examination and judgment, hoping that when you have arrived at a sure decision you will communicate it to me in your wonted friendliness and kindness, partly in order that the truth, which you have ever fearlessly reported, may come to light, partly that thereby the fame of your name may be further increased: and this I promise you to do as long as my hands, which were trained by you, can wield a knife. More I will not write, lest I become tedious; farewell, and do not cease to cherish your former pupil.

Padua, 7 July 1643.

Your Highness's most devoted
Io. Geor. Wirsung

(Rev. SCHIRMER, 1893, p. 12–14)

A dispute as to priority developed between HOF(F)MANN and WIRSUNG. Of historical importance is a communication from Bartholinus, who, as a witness of the discovery of the pancreatic duct, writes in his *Anatomia reformata* (1651):

> "The pancreatic excretory duct, never previously described by anyone, was first discovered in Padua, in my presence, at the beginning of March 1642 by JOHANNES GEORG WIRSUNG, an extremely circumspect anatomist, whose life was extinguished by a cruel fate."

The debate on the pancreatic duct was inaugurated by Wirsung's teachers: JOHANNES RIOLAN and JOHANNES VESLING.

RIOLAN published his written reply in his *Opera anatomica* (1649) and spoke of an "admirable discovery" which stimulated him to further anatomic studies. He himself, however, was unable to find the duct depicted in the figure because of "a lack of hanged men". But he trusted WIRSUNG and supported the view that the pancreas might be a form of filter for the liver and spleen in which the chyle was purified, should this not have taken place in the glands of the mesentery. RIOLAN unequivocally denied that the pancreas was a cushion for the stomach or a support for the veins.

JOHANNES VESLING (1598–1649), professor of anatomy and botany in Padua, already mentioned in 1647 in his work *Syntagma anatomicum* that WIRSUNG had described a duct of venous structure in the pancreas, which opened in common with the ductus choledochus into the duodenum. VESLING found it particularly interesting that the pathway was sometimes double. He also published an illustration of his findings and expressed the supposition that an obstruction of the duct must lead to severe damage to the liver and spleen. A widespread view was that the excretory duct was a large chyliferous vessel, and VESLING also subscribed to the view that the pancreas filtered the chyle and retained residues. The anatomists saw in the duct one of the chyliferous vessels discovered by ANSELLIE in 1627, and in the "pancreas Anselli" a convoluted gland with lymph-vessels.

With the discovery of the pancreatic duct, the anatomic dogma of the pancreas as a supportive and space-occupying organ was overturned, while at the same time a decade-long dispute on the problem of this duct was precipitated, a dispute which involved both anatomists and physiologists.

3. The results of research up to the foundation of microscopic anatomy

The Copenhagen anatomist, THOMAS BARTHOLIN (1616–1680), was one of the first to side with the recognition of WIRSUNG's discovery. As stated above, he had himself as a student experienced the moment of the inital discovery of the "ductus Wirsungianus". In his famous *Anatomia reformata* (1651), BARTHOLIN tells the story of the discovery of the pancreatic duct and of the results of his research thereon:

"Besides these (vessels), it (the pancreas) has yet another, membrane-like duct, extending strangely almost cross-wise or transverse in relation to the length of the pancreas, which was not described by anyone before this and was first discovered in Padua when we were studying there in 1642 by JOH. GEORG WIRSUNG, an energetic anatomist who lost his life by a bloody deed; of marked thickness and with strong walls. That it was known to FALLOPIUS I do not believe. True, he speaks of small ducts which end in the pancreas and in the vicinity of the glands; but as this duct is only solitary, so he saw numerous dark milky veins which are distributed in the pancreas, the mesentery and the other glands. It is usually only one, although is may be observed doubled on itself in parallel course. It is short at the usual place and wider underneath this. Its orifice opens widely into the duodenum by the entrance of the bile-duct, with which it sometimes combines in the same opening; but more often, as I myself perceived with the discoverer, as a separate but adjacent orifice. The valve which is situated in front of the duct and looks outward does not allow a sound to be inserted from the duodenum into the new duct; therefore, if in a living animal a ligature is applied adjacent to the intestine, a swelling develops; and if it is applied still deeper the animal dies, if we are to believe JAK. BACCIUS, for this experiment is very difficult; for before this obstructed duct is divided, that is to be ligated the animal dies. From there it creeps through the antire body of the pancreas, giving off unnumerable branches on both sides, until it gradually disappears towards the spleen in narrow but straightly-patterned rami. However, it does not enter this organ, although FOLIUS asserts, contrary to me, that

he has seen it to do so. Probably this was extraordinary and should not have happened, because the branches grew through a normal weakness before they came into contact with the spleen and obliterated the concavity against the bowel. In this receptacle there is no visible juice, only the probe is usually moistened with yellowish biliary juices, and the walls are covered with this same fluid, so that the bile seems to be arrested here according to the usual natural laws; this has also been seen by our friend JOH. von HORN in Venice with his own eyes, when the gallbladder is distended in jaundice."
(Rev. SCHIRMER, 1893, p. 20–22)

BARTHOLINUS, after exhaustive studies of the pancreas, refuted the error that the "ductus Wirsungianus" was a large chyliferous vessel. It is interesting, from the viewpoint of the history of science, that the term *'fermentatio'* was already used by him. At this time, too, a clear depiction of the pancreas and its pancreatic duct was supplied by an Oxford friend of Harvey's, NATHANIEL HIGHMORE (1613–1684) in his *Corporis humani disquisitio anatomica* (The Hague 1651). From both the anatomic and artistic aspects, it offers one of the best representations of the pancreas of this period.

The debate on the role of the pancreas as a chyliferous vessel was also continued by the Rotterdam anatomist, JACOB DE BACK (dates unknown, doctoral dissertation 1660). In his *Dissertatio de Corde* (third edition, Rotterdam 1660), he wrote:

"To what end, I ask, is the chyle produced? Surely not so as to provide the pancrease with nutrition. By no means; for this fluid is unsuited for nutrition: further, the pancreas receives from the celiac branch arteries adapted for this purpose, which are much larger than required by its small size."

In the same year (1660), the versatile doctor FRANS DE LA BOE, known as SYLVIUS (1614–1672), submitted a classification of the glands in his text *De Lienis et Glandularum usu* in two main parts: *Glandulae conglomeratae* and *Glandulae conglobatae.* He included the pancreas in the first part. The importance of the pancreas in physiology is discussed in the chapter on iatrochemistry. Its classification as a gland was also adopted by the polyhistorian NIELS STENSEN (1638–1696) in his text *De musculis et glandulis observationem specimen* (Amsterdam 1664). He particularly regretted that the glands had hitherto been neglected organs in anatomy, the *"summum conditoris artificium"*. As a comparative anatomist, he enriched the understanding of the pancreas and wrote, in the chapter *Ductus Wirsungianus:*

"An observation made in birds serves to illustrate the Ductus Wirsungianus and also clarifies the use of the liver. In different types of birds which were opened, I have seen a double pancreatic duct, which likewise resembled the bile-duct."

In the manner of the time he considered the glands as "sieves", through which the blood was driven by the force of heat through the pores into the capillary vessels of the lymph-ducts. The gland secretions derived from the arterial blood.

"All lymph-ducts which are adjacent to the gland clusters pour their contents into certain body cavities." (Rev. SCHÖNWETTER, 1968, p. 17)

A special work by BERNHARD SWALWE (d. 1680), entitled *Pancreas adornante sive pancreatis et succi ex eo profluentis commentum succinctum* (Amsterdam 1667) dealt thoroughly with the anatomy of the duct:

"The opening of this duct to the right of the pancreas is fairly large. But only if it has entered the bile-duct and so ended at the usual entrance into the bowel, approximately four fingerbreadths below the pylorus. In most cases, this duct and the ductus choledochus soon after their junction have only one opening and only one orifice into the duodenum, if we regard this as the lower part of the duodenum or the upper part of the jejunum; it is always separate and different, sometimes duplicated; at one time distant from the papilla of the bile-duct, at another close to it, at yet another joined with it . . ." (Rev. SCHIRMER„ 1893, p. 23)

One of the most artistically accomplished anatomical plates of the pancreas is provided by GODEFRIDI BIDLOO (1649–1713) in his *Anatomia humani corporis* (1685). In 1706, he founded the military hospital in Moscow, the first medico-surgical school in Russia at that time. The illustration of the human pancreas with its excretory duct was drawn by the Dutch painter GERARD DE LAIRESSE.

In the 17th century, various spicilegia (*spiciligium* = discourse) were published which were devoted mainly or almost exclusively to morbid anatomy. Thus, THEODOR KERCKRINGIUS (1640–1693) in his *Spicilegium anatomicum* (1670) reported on the *Ductus pancreaticus foetus parenchymate denudatus* (p. 149). Various additional information about the pancreas was now supplied from pathology, which separated itself from anatomy as an independent discipline at this time. However, in the context of our topic, it is not possible to deal in more detail with the extensive material of the pathologic studies of the 17th century.

With the foundation of microscopic anatomy by the Bolognese anatomist MARCELLO MALPIGHI (1628–1694), a new era in research into the anatomy and physiology of the glands was ushered in. Whereas microscopists hitherto, in their delight at the discovery of a previously invisible world, communicated their findings without any sort of system. MALPIGHI in 1666 published his views on the structure and function of the glands under the title *De structura viscerum* (this appeared in the *Opera omnia,* Leiden 1687). According to MALPIGHI:

". . . the acinar glands, of which the pancreas and thymus can be taken as examples, are subdivided into portions and small parts which are themselves assembled into glandular lobes, as I have seen in the thymus of the ox. From these lobules a considerable vessel takes its origin, into which the smallest cell-component of the gland empties its excreted juice in a special cavity and for a special purpose." (Rev. SCHÖNWETTER, 1968, p. 12).

This most significant pronouncement about the pancreas renders the first histologic findings and is thereby of scientific historical value. MALPIGHI even claimed – like SWAMMERDAM – to have seen an organ similar to the pancreas in insects.

After the discovery of the circulation of the blood by HARVEY in 1628, and together with the morphologic line of research which advanced to microscopy, such discussions about the pancreas developed in a more physiologic manner. After the discovery of the duct, the *anatomia animata* explained the pancreas as an organ of blood formation. Here, too, we see the smooth transition from Galenic medicine with the concept of the liver as a blood-forming organ, into which ASELLI would have the chyliferous vessels open. Now there was added the beginning of research into the physiologic aspects.

Summary

The historical development of the morphologic study of the pancreas from VESALIUS to KERCKRING is discussed. Beginning with a sketch of the scientific picture of the Renaissance, the concepts of ANDREAS VESALIUS about the pancreas are studied. It is shown that his views on this organ still bear Galen's imprint. VESALIUS, the founder of modern anatomy, made no individual contribution to explanation of the pancreas, nor was any decisive advance made during the century after the appearance of Vesalius's *Fabrica.* It was only the discovery of the pancreatic duct (major and minor) by WIRSUNG in 1642 that led to an understanding of the glandular function of this organ, aided by his discovery of the pancreatic juice. Of course, this information became known only gradually. THOMAS BARTHOLIN was the first, in his *Anatomica reformata* of 1651, to use the term *fermentatio* in connexion with the description of the pancreas and the "ductus Wirsungianus".

Knowledge about the comparative anatomy of the pancreas based on Wirsung's discovery was especially expanded by NIELS STENSEN (1664), who dissected mainly birds for this purpose.

In 1667, SWALWE described the common opening of the pancreatic duct and the common bile-duct into the duodenum, while KERCKRING (1670) reported on the pancreatic duct in human fetuses, but for the time being there were no further decisive advances in knowledge of the structure and function of the pancreas.

The breakthrough was made with Wirsung's discovery, through which Galen's concept that this organ functioned as a support for the stomach was overcome.

References

ASELLI, G., De lactibus seu lacteis venis, quarto vasorum mesaraicorum genere, novo invento dissertatio, Mailand 1627 und Leiden 1640.

BACK, I. DE, Dissertatio de corde. Roterodami 1660, Vol. 3.

BARTHOLINUS, TH., Anatomia reformata. Lugduni Batavorum 1651.

– Anatome. Ex omnium veterum recentiorumque observationibus. Lugduni Batavorum 1673.

BAUHIN, C., Institutiones anatomicae virilis et mulierbris historiam exhibentes. Basel 1609.

BERTINI, G., Campani medicina. Basileae 1587.

BIDLOO, G., Anatomia humani corporis centum a quinque tabulis per artificios. Amstelodami 1685.

BOE, F. DE LE, Disputatio medica de spirituum animalium in cerebro cerebelloque confectione per nervos distributione atque usu vario. Leidae 1660.

– De lienis et glandularum usu. Leidae 1660.

BROCKSTEDT, H., Vesals Anschauungen über die Drüsen. Inaug.-Diss., Kiel 1968.

CARPI, B. DA, Commentaria super anatomia Mundini, Bologna 1521.

CHOULANT, L., Graphische Incunabeln für Naturgeschichte und Medizin. Leipzig 1858.

COLOMBO, R., Anatomia, das ist sinnreiche, künstliche begründete Aufschneidung. Deutsch. Übers. von I. A. SCHENK, Frankfurt/M. 1609.

ESTIENNE, CH., La dissection des parties du corps humain. Paris 1546.

FALLOPPIO, G., Observationes anatomicae. Coloniae 1562.

GALENUS, C., De usu partium corporis humani. Venetiae 1565.

HAESER, H., Lehrbuch der Geschichte der Medizin und der epidemischen Krankheiten. 3 Bde. Jena 1875/82.

HALLER, A. VON, Elementa physiologiae corporis humani. Tom. 1–5, Lausanne 1757/63, Tom. 6–8, Bern 1764/66.

HIGMORE, N., Corporis humani disquisitio anatomica, Hagae Comitis Oxon 1651.

KERCKRINGIUS, TH., Spicilegium anatomicum. Amstelodami 1670.

MALPIGHI, M., Opera omnia. Leiden 1687.

PICCOLOMINI, A., Anatomicae praelectiones. Rom 1586.

PLATTER, F., De corporis humani structura et usu, tabulis methodice explicati. iconibus acute illustrati, Basel 1583.

RIOLANUS, J., Opera anatomica. Paris 1649.

SCHIRMER, A. M., Beitrag zur Geschichte und Anatomie des Pankreas. Diss., Basel 1893.

SCHÖNWETTER, H. P., Zur Vorgeschichte der Endokrinologie. Med. Diss., Zürich 1968.

STENONIS, N., De musculis et glandulis observationem specimen cum epistolis duabus anatomicis. Amstelodami 1664.

SWALWE, B., Pankreas pancrene, sive pancreatis et succi ex eo profluentis commentum succinetum. Amstelodami 1667.
VESALIUS, A., De humani corporis fabrica libri septem. Basileae 1543.
VESLING, J., Syntagma anatomicum. Patavii 1647.

in: *Anatomischer Anzeiger 138, Jena (1975) 11–25.*

On the Development of Anatomical Research on the Pancreas from Vesalius to Bichat

Part II: from Borelli to Bichat

by HANS-MICHAEL DITTRICH and HERWIG HAHN von DORSCHE

Abstract

This study deals with knowledge of the pancreas from the 17th to the 19th centuries. The investigations of Brunner in 1689 were a landmark: he described the symptoms of diabetes mellitus in pancreatectomized dogs but did not make the actual diagnosis. Another culminating point was the tissue system described by Bichat in 1800. However, knowledge of the histology of the pancreas during this period was very minor.

Introduction

According to *Bernal* (1967), 17th-century science showed a "homogeneity that stemmed from a threefold root: personalities, concepts and applications". The anatomists of that time were "virtuosi" in the truest sense of the word, i.e. their creative achievements were produced in different sectors of science. A basic unifying factor in the concepts of the physicians was the working method which, by its nature, had a mathematical bias. It was even held by some that the operation of the various glands of the body could be explained by the relative momentum of their particles which was thought to depend on the angles at which their secretions were secreted. A further typical feature was that the anatomists applied themselves to the technical problems of their time. With these three characteristics, 17th-century science made a radical break with tradition. In medicine new problems concerning the concept of life were tackled in the 17th century. In principle, as at present, there were two schools in opposition to the Alexandrian school: iatrophysics with its biophysical slant and iatrochemistry with its biochemical angle.

1. Contributions of iatrophysics to investigation of the pancreas

Iatrophysics with its biophysical slant, which applied experimental quantitative methods to physiologic processes and endeavoured to account for all the vital functions by pure mechanics, enlarged our knowledge of pancreatic function in its own specific way. The Galenic teaching concerning "digestiones" was superseded thereby. In the light of corpuscular/physical reasoning, the lymph and blood vessels were conceived as a delicate system of pipes and interconnected filters. Italy was the home of iatrophysics, which dealt with various matters relating to digestion and respiration and also to the physiology of the brain and nerves. Bone, muscle and joint function were studied from mathematical/physical angles, applying the principles of levers.

The Italian mathematician, physicist and physiologist *Giovanni Alfonso Borelli* (1608–1679) investigated the structure and function of the glands, applying mechanical principles. In his standard physiologic work *De motu animalium* (written as early as 1662) he wrote on this subject:

> "It cannot be denied that some glands are the places where certain fermentative juices which serve the animal economy in the digestion of food, the formation of chyle, blood and spirit are formed. On the other hand, it does not seem credible that all glands should be places for the storage and formation of fermentative juices because the gland lobules appear to have the same purpose as the clods in which the capillary roots of plants are spread out and are closely surrounded by them . . . " (transl. Schönwetter I, 1968, p. 13).

The iatrophysicists saw the glands and the pancreas, too, as a kind of "sieve". The most significant aspect of this school nevertheless was that they called for and practised experimentation as the basis of scientific research. They thus laid important foundations for glandular research and helped to oust speculative thinking. To be sure, the technical prerequisites were in many ways inadequate yet in the second half of the 17th century basic discoveries were made concerning the detailed structure of the glands.

2. Contributions of iatrochemistry to investigation of the pancreas

In opposition to the absolutist school of iatrophysics, there was iatrochemistry which aimed at extending the old humoral teaching scientifically. They interpreted the chemical transformations that take place in the body by analogy with the fermentation process as *"fermentatio"*. Studies of the process of digestion by precise observations and experiments led to further insight into the vital processes.

Investigation of the pancreas as reflected in iatrochemistry bore a typical stamp and was greatly advanced by the interest taken in the glands. Apposite statements concerning glandular function existed from antiquity. *Galen* was already talking of intestinal glands which released a saliva-like juice (*De semine*, Lib. II). *Vesalius* described them according to the sectores: supporting function, filling, protective and secretory functions. By the term "fleshy" he intended rather to describe the nature of the tissue. The vessels were thought to be the actual substrate for the glandular structure. The complete revolutionizing of anatomy by *Vesalius* and the discovery of the circulation of the blood by *Harvey* led to the systematic investigation of the glands from the mid–17th century onwards.

In the year 1654 there appeared in London the *"Anatomia hepatis"* of *Francis Glisson* (1597–1677) in which he gave an account of his views concerning the glands and their functions. As he was the first to attempt a rational classification of the different types of gland, a few speculative elements still crept in. For all that, he had already correctly recognised their secretory activity:

> "One thing is certain: all glands have a common task, to produce some secretion or other."

The lectures on the theme *"Glandularum totius corporis examinatio"* (1652) gave rise to the *"Adenographie"* (1695) of *Thomas Wharton* (1614–1673), the first major work relating to glands. He thought that their main function was closely connected with the nerves:

> "The glands do not serve the blood so much as the nerves."

Thus the concept of a blood-building function that had gained wide acceptance since the discovery of the pancreatic duct was superseded. *Wharton*'s work contained a detailed description of the different glands, including the pancreas. He construed it as a storage organ for nerve fluid and already conjectured that besides the main pancreatic duct there might exist several accessory ducts which also opened into the duodenum.

In 1660 *François de la Boë* or *Sylvius*, the founder of the iatrochemical school, dealt in the first and second *"Disputatio medica"* with the physiologic processes in the intestinal canal. In these works he attached the greatest importance to certain acid and alkaline particles in the degradation of food by the digestive juices – including those of the pancreas – and wrote: "That the natural pancreatic juice differs not at all or very little from saliva."

The therefore thought that the succus pancreaticus was acidulous. The pancreatic juice would combat the bile in the duodenum and thereby separate the waste from the chyle. *Sylvius* even described pathologic conditions of the pancreatic juice and connected it with the fermentation that took place in the stomach and intestine. His pupil *Regnier de Graaf* (1641–1673) had already, as a student, written the *"Tractatus anatomico-medicus de succi pancreatici natura et usu"* (Leiden, 1663) in which he stated *"succus noster, a nobis prima detectus"* (our juice, first discovered by us). In 1664 he once again in his *"Disputatio medica de natura et usu succi pancreaticis"* tackled the question of the function of the pancreas, starting with iatrochemical experiments. With the aid of pancreatic fistulas, which he created in live dogs who had previously eaten nothing for a long time, he endeavoured to prove the theory of his teacher, *Sylvius*, concerning the mixture of the "acid pancreatic juice" with the "alkaline bile". In a sailor who had died suddenly and whom *de Graaf* opened up while still warm, he found the pancreatic juice so "pleasantly acid in taste" as he had never found it in dogs. In the same year (1664) he introduced a quill into the pancreatic papilla, which was, however, not described until 1720 by *Abraham Vater* (1684–1751).

3. The pancreas/diabetes experiments of *Johann Conrad Brunner*

When the pathologist *Théophile Bonet* (1620–1689) in his *"Sepulchretum anatomicum sive anatomica practica"* (Geneva, 1679) expressed the thought *"Succus pancreaticus plurimos morbos facit"*, he was probably not thinking of the close connection between the pancreas and diabetes mellitus. At that time the debate over the significance of the pancreatic juice was too concerned with the vital process of digestion and explained this incidentally as "rendering the bile effervescent with pancreatic juice". Some authors maintained that in the absence of pancreatic function another organ was capable of taking this over, too.

In the light of such assumptions the opponent of iatrochemistry, *Johann Conrad Brunner* (1653–1727), began from 1673 to 1683 to undertake extirpation of the pancreas in live dogs. As the experimental animals survived, he at first concluded that the pancreas could not have the vital importance that was assigned to it. He even saw in this a refutation of the teaching of fermentative function, as set out by *Sylvius*. Because many of *Brunner*'s contemporaries did not agree with but even attacked his experimental physiologic research, he felt obliged to conduct further tests on live dogs. On 6th October 1685 he removed the pancreas from a hound and wrote about this experiment in his work *"De Experimentis circos Pancreas novis confirmatis"*:

". . . Then I tied the duct off firmly at its outlet and first divided the upper part of the branch from the stem, removed a portion and shortened it carefully, so that later after disposal of the bond it could not grow together again, as has always occurred otherwise. Then (I detached), too, the lower part together with the mass of the pancreas from which a secondary, lateral and minute duct led to the bile duct.

Cutting off the upper portion of the pancreas is ruled out first, by the internal connections with the intestine, then by the abundance of vessels carrying blood, and then by the inaccessible position where it lies, which is too remote to be reached with the knife. Nor is it necessary.

I could therefore think that the pancreas had been deprived of any connection with the intestines and that the route linking them was interrupted; I applied warm liquid lard to the area of the wound, coated it there with and replaced it as carefully as possible in the abdomen. I sewed up the wound and applied the same salve to it. I finally freed the dog from its fetters and let it loose." (transl. Zimmermann, 1944, p. 117)

In this experiment *Brunner* achieved complete disconnection of the exocrine portion of the pancreas. The extirpated portion of the pancreas was "seven thumbs long and one and a half wide". He kept a diary in the form of a case-history of the course of the dog's postoperative condition and unwittingly discovered the three cardinal symptoms of diabetes mellitus: polydipsia, polyuria and polyphagia. *Wolf–Heidegger* (1939) therefore called him the "true discoverer of pathologic/physiologic connections . . . which, with their symptoms, forge the link between diabetes and the pancreas".

Here, however, his anatomical findings in pancreatectomized dogs are of more interest to us. On this subject *Brunner* wrote as follows:

"The lower part of the pancreas, which might be called its tail, was completely missing (see letters c. c. c.) as it had been duly cut away. The upper part, however, was withered and dried and, strange to say, only as long as a middle finger and scarcely as wide as the little finger (the "ear finger") and as thick as the penholder with which I am writing this (letters d. d. d.), and otherwise hard and granular, as I had already observed before in the third of my experiments.

The opening of the pancreatic duct allowed the passage of a peg from the intestine as far as a finger's breadth (letter f.), namely in front of the ligature made earlier in the experiment in the place where there was a healthy mass about the size of a walnut (letters e. e. e.); I could not introduce a peg or blast of air any further.

I attempted to trace the pancreatic duct in the dried-up portion or rather in the cadaver of the pancreas but I found it had hardened blind, exceptionally thick and impenetrable (letters g. g. g.) especially at the spot where the ligature had once been applied. Indeed, a very strong callosity would almost have shattered the knife (letter h.). As these details can be better shown in pictures than they can be described, it will be advantageous to represent the whole matter pictorially." (transl. Zimmermann, 1944, pp. 120/121)

A review of the research epoch of *"Anatomia animata"* enables us to establish that all the findings led to a greater knowledge of the unity of form and function of organs. This applied to the pancreas, too. Iatrophysics and iatrochemistry boosted the use of inductive methods and led to the introduction of more quantitative measurement in research. The previous morphologic findings were significantly expanded therby. The scientific advances clearly went hand in hand with the development of the range of instruments an the refinement of investigative technique. Nevertheless the path to deeper insights into the structure and function of the pancreas was still blocked as before. Further important steps were required to improve the preconditions for the systematic investigation of the human body, too.

4. Aims and results of research on the pancreas in the 18th century

4.1 The development of investigative technique

The 18th century anatomists who made detailed studies of the pancreas used macroscopic and microscopic methods of examination in order to gain a deeper understanding of the structure and function of this organ. In the sector of *macroscopic methods* injection technique was further developed. In the Baroque era, for which bizarre forms held a special appeal, this method of preparation was widely used. *William Hunter* (1716–1783) introduced liquids into the vascular system in order to preserve material. He thus inaugurated the method of preservation that is nowadays in general use. *Hunter* used oil of turpentine which is, of course, not very suitable for this purpose (*Schmeidel,* 1938). For the preservation of material, 18th-century researchers endeavoured to discover cheap, water-soluble preserving agents. For this purpose, corrosive sublimate and zinc chloride, in particular, were used. The Parisian anatomist *Pierre Augustin Béclard* (1785–1825) was the first to make use in corpses of the preservative effect of corrosive sublimate that had been discovered by his fellow-countryman *François Chaussier* (1746–1828). Since *Boyle* alcohol had played a leading role as a preservative for organ preparations.

In the field of *microscopic methods* progress was dependent on the perfection of microscope technology. In the 18th century the considerable initial successes of the microscope-users soon came up against the limits imposed by the state of development of the optical apparatus. Because the technique of vascular injection and infusion with coloured liquids, air, mercury and stains plainly led to more discoveries than microscopy, the latter was generally practised only for "visual entertainment". Nevertheless, this century witnessed some improvements in microscope technology, too. Among these were the illuminating mirror of *Hertel* (1712) and the swiveling saddle bracket. At that time both transmitted and incident light were used. In the year 1757 the Parisian optician *Charles Chevalier* invented achromatic systems. Owing to the state of development of the technology, microscopy underwent a period of stagnation in the 18th century. It did not recover from this until the 19th century when, apart from an improvement in optics, methods of cutting and staining sections were introduced and allowed effective histologic studies to be carried out (*Dittrich*, 1971).

4.2 Research on the pancreas in the 18th century

Because research in the 18th century yielded no basic new findings owing to the stagnation of microscopy, medical historians have not hitherto paid enough attention to this period. Thus in *Schirmer* (1893) and *Schadewaldt* (1964) we find only a few relevant references. However, if we examine the medical works of that time systematically, we can discern two developmental trends that paved the way for research on the pancreas:

1. the route to refinement of morphology and the evolution of histology and

2. differential studies on the physiology of the pancreatic juice in conjunction with the digestive process.

In view of our subject, we concentrate more on the morphologic/histologic investigations of the pancreas. An important contribution to the morphology of the pancreas was made in the early 18th century by the Italian physician *Giovanni Maria Lancisi* (1654–1720) in his work *"Tabulae anatomicae Bartolommei Eustachii"* (Rome, 1714). In it he published a diagram by *Eustachius*, thus forging a deliberate link with the 16th-century tradition of anatomy. Even for its period this work is more concerned with scientific history. Its significance lies in the fact that it kept interest in the pancreas alive. Another work similar in character was the *"Theatrum anatomicum"* (1717) of the Genevan physician *Jean-Jacques Manget* (1652–1742) who based it mainly on the findings of *de Graaf* and *Brunner*. The Wittenberg Professor of Anatomy *Abraham Vater* (1684–1751) in his *"Dissertatio anatomica"* (1720) was the first to describe the major duodenal papilla where, as a rule, the main efferent duct of the pancreas opens, together with the common bile duct, into the duodenum. It was not until over three-quarters of a century after the discovery of the pancreatic duct by *Wirsung* that the junction was described in detail, although in the meantime many anatomists and physiologists had already dealt with it more fully.

The first eminent anatomist in Louvain was *Philip Verheyen* (1648–1710). His biographer, van Raemdoncke, called him the "Vesal des Landes von Waes" (Vesalius of Waasland). In an "Anatomie oder Zerlegung des menschlichen Leibes" (Anatomy or dissection of the human body) (1699) he also discussed in Chapter XIII "of the pancreas" (pp. 115–118) the anatomy of the pancreas. Concerning the anatomy of this organ he observed as follows:

> "This pancreas is composed of innumerable small glands, each of which is so hard and firm that, when it is separated, it holds its shape but because they are arranged too closely together, the pancreas that is formed by them is softer and more extensive than many other glands.
>
> These glands are held together first by vessels, then, too, according to the testimony of R. de Graaf, by special membranes with which each is endowed. These are all surrounded by a fairly strong skin, originating from the intestinal skin in such a way that the whole pancreas is held fast in its place."

As regards the function of the pancreas *(officium pancreatis)*, however, *Verheyen* still took the old Vesalien view of this "composite" gland as a cushion:

"The business of the pancreas is, whenever a portion is ingested, to remove supposed moisture from the blood through its glands and to discharge suchmatter through its whole entity into the intestines. It is also thought that the pancreas serves the stomach instead of a support and so prevents the stomach when it is overextended from pressing too hard upon the vertebrae."

By means of his own observations he established that the taste of the glandular secretion had a "pleasant acidity", "above all, however, like an acid salt". Moreover, he subscribed to *de Graaf's* concept, according to which the efferent duct in man and in several animals was a double or sometimes even triple duct.

An importance advance in research on the pancreas was the first reference to the diverticulum and perhaps, too, to the accessory pancreas by the anatomist *Johann Heinrich Schulze* (1687–1744). In his autopsy report, which was published in the *"Acta naturae curiosorum"* of the "Leopoldina" German Academy of Naturalists (Halle, 1727, vol. 1), the following appears:

"In the stomach and in the spleen, apart from the fact that they were somewhat displaced, I observed nothing special; nor in the intestines, except that the ileum had, four thumb's breadths before the cecum, an extraordinary appendage equal in length to the top joint of the ring finger, the base being twice as great as the width of the intestine itself but tapering immediately, and the apex being, as it were, crowned by a glandular papilla." (transl. Schirmer, 1893, p. 69)

The leading anatomist of the 18th century in France and one of the most influential altogether, *Jacob Beningue Winslow* (1669–1760), a great-nephew of Niels Stensen, dealt with the pancreas in his work "Exposition anatomique de la structure du corps humain" (Paris, 1732) and there coined the term "petit pancréas" (accessory pancreas). The German translation (Berlin, 1733) reads as follows on the subject:

"For many years I have found in man that the thick end of the mesenteric gland at the place where it is attached to the bend of the duodenum forms a sort of extension which rests against the succeeding portion of the intestine below. Upon examination I found there a singular mesenteric gland duct which divided into branches like the large duct and which bent towards the end of the large one, crossed the latter and then penetrated the duodenum and debouched into the end of the large duct. I call this portion the little pancreas."

In the work "Anatomische Tabellen mit 27 Kupfern" (Leipzig, 1741, 4th ed.) by *Johann Adam Kulmus* (1689–1745) we find an engraving of the pancreas which, in regard to depiction, resembles that of *Verheyen*. In his brief explanation *Kulmus* uses, in essence, only the previous knowledge concerning the pancreas, and this applies especially to the anatomy. The "succus pancreaticus" he declares "separates from the blood" (p. 100). The gland is said to resemble a "dog's tongue" (cf. *Winslow*).

At this time there was published, too, in the year 1775 the work *"Anatomici summi septemdecim tabulae"* of Michael Girardi (1731–1797), the favourite pupil of *Morgagni*. The splendid plates had been produced as early as 1722 to 1728 with the assistance of the artist of note *Giovanni Battista Piazzetta* but they had not been published owing to the untimely death of *Santorini*. *Santorini* recognised that the accessory duct of the pancreas must be regarded as a standard attribute of that organ. Thus the previous conjectures of earlier researchers were confirmed as fact. As *Santorini*'s publication was unknown, this is only hinted at in the works of the 18th-century anatomists. The anatomist *Justus Christian von Loder* (1753–1832), who had been active in Moscow since 1809, considered the relevant diagram so valuable that he included it in his *"Tabulae anatomicae quas ad illustrandam humani corpus fabricam"* (1803), a work which collected together and arranged systematically the anatomical diagrams familiar up to then insofar as they reproduced the factual conditions. *Santorini* (1681–1737) wrote concerning the accessory duct, inter alia, as follows:

"This second pancreatic duct makes it way, as it is situated almost crosswise and its free origin arises from the crosswise part, with the addition of many small branches to the main duct and opens into it." (transl. Schirmer, 1893, p. 31)

This discovery, however, went unnoticed by the contemporary anatomists. The presence of two ducts was not conclusively demonstrated until 1851 by the Parisian surgeon *Aristide Auguste Verneuil* (1823–1895) and in 1856 by the French physiologist *Claude Bernard* (1813–1876).

The Berlin anatomist and botanist *Johann Christian Andreas Mayer* (1747–1801) dealt in his "Beschreibung des ganzen menschlichen Körpers" (1783/1794) with the anatomical, histologic and physiologic aspects of the knowledge relating to the pancreas. In doing so he compared the gland with a pyramid and wrote about its structural composition:

"The gland consists namely of separate pieces or grains which are joined by solid cellular tissue and which can be separated by the anatomical knife, but still more so by maceration, into ever smaller grains. In the smallest grains an injection shows an amazing complexity of blood vessels although it is difficult to determine whether they occupy only the surface of the grain or whether they penetrate into its inmost core, thus leaving no hollow space. Out of each granule, be it never so small, issues a fine little efferent duct which contains the juice secreted therein; several similar vessels unite, forming ever larger branches and finally all terminate in the pancreatic duct, which is called Wirsung's duct."

In his histologic investigations, *J. C. A. Mayer* found "the utmost similarity with the salivary glands", at the same time, stressed the similarity of the secretion with saliva, writing: "The pancreatic juice is saliva." He published an illustration of the pancreas in his work "Anatomische Kupfertafeln nebst dazugehörigen Erklärungen" (Vol. 3, 1783–1788) and even added a diagram of the structure of the gland.

If we review the achievements of anatomy in the investigation of the pancreas in the 18th century, we have to record that during this period no essential insights were gained; however, this should not delude the medical historian into declaring the whole century to be a period of stagnation. As shown by the examples presented in this study, despite all the handing down of illustrations of the pancreas in the anatomical works, isolated new discoveries were made. This demonstrates that there was undoubtedly a certain continuity in the investigation of the pancreas. The most important achievements were based on the refinement of anatomical illustration and the developmental studies.

Closely bound up with the anatomical studies, the 18th century also made significant contributions relating to the *physiology* of the pancreas. Physiology gradually began to evolve into an independent discipline. The sharpest stimuli for this came from physics and chemistry. In any case, the general biological concepts were still saturated with vitalistic ideas, a state of affairs which was not outgrown until the 19th century. Physiological knowledge reached its zenith with the greatest medical polymath *Albrecht von Haller* (1708–1777) in his *"Elementa physiologiae corporis humani"* (vol. 1–5, Lausanne, 1757/63, vols. 6–8, Berne, 1764/66). In his article on digestion he accorded great importance to the saliva. In his opinion, the pancreatic juice, like the saliva, aided the decomposition of food. *Samuel Thomas Sömmerring* (1755–1830) translated this work and in 1798 introduced the name "Bauchspeicheldrüse" (= pancreas) (literally, "abdominal salivary gland") which has remained current in German literature until the present day. *Haller* glimpsed parallels between the structure of the oral salivary gland and the pancreas. The secretion of the juice was seen – as by *J. C. A. Mayer* (1786), for example – to be caused by the circulation of the blood, nerve forces, the pressure of the stomach and that of the duodenum when it moved.

If we wish to describe the state of physiologic knowledge at that time, we can concur with the assessment of the anatomist and physiologist *Friedrich Hildebrand* (1764–1816) who wrote on this subject as follows:

"There are some organs . . . whose purposes are completely unknown to us; others of which we are able to determine the remote and specific purpose but are in doubt as to the immediate (purpose) and remain so as to how they achieve either of these. Among these we must still count the pancreas, too, irrespective of all that was stated about it in the 17th century. It may perhaps be time to have another look at the organ that has been so little regarded by physiologists since that time, now that the field of chemistry has been so considerably extended and it has been so fruitfully applied to the physical aspect of the body."

5. On the state of histology in Bichat's time

In the history of science *Marie François Xavier Bichat* (1771–1802) is generally honoured as the founder of histology. His works "Traité des membranes en général et de diverses membranes en particulier" (Paris, 1800) and "Anatomie générale appliquée à la physiologie et a la médecine (Paris, 1801) described for the first time the form and physical and physiologic characteristics of all the tissues in the human body – even with regard to their function – at different ages. *Bichat* used various methods for his studies. In addition to dissection, he used boiling, maceration, desiccation and treatment with acids, alkalis and alcohol. He told his pupils: "A few dissections will enlighten you more than twenty years of observing symptoms." He never used a microscope, however, because he thought that it would produce only false images. *Bichat* regarded it as a "quantité négligeable" and expressed his view of the use of microscopy as follows:

"Altogether it seems to me as though physiology and anatomy have as yet reaped no special gains from microscopes; for if you observe in the dark, each one sees in his own way, nay in accordance with his prejudices."

In his works, moreover, we find no illustrations because they, too, in his opinion, would only reproduce the facts in a misleading way.

Owing to the inadequate strength and imprecise focus of the first lenses, histology was still a long way from really fathoming the elements of animal or human bodies. In these conditions histology nevertheless developed into an independent biological/medical discipline. *August Franz Josef Karl Mayer* (1787–1865) coined the term histology in the year 1819. The further evolution of histology was dependent above all on improvements in the optical equipment of microscopes and in the methods of cutting and staining sections.

If we examine the works of *Bichat* with a view to discovering traces of research on the pancreas, we find that he devotes no separate chapter or article to the pancreas. In his work "Traité des membranes . . ." (1800) he discussed the physiologic/anatomical aspects of the mucous membranes in man and, in doing so, described the organs that had to be dissected (stomach, gall bladder, intestine) without any mention of the pancreas. Nonetheless *Bichat*'s work is a milestone in the history of histology. Any analysis of anatomical and histologic matters in the light of scientific history must therefore examine and compare the discoveries before and after *Bichat*.

Bichat himself was a vitalist and had endeavoured to maintain close contact with physiology. Whereas *Giovanni Battista Morgagni* (1682–1771) had located the seats of disease in the individual organs, *Bichat* was now looking for these in the tissues. He differentiated between 21 different tissues in the human body, namely eight "common" tissues and 13 "special" tissues. As these, on the one hand, occurred together as part of one and the same organ and, on the other hand, occurred in different organs, he was able with this systematic scheme to lay an important foundation stone in relation to systemic diseases. At the same time he understood in large measure how to adopt the best from his predecessors, such as *C. F. Wolff, G. Stahl* or *Buffon*, and to base his own research on it. Up to the 1830s *Bichat*'s histology prevailed in zoology and medicine with some modifications. The idealistic elements of his vitalism were superseded by the ideas of *François Magendie* (1785–1855) and *Claude Bernard* (1818–1878). His tissue classification was, however, developed further by *I. A. M. Fr. Comte* (1798–1857) who also considered structures as the essence of a living organism. The anatomist *Karl Asmund Rudolphi* (1771–1832), who worked in Greifswald from 1793 to 1820 and then pursued his career in the newly-founded University of Berlin, brought about a major advance with his readily grasped tissue classification, as did *Jacob Henle* (1809–1885), although his system of tissue classification is cumbersome.

Bibliography

BERNAL, J. D., Die Wissenschaft in der Geschichte. 3. Aufl. Dt. Verl. d. Wiss., Berlin 1967.

BICHAT, M. F. X., Traité des membranes en général et de diverses membranes en particulier. Paris 1800.

– Abhandlung über die Häute. Aus dem Französischen übersetzt von C. F. Dorner, Tübingen 1802.

– Anatomie générale, appliquée à la physiologie et à la médecine. Tom. I, II, Paris 1801. Deutsch von C. H. Pfaff. Leipzig 1802.

BOË, F. DE LA (SYLVIUS), Disputatio medica de spirituum animalium in cerebro corebelloque confectione per nervos distributione atque usu vario. Leidae 1660.

BONET, TH., Sepulchretum anatomicum sive anatomica practica. Genf 1679.

BORELLI, G. A., De motu animalium. Pars II. Lugduni Batavorum 1717.

BRUNNER, J. C., De experimentis circa pancreas novis confirmatis. Miscellanea curiosa sive Ephemeridum Medico-Physicarum Germanicarum Acad. Imp. Leopold. Natur. Curios. Dec. II, Annus VII, 1688. Norimbergae 1689.

DITTRICH, M., Hauptetappen der mikroskopischen Forschung. Jenaer Rdsch., Halle (Saale) 16, 211–216 (1971).

GIRARDI, M., Jo. Dominici Santorini anatomici summi septemdecim tabulae quas nunc primum editatque explicat iisque alias addit destructura mammarum et de tunica testis vaginali Michael Girardi. Parma 1775.

GLISSON, F., Anatomia hepatis. London 1654.

GRAAF, R. DE, Tractatus anatomico-medicus de succi pancreatici natura et usu. Lugduni Batavorum 1663.

– Disputatio medica de natura et usu succi pancreatici. Leidae 1664.

HALLER A. VON, Elementa physiologiae corporis humani. Tom. 1–5, Lausanne 1757/63, Tom. 6–8, Bern 1764/66.

HILDEBRANDT, F., Über den Zweck des Pankreas. In: Abhandlungen der Physikalisch-Medicinischen Societät zu Erlangen. 1. Band. Frankfurt am Mayn 1810.

KULMUS, J. A., Anatomische Tabellen mit 27 Kupfern. Leipzig 1741.

LANCISI, G. M., Tabulae anatomicae Bartolommei Eustachii, Tom. 10. Rom 1714.

LODER, J. CH. von, Tabulae anatomicae quas ad illustrandam humani corporis fabricam. Vimariae 1803.

MAYER, J. C. A., Anatomische Kupfertafeln nebst dazugehörigen Erklärungen. Berlin, Leipzig, Heft 1–4, 1783–1788, Heft 5–6, 1794.

– Beschreibung des ganzen menschlichen Körpers, mit den wichtigsten neueren anatomischen Entdeckungen bereichert, nebst physiologischen Erläuterungen. Berlin, Leipzig 1783/94.

MORGAGNI, G. B., De sedibus et causis morborum per anatomen indagatis. Libri quinque. 1761 (Leipzig 1827/29).

SANTORINI, J. D., Anatomici summi septemdecim tabulae. Hrsg. von M. GIRARDI. Parma 1775.

SCHADEWALDT, H., Das Pankreas in der Geschichte der Medizin. Stuttgart 1964.

SCHIRMER, A. M., Beitrag zur Geschichte und Anatomie des Pankreas. Med. Diss., Basel 1893.

SCHMEIDEL, G., Methoden zur Konservierung von Organen und ganzen Organismen. In: Handbuch der biologischen Arbeitsmethoden. Hrsg. v. E. ABDERHALDEN. Abt. VII, T. 2. Springer, Berlin, Wien 1938. 427–460.

SCHÖNWETTER, H. P., Zur Vorgeschichte der Endokrinologie. Med. Diss., Zürich 1968.

VATER, A., Dissertatio anatomica qua novum bilis diverticulum . . . proponit. Wittenberg 1720.

VERHEYEN, PH., Anatomie oder Zerlegung des menschlichen Leibes. 1699. Aus dem Lateinischen übersetzt von Th. Fritschen. Leipzig 1722.

WHARTON, TH., Adenographia sive glandularum totius corporis descriptio. London 1695.

WINSLOW, J. B., Esposition anatomique de la structure du corps humain. Paris 1732. Deutsche Übersetzung Berlin 1733.

WOLF-HEIDEGGER, G., Johann Conrad Brunner. In: Große Schweizer Forscher. Hrsg. v. E. FUETER. Atlantis-Verlag, Zürich 1939, 84–85.

ZIMMERMANN, O. CH., Die erste Beschreibung von Symptomen des experimentellen Pankreas-Diabetes durch den Schweizer Johann Conrad Brunner (1653–1727). Med. Diss., Basel 1944.

in: *Anatomischer Anzeiger 143, Jena (1978) 21–38.*

From the History of Diabetes with Particular Reference to the Pancreas

by ERICH EBSTEIN

Motto: Historical studies are a very important part of scientific education (*Mach*, Principles of the science of heat)

In his "Prolegomena to the introduction of insulin therapy for Diabetes mellitus" (Schweizer med. Wochenschrift, 1923, No. 35) *Hermann Sahli* has recently expressed the view openly that: "Once again we have here a typical, instructive example from the history of medicine which shows how an important invention or discovery can sink into complete oblivion again if it is not adequately worked through, so that with the loss of intellectual energy it does not reemerge until after a period of years when it is then brought to fruition through more consistent work. The history of medicine and of inventions and discoveries in general contains many such examples."

Although the pancreas was already known to the school of Hippocrates and to *Galen*, great thirst and gangrene of the foot in-vivo were first described by *Lieutaud* (1703–83) on the basis of autopsy findings of a scirrhous pancreas (observat. 108, cited from *Wolff*, II, 725). *Lieutaud* did not bring these pathologic symptoms into any direct relationship with the pancreas however (*Wolff* II, 758).

Comments about the *hereditary relationships* in diabetes seem to me to be particularly striking and in advance of their time.

Thus *Wilhelm Rondelet* (1507–66) observed that Diabetes mellitus passed from father to son:

"Ego ter vidi in filia et patre, quasi morbus esset hereditarius, vel potius, quia erant ejusdem temperamenti, sollicet biliosi."

In the 17th century the London physician *Richard Morton* (1635–98), who classified diabetes under the heading of Phthisis (*Phthisiologia, libri* III, London 1689) had already made the observation that kinship, familial predisposition can play a role in this: for in one case father and son suffered from this disease, whilst in another three siblings succumbed to it. In the 18th century Professor *Jacob Friedrich Isenflamm* from Erlangen (1726–93) was able to describe a family in which all 8 children died from diabetes in the 8th to 10th year of life (the parents were apparently healthy).

The *actual* history of the pancreas first commenced in about the middle of the 17th century. To the German anatomists of the Middles Ages the pancreas appeared to be "Eyttelfleisch", i.e. made up completely of flesh, i.e. consisting of glandular substance. It has also been called:[1] abdominal gland, large gastric gland, paunch-thymus, mesenteric gland, small back of the stomach *(M. Höfler).*

In 1642 *Georg Wirsung,* who was born in Bavaria and who was studying in Padua at that time, discovered the excretory duct of the human pancreas after *Moritz Hofmann* the elder (1621–98) had discovered this somewhat earlier in the turkey-cock and had shown it to *Wirsung.* In 1643 *Wirsung* – according to *Hyrtl* – was killed in a duel with a Dalmatian count. *Hofmann* became professor of anatomy in Altdorf, where his discovery was celebrated every year for many years by the doctors and students by a banquet (*Haller,* Bibl. anatom., Vol. 1, 416). *Wirsung* had not written anything about his discovery but instead had merely sent an illustration of the duct to the Paris Academy *(Hyrtl).* Both *Hofmann* and *Wirsung* initially thought that the pancreatic duct was a chylous vessel. (The letter which *Wirsung* sent to *Riolan* the younger about his discovery has been printed and translated by *Schirmer* op. cit., p. 12–14.) It was *Thomas Bartholinus* (died 1680) who decuded the real function of the excretory duct from the valve to be found at its opening (cf. *Kurt Sprengel,* Vers. einer pragm. Gesch. d. Arzneikunde, 1801, Part 4).

In 1664 the Delft physician *Regnerus de Graaf* made his observation about the pancreatic juice, in that he introduced a cannula into the pancreatic duct of a living dog and observed, albeit erroneously, that this showed an acid reaction. In his *Bibl. anatom.* I, 523 *Haller* had already expressed the opinion that *Graaf* must presumably have obtained acid gastric juice as well. In any event the title page of *R. de Graaf*s work: *"De succi pancreatici natura et usua"* shows an autopsy table on which a human cadaver is being dissected, and in the immediate vicinity a dog with an abdominal fistula, in which a bottle intended for the collection of the pancreatic juice is clearly visible. Besides this there are birds, fishes etc. lying on the ground and in the back-

[1] Lay German terms just transliterated – no equivalents in English.

ground an open chamber is seen in which an old, sick man lying in his bed is a spectator of the varied goings on. The title-page illustrates very clearly however that practical medicine, pathological anatomy and animal experimentation belong together (cf. *Wilhelm Ebstein,* Der medizinische Versuch, etc., Wiesbaden 1907, p. 53). *R. de Graaf can be described as a modern researcher like Pavlov.*

In the year 1683 the Swiss physician *J. Conrad Brunner* published: *Experimenta nova circa pancreas* etc., in which he ligated the excretory duct of the gland or completely extirpated the organ in the dog. *Brunner* had acquired the technique when he was studying under *Duverney* in Paris (1683). The operated animal survived and he observed – as did also *Bohn* – that the juice did "not show an acid" reaction.

Incidentally, *Muralt* who studied under *Sylvius* in Leiden, had already established this fact, in that he had collected the secretion from the dog and on tasting it found it *"sine sapore"*.

"Idem mihi testimonium celeberrimi Medici Leydensis exhibebunt, qui succum pancreaticum die 22 Julii 1667 Lugdun. Batav. à D. D. Regnero de Graaf, *in aedibus Clarissimi Sylvii collectum, mecum gustarunt" (Vademecum anatomicum, p. 46; also* Haller, *Elementa physiologiae VI, 450 (cf.* Brunner and Muralt, *"From the letters of eminent Swiss doctors etc. p. 28/29, Basle, 1919).*

To come back to *Lieutaud's clinical observation described above, with his autopsy findings on the pancreas, this is all the more remarkable since Morgagni* (d. 1771) and *Valsalva* (d. 1723) did *not* carry out *any* autopsies on diabetic patients (*F. Falk,* p. 89).

According to *Morgagni,* diabetes mellitus still belongs to the *Morbi incertae sedis.* He mentions it amongst the abnormalities of the urine-secreting organs.

Lancisi (died 1720) also thought of diabetes as a disease of the kidneys, in which he claimed to have seen a noticeable change in consistency: *"Renes omnino flaccidi, plicabiles ac ductiles"*. *Willis* (died 1675), who recognised the sweet taste of the urine, saw diabetes above all as a blood disease, ultimately induced through abnormal nervous influences, which also explained the nervous symptoms of the disease. (*De medicamentorum operationibus.* Sect. IV, chap. III.)

Here we see a modern way of looking at things again!

The Liverpool physician *Matthew Dobson,* who in 1776 demonstrated that the sweetness of the urine and blood serum in diabetes is due to sugar (Med. Obst. & Inq., London 1776, V,

298–316), considered the cause of the disease to be disorder of digestion and assimilation and classified diabetes as a general systemic disease ("Disease of the system in general").

John Rollo (Cases of the Diabetes mellitus, London 1798, p. 384) claimed to have found changes in the renal vessels ("an increase of the vascular structure") as the sole and inconstant autopsy finding, whereas *Richard Mead* (died 1754) on autopsy of diabetics frequently found something of a fatty tumor in the liver: *"semper inveni in hepate steatomatosi aliquid, isti non dissimile visum materiae, quae saepe in ictero confirmatiore per alvum dejicitur, sed consistentiae quam haec durioris"* (*Exposit. mechanic. venenorum.* Tent. I *de vipera*, p. 40).[2]

The oldest case of the coincidence of pancreatic conditions with diabetes mellitus concerns a lithiasis in the pancreas.

In 1788 *Cowley* reported on a 34-year-old, very corpulent diabetic man who had taken to drink, in whom at autopsy the pancreas was found to be filled with small stones, up to the size of a pea, firmly embedded in the substance of the gland (cf. *Heiberg*, Handbuch, p. 212).

Meanwhile *Sömmerring* had added the name *"abdominal salivary gland"* to the old one of the pancreas in 1796 (*Wolff*, II, 749), which it has retained to this day. This indicated the role of the gland in digestion.

Magendie in his *Textbook of Physiology* (Paris, 1816) had still expressed the view that it was not possible to say "what the purpose of the pancreatic juice actually is".

After *Tiedemann* and *Gmelin* (Die Verdauung, Heidelberg, 1826, I, 25) had once again established the *alkalinity* of the pancreatic juice and *Leuret and Lassaigne* had described it as being like saliva, it was left to *Johann Nepomuk Eberle* (b. 17. 1. 1798 in Buch in Vorarlberg, d. 18. 12. 1834 in Würzburg) to establish the effects of the pancreas on starch and fat in his epoch-making work, as *Kölliker* called it. This appeared in Würzburg in 1834 and carried the title: *"Physiologie der Verdauung nach Versuchen auf natürlichem und künstlichem Wege"*.[3]

On the basis of these experiments *Eberle* (op. cit. p. 76, 244, 251) was able to come to the conclusion: "Consequently the

---

[2] The passage is not mentioned by *Claude Bernard*, *Senator* and *Frerichs*, but it is by *Salomon*, 1871, p. 60 and by *F. Falk* (1887), p. 89.

[3] "Physiology of digestion on the basis of experiments by natural and artificial methods".

pancreatic juice is able to absorb fat in a very finely dispersed state and to form a kind of emulsion with this".

In 1836[4] *Purkinje and Pappenheim* and, not until 10 years later (1846), *Claude Bernard* emphasized its property of splitting fats. Meanwhile *Bouchardat* and *Péligot* in the year 1838 (Annales de chimie et pharmacie, Vol. 68, p. 206–211) had established the identity of grape- and urinary-sugar.

The *Trommer-Milscherlich*-test of 1841 and also those of *John Moore* and *Heller* (1844) placed valuable aids for the clinical diagnosis of diabetes in the doctors' hands, to which were added the construction of the first Mitscherlich polarisation apparatus in 1847 and the fermentation test in 1850, which *Francis Home* had already introduced as a clinical method of investigation in 1780.

The Parisian hygienist and chemist *A. Bouchardat* (1806–86[5]) already mentioned, not only discovered the diastatic action of the pancreatic juice, together with *Sandras* in 1844 (Comptes rendus de l'Académie 20, 1085), and isolated pancreatin – simultaneously with *Valentin* (*v. Lippmann,* Zeittafeln 1921, p. 28) –, but he was also the first to teach that *diabetes comes about through a disease of the pancreas.*

Although *Bouchardat* found the pancreas to be unaltered in many cases, he found himself forced to assume that only functional changes were present in it in certain circumstances. Thus the concept of *pancreatic diabetes* was created. In fact the suggestion that this should be extirpated was already expressed at that time.

This achievement, which brought the pancreas into a close relationship with diabetes, was pushed into the background however in the year 1849 through *Claude Bernard's* "pigûre" or sugar-puncture. He showed, to use his own words, "that the nervous system has a direct influence on the amount of sugar which passes into the blood", and "taught how to induce artificial diabetes at will: puncture made into the fourth ventricle of an animal loated its blood with an excess of sugar, which also passed into the urine; the animal was diabetic".

It was the 33 year old *Rudolf Virchow* (in the year 1854) who expressed the idea that the pancreas "did not merely secrete

---

[4] According to *Schirmer* 1839 (op. cit. p. 42).

[5] *Bouchardat* (born 1806, died 7th April 1886 in Paris) was at first the chief pharmacist at the Hospital Saint-Antoine and the Hôtel-Dieu in Paris, and finally Prof. of Hygiene there (H. Griesbach, Propädeutik., Leipzig 1915, Vol. II, p. 213).

externally but also internally into the blood", using these words, and who thereby assumed its internal secretion (Virchows Archiv 7, 580).

Meanwhile, in the clinical diagnosis of diabetes *E. Brand* (1850) had brought attention to the aroma of apples in the mouth, the cause of which was recognized by *Petters* in 1857 as acetone. Moreover *Böttger* in 1857 and Almén in 1867 had made known their reduction sugar test in the urine with alkaline bismuth salts.

After *Willy Kühne* had demonstrated a protein-splitting enzyme in the pancreas in 1867, which was first given the name trypsin in 1877, Virchow's friend *Paul Langerhans* described the "islets" which were later named after him in his Berlin Dissertation in 1869, but these were not to play a role until very much later. In the following years *Bouchardat* had gained his experience with the treatment of diabetes during the siege of Paris, which he summarized in his work in 1875 along the lines: "to eat as little as possible". Specifically he emphasized:

"During the rigors of the siege of Paris I saw the sugar disappear from the urine of patients who were on almost complete abstinence from meat and, it has to be said, whose total diet was far from being adequate".

In the 80's (1880) *Armanni* and in 1881 *Wilhelm Ebstein* pointed out the glycogen infiltration of the renal epithelial cells which was occasionally found, and the presence of cylinders in coma. In 1882 *Legal* published the test for acetone and in 1883 *von Jaksch* isolated the acetoacetic acid in the urine, which *Karl Gerhardt* had taught how to detect in 1865. In 1884 *Külz* found betahydroxybutyric acid.

The discovery of phloridzin diabetes by *J. von Mering* (Ztbl. für innere Medizin 1886, p. 185–189) in the year 1886 followed the studies of *Mering* and *Minkowski* (Zentralbl. für klin. Med. 1889), which had demonstrated the fact that sugar is artificially produced in the urine after extirpation of the pancreas. *De Dominici* in Italy had come to the same findings at the same time.

Dutil (B. kl. W. No. 14) had observed sugar which appeared in the urine after the ingestion of 125 g syrup in pancreatic cancer in 1889.[6]

---

[6] In 1818 *Krimer* had tried to induce diabetes by feeding buckwheat to animals.

Also in 1889 *Vasalle* (*Carly Seyfarth*, Neue Beiträge zur Kenntnis der Langerhansschen Inseln,[7] p. 53, Jena, 1920) had reported that after ligature of the excretory ducts the secretory pancreatic parenchyma had disappeared, whereas numerous groups of islets remained.

Such lines of thought reappear over the next few years causing the pancreas to become the focal point of research.

In 1892 *Minkowski* occasionally expressed the view (b. kl. W., No. 5), that the pancreas "produces something which is also involved in the destruction of sugar". *Minkowski* had recently related this "something" to insulin (D. m. W., 1923, No. 34).

There was still a great deal of work to be done before then however. Whereas *Hansemann* (1894) considered the granular atrophy of the gland parenchyma of the pancreas to be a specific disease of diabetes mellitus (Z. f. kl. Med., Vol. 26), the Edinburgh physiologist, *Schäfer*[8] attributed the diabetes to a decline of islet secretion in the pancreas (British Medical Journal 1895).

Attention was not directed towards the islets of Langerhans however until 1900 through the work of the American, *Opie* (John Hopkins Hospital Bulletin, September), while these were then measured in 1906 by *K. A. Heiberg* in Copenhagen (Anatom. Anzeiger) using his microscopic method. *Weichselbaum* started investigations into the same subject in 1908 (Wien. Akademie, Vol. 117, 119).

At this point a few comments will be included – in tabulated form – on the history of *Kussmaul's respiration,* especially in diabetes and uremia. These also show long it took not only for attempts at therapy but also for the clinical-diagnostic clues to emerge.

The history of Kussmaul's respiration, in particular in diabetes and uremia

In 1854 *Th. von Dusch* (Jahrb. f. rat. Med., Vol. 4) discussed the question of whether the accelerated but deep respiration, without rhonchi, of a girl with diabetes who died from this in a coma, was to be related to the diabetes or to the uremia.

[7] "New Contributions to our Knowledge about the Islets of Langerhans".

[8] According to *Minkowski* it was *Lépine* who first used the expression coined by *Brown-Séquard* "Internal secretion" for the function of the pancreas in the utilization of sugar.

In 1868 *Pribram* and *Robitschek* (Vierteljahrsschr. f. prakt. Heilkunde, 1868, p. 202, Comment): "Some time ago we had an opportunity to observe the last days of life of a diabetic, who, besides very great acetone formation which constantly increased up until death, also presented with all of the symptoms (conjunctival injection, sopor, alternating with delirium, *very forced deep respiration with completely normal behaviour of the lungs)* which one generally and specifically only finds to this extent in cholera-typhoid, in whom moreover a uremic infection, with copious excretion of urea via the urine and no detectable urea content in the blood could definitely be excluded, and there was no other explanation for the terminal symptoms described than massive acetone formation".

In 1874 *Adolf Kussmaul* (Deutsch. Arch., Vol. 14, p. 1 ff.), in his paper: "On a peculiar form of death in diabetics", referred to a "peculiar dyspnoea which preceded and then accompanied a comatose state", which he described as *"great respiration"*, and to which he attributed the "most important role" in the disease picture of his three cases.

In 1877 *Botho Scheube* published two cases from the *Wunderlich* hospital (Archiv. d. Heilkunde, *18*, p. 389), that had definite *uremia* with *Kussmaul's* respiration (confirmed by Strümpell in 1884 in the 1st edition of his textbook).

In 1883/84 *Frerichs* argued strongly against this equating of 'Coma uraemicum' with 'Coma diabeticum' (Z. f. klin. Med., Vol. 6) and "Über den Diabetes", 1884, page 112): "The symptoms are not the same; there are essential differences, as just a fleeting glance at the disease pictures shows".

In 1883 *von Jaksch* (Verh. des Kongr. f. innere Med., p. 270, and Wien. med. Woch., p. 473) was the first to report on the occurrence of "great respiration" in *cancer patients.*

In 1884 *Senator* (Z. f. kl. Med., vol. 7, p. 235) reported on *Kussmaul's* respiration in various severe pathological states.

In 1884 *Riess* (Z. f. klin. Med., Vol. 7, Supplement p. 34) observed this form of respiration in cases of severe cerebral anemia. Five of his cases were nephritic, but despite this *Riess* related the Kussmaul respiration to the anemia and not to the uremia.

In 1884 *Litten* (Z. f. klin. Med., Vol. 7, Suppl. p. 81) described the same form of respiration in 'Coma dyspepticum', and then it was similarly noted in various intoxications.

In 1902 *Fr. Pineles* (Wien. klin. Rundschau, 1902, No. 16) reported on 'Coma dyspnoicum' in uremia and established once again the occurrence of Kussmaul's respiration in *uremic coma.*

In 1904 *Wilhelm Ebstein* (Dtsch. Arch. f. klin. Med., Vol. 80, 589–601) drew attention to: "*Cheyne-Stokes*' respiration in 'Coma diabeticum' and *Kussmaul's* 'great respiration' in uremia".[9]

In the year 1907 *Zuelzer* was the first to point out (Konress für innere Medizin. D. med. Woch., 1908, No. 32, and Z. f. exp. Pathol. und Ther., 1908, V. 307), that the parenteral administration of pancreas extracts not only prevented adrenaline-glycosuria, but also reduced in particular the acidosis both in experimental pancreatic diabetes and in human diabetes. The actual principle of insulin had thus already been found 16 years ago, as *Sahli* (op. cit.) has quite rightly emphasized. *Zuelzer* did not achieve any practical success however with his hormone produced from dog- and horse-pancreas.

In remained for two young Canadian doctors to find the solution to the problem. For in 1922 *Banting* and *Best*, the one a young doctor, the other still a student in Toronto, Canada, produced a pancreatic extract which was virtually free of trypsin – whilst their teacher *Macleod* was in Europe – by tying off the pancreatic duct for a fairly long time. After 8 weeks the islets of *Langerhans* were still functioning (Journal of Laboratory and Clinical Medicine 7, 251 and 464, 1922 and American Journal of Physiology, Vol. 59, 1922, p. 479).

Macleod produced extracts from the pancreas of fishes (thornback and ray) and showed a typical fall in the blood-sugar level through the injection of these into rabbits. The dependency of sugar metabolism on the islets of Langerhans had thus been proven (Journal of Metabolism Research 2.H., 2, 1922; cf. also *H. Staub*, Klin. Wochenschrift 1923, with numerous literature references; 1924 published in book form by Jul. Springer).

In connection with these experiments of the two young researchers, *Banting* and *Best, Sahli* again made the telling remark: "Thus ignorance of the history of medicine occasionally has advantages, through the unprejudiced approach to the problem, although it is far more often the case that such ignorance has very great disadvantages. How many discoveries have had to be made over again twice or three times before they finally gained a foothold, because they were initially ignored".

---

[9] Cf. *Erich Ebstein*, Zur Vorgeschichte des Coma diabeticum. Wien. klin. Woch., 1912, No. 23, and *Karl Pichler*, Zur Geschichte der großen Atmung, Zbl. f. innere Med., 1921, No. 37.

The history of diabetes, as I have described it with particular reference to the pancreas and the internal secretion, goes back about 2 1/2 centuries.

This small but important excerpt from the development of clinical diagnosis, based on historical principles, which I have pursued for many years now, also demonstrates once again how much work is needed, both on the part of theory and of practice, if one is to arrive at the present-day state of the problem. Let us hope that the present formulation of the question, the ultimate objective of which is the cure of diabetes, may finally lead to a solution.

This excerpt of historical research confirms the saying of *Emil Fischer:* "Science is not abstract, but rather, as the product of human work its development is linked with the individual characteristics and the fate of those who devote themselves to it".

Literature

Arnozan, Pancréas. A. Dechambre, Dictionnaire encyclopédique des sciences médicales. Bd. 20 (Paris 1884), S. 102–180.

Baumel, Pancréas et diabète. Montpellier médical 1881.

Bérard und *Colin*, Mémoire sur l'exstirpation du pancréas. Acad. de médicine 1858.

Bouchardat et *Sandras*, Compt. rend. de l'Académie des Sciences. Bd. 20 (1845).

Claessen, Die Krankheiten der Bauchspeicheldrüse. Köln 1842.

Cowley, London medical Journal. Sammlung auserlesener Abhandlungen. 13. Bd. 1789 S. 219 (zitiert nach Claessen a. a. O.).

Diamare, Internationale Monatsschrift XVI (1899).

J. N. Eberle, Physiologie der Verdauung. Würzburg 1834.

Edmund O. von Lippmann, Zeittafeln zur Geschichte der organischen Chemie. Berlin 1921.

Erich Ebstein, Entwicklung der klinischen Harndiagnostik. Leipzig (G. Thieme) 1915.

Wilhelm Ebstein, Über die Lebensweise der Zuckerkranken. 3. Aufl. Wiesbaden 1905.

W. Ebstein, Über Drüsenepithelnekrosen beim Diabetes mellitus mit besonderer Berücksichtigung des diabetischen Coma. Dtsch. Arch. f. klin. Med. Bd. 28. S. 143–242.

Wilhelm Ebstein, Die Toxintheorie des Diabetes mellitus. Dtsch. med. Woch. 1900. Nr. 10.

F. Falk, Die pathologische Anatomie und Physiologie des Joh. Bapt. Morgagni. Berlin 1887. S. 89.

Alfred Gigon, Neuere Diabetesforschungen. Ergebnisse der inneren Med. Bd. 9 (1912).

Chr. Fr. Harleß, Über die Krankheiten des Pankreas. Nürnberg 1812.

K. A. Heiberg, Die Krankheiten des Pankreas. Wiesbaden 1914.

K. A. Heiberg, Der gegenwärtige Stand der Pathologie und Prophylaxe des Diabetes mellitus sowie die Therapie des Frühstadiums. Halle a. S. 1914 (mit Literatur).
M. Höfler, Krankheitsnamenbuch. München 1899. S. 103 und 525.
Isenflamm, Versuch einiger praktischer Bemerkungen über die Eingeweide. Erlangen 1784. S. 168–169. (Vgl. Heiberg 1914, S. 315).
Lancereaux, Du diabète maigre. Union médicale 1880.
Landois-Rosemann, Physiologie des Menschen. Berlin und Wien 1905. S. 354.
Lapierre, Diabète maigre et pancréas. Thèse de Paris 1879.
Lépine, Le diabète sucré. Paris 1909.
Lieutaud, Zitiert nach Wolff, Die Lehre von der Krebskrankheit. Bd. 2. S. 752. Jena 1911.
Ralph, H. Major, The treatment of Diabetes mellitus with Insulin. Journal of the American med. Association vom 2. Juni 1923.
O. Minkowski, Zur Insulinbehandlung des Diabetes. Dtsch. med. Woch. 1923. Nr. 34.
R. Morton, zitiert nach Salomon a. a. O.
Popper, Das Verhältnis des Diabetes zu Pankreasleiden und Fettsucht. Österreich. Zeitschr. f. prakt. Heilkunde 1868. XIV, 193–196.
H. E. Richter, Grundriß der inneren Klinik. Bd. 2 (3. Aufl.). Leipzig 1856. S. 464 f.
W. Rondelet, Zitiert nach Salomon.
Ruehle, Pankreasveränderungen bei einem Diabetiker. Berl. klin. Woch. 1879.
H. Sahli, Schweizer med. Woch. 1923. Nr. 35.
Max Salomon, Geschichte der Glykosurie. Leipzig 1871 (aus Arch. f. klin. Med. Bd. 8).
S. Th. Sömmerring, Eingeweidelehre usw. Frankfurt a. M. 1796. S. 156 f. (Hier scheint der Name Bauchspeicheldrüse zum ersten Mal aufzutreten.)
Alfred Max Schirmer, Beitrag zur Geschichte des Pankreas. Basel 1893, bes. S. 42 f.
Schulze, Archiv für mikroskopische Anatomie. Bd. 56 (1900).
H. Staub, Insulin. Berlin, J. Springer 1924.
H. Strauß und *M. Simon*, Über Insulinbehandlung bei Diabetes. Arch. f. Verd. Bd. 32 (1923), S. 89–124.
Tiedemann, Meckels Archiv. Bd. IV. S. 403.
Julius Wolff, Die Lehre von der Krebskrankheit. Jena 1911. Bd. 2.

From a lecture given on 18 September 1923 in Bad Steben on the occasion of the 16th General Meeting of the German Society for the History of Medicine and Natural Sciences.

in: *Archiv für Verdauungskrankheiten 33 (1924) 215–226*

First Steps in Claude Bernard's Discovery of the Glycogenic Function of the Liver

by Mirko Dražen Grmek

The Archives of the *Collège de France* in Paris are in possession of a very large and impressive collection of the notebooks, laboratory journals, and other scientific manuscripts of Claude Bernard. These papers are now classified and available for scientific research.[1] Some notebooks and papers give significant documentary information on Bernard's philosophical background and his position between the materialistic doctrine and the vitalistic conception of life.[2] For the historian of science, however, more interesting perhaps are Bernard's laboratory journals and day-by-day reflections on physiological problems.[3] In his famous *Introduction*[4] he accords to his own discoveries the dignity of

---

[1] M. D. Grmek, *Catalogue des manuscripts de Claude Bernard. Avec la bibliographie de ses travaux imprimés et des études sur son œuvre. Avantpropos par M. Bataillon et E. Wolff. Introduction par L. Delhoume et P. Huard.* Paris: Collège de France and Masson & Co., 1967, 419 pp.

[2] Cf. C. Bernard, *Philosophie. Manuscrit inédit. Texte présenté par Jacques Chevalier.* Paris: Hatier-Boivin, 1937, XIV, 63 pp. See also M. D. Grmek, "Quelques notes intimes de Claude Bernard," *Arch. Intern. Hist. Sci.*, 1963, 16, pp. 339–352. Many important materials are still unpublished. Thus, for example, in the first draft of his acceptance address upon his election to the Académie Française, Bernard expresses some very interesting thoughts which in fact were not intended to be disclosed publicly, and which subsequently were omitted from the final lecture.

[3] Only a small part of these journals is published. The so-called "Cahier rouge" represents a curious mixture of "philosophical" and technical notes; *cf.* C. Bernard, *Cahier de notes 1850–1860. Présenté et commenté par M. D. Grmek; preface de R. Courrier.* Paris: Gallimard, 1965, 315 pp. In one of my recent publications I have used Bernard's manuscripts for a detailed analysis of the genesis of an important scientific concept with complicated "philosophical" involvements; see "Evolution des conceptions de Claude Bernard sur le milieu intérieur," *Philosophie et méthodologie scientifique de Claude Bernard.* Paris: Masson & Cie, 1967, pp. 117–150.

[4] C. Bernard, *Introduction à l'étude de la médecine expérimentale.* Paris: Baillière, 1865, 400 pp. *An Introduction to the Study of Experimental Medicine. Translated by H. Copley Greene, with an Introduction by L. J. Henderson and a Foreword by I. B. Cohen.* New York: Dover, 1957, 226 pp.

paradigms. Thus a detailed study of all the steps in his creative activity is a necessary condition for acceptance of his findings as epistemological examples. An analysis of his laboratory journals reveals in many cases an important historical inconsistency. On the one side, his original manuscripts suggest a very complicated gradual development of his discoveries, while on the other side, his published works show a tendency toward a secondary rationalization, that is, a very strong *post hoc* simplification of facts. If the examples quoted in his *Introduction* are all logically consistent, many of them are chronologically incorrect and simplified to the point that some very important steps are masked.[5] I will try to illustrate this point by an example which seems minor at first glance, but which actually is of extremely great importance in Bernard's research work. The unexpected result of one experiment changed the whole direction of his investigation of the destination of sugar in animal organisms.

When he began his experiments with sugar, Bernard shared the view of Dumas and Boussingault that it was formed by green plants, introduced in animals by alimentation, and destroyed in them by a special process of combustion.[6] Animals were supposedly able only to break down sugar supplied by vegetables. Bernard accepted Liebig's opinion that sugar was the fuel of life, and he believed that the action of combustion took place either in the lungs (Lavoisier's initial hypothesis) or in the general capillaries (hypothesis of Lagrange and Hassenfratz). In 1843 Bernard discovered that an animal organism could directly utilize only sugars of the so-called "second species" (for example, grape sugar) and that sugars of the "first species" (cane sugar), when injected into the blood of animals even in very weak doses, passed into the urine. He noted, too, that gastric juice could transform cane sugar into a form capable of assimilation, that is, of destruction in the animal organism.[7]

The next step in Bernard's work was later summarized by him in the following way:

---

[5] *Cf.* M. D. Grmek, "Examen critique de la genèse d'une grande découverte: la piqûre diabétique de Claude Bernard." *Clio Medica, 1* (1966), 341–350.

[6] J. B. Dumas and J. B. Boussingault, *Essai de statique chimique des êtres organisés.* 3d ed. Paris: Fortin, Masson et Cie, 1844. – *The Chemical and Physiological Balance of Organic Nature.* London: J.-B. Baillière, 1844; New York: Saxton, 1844.

[7] C. Bernard, *Du suc gastrique et de son rôle dans la nutrition. Thèse pour le doctorat en médecine.* Paris: Rignoux, 1843, 34 pp.

There upon I wished to learn in what organ the nutritive sugar disappeared, and I conceived the hypothesis that sugar introduced into the blood through nutrition might be destroyed in the lungs or in the general capillaries. The theory, indeed, which then prevailed and which was naturally my proper starting point, assumed that the sugar present in animals came exclusively from foods, and that it was destroyed in animal organisms by the phenomena of combustion, i.e., of respiration. Thus sugar had gained the name of *respiratory nutriment*. But I was immediately led to see that the theory about the origin of sugar in animals, which served me as a starting point, was false. As a result of the experiments which I shall describe further on, I was not indeed led to find an organ for destroying sugar, but, on the contrary, I discovered an organ for making it, and I found that all animal blood contains sugar even when they do not eat it. So I noted a new fact, unforeseen in theory, which men had not noticed, doubtless because they were under the influence of contrary theories which they had too confidently accepted. I therefore abandoned my hypothesis on the spot, so as to pursue the unexpected result which has since become the fertile origin of a new path for investigation and a mine of discoveries that is not yet exhausted.[8]

This famous text emphasizes an invaluable general recommendation. But in some details it seems quite vague, even to the point of obscurity. With his sentence "But I was immediately led to see . . ." Bernard gives the impression, and wrongly so, that he changed his mind very quickly after the beginning of his experiments on sugar destruction in an animal organism. And what is more important, he does not really explain why – at which, concrete occasion – he abandons the prevalent theory. Curiously enough, he never really elucidated this point,[9] and in his funda-

---

[8] C. Bernard, *An Introduction. Transl. by H. C. Greene, New York:* Dover, 1957, pp. 163–164.

[9] It is only in his thesis for the doctorate in science that Claude Bernard gives some valuable information concerning the first steps of his discovery of the glycogenic function of the liver. He states that his aim was to follow closely the sugar which was absorbed from the food. He wanted to know if it was destroyed in traversing the liver; then what happened after the passage of the blood stream with sugar through the lungs, and so on. For this purpose a dog which had been fed on carbohydrate food for seven days was killed during the digestion, and Bernard was able to show that the blood of the hepatic veins, where they join the inferior vena cava, contained a large amount of glucose. This seemed to be an experimental proof that the liver did not destroy the sugar. As a counter-proof, Claude Bernard performed a similar experiment on a

mental publication on the discovery of the glycogenic function of the liver, he presented his experiments without chronological order, without dates, and following a logical development completely independent of the historical linkage of his experiments and the real evolution of his thought.[10]

He was not "immediately led to see that the theory about the origin of sugar in animals . . . was false," because he started his experiments in 1843, increased their number and perfected them from 1844 to 1847, and finally understood that he was on the wrong track in August 1848. His notebooks contain descriptions of large numbers of experiments concerning the search for the location and mode of destruction of carbohydrates after ingestion, intravenous injection or other introduction into an animal organism.[11] These experiments have never been published because Bernard was fully aware that they brought forward nothing new and represented only a failure. The positive side of all of this lengthy previous work is that Bernard elaborated – with his friend, the young chemist Charles-Louis Barreswil (1817–1870) – on the chemical testing of sugar, further that he understood better the first phases of the digestion of starch, and that he observed the influence of the nervous system on the presence of

---

dog which had been fed exclusively on meat, and to his surprise found again that the blood of the hepatic veins contained a considerable amount of sugar, although there was no sugar in the intestines. He found also that "the blood of the portal vein contains no sugar before it enters the liver, whereas on leaving that organ the same blood contains considerable amounts of glucose." *Cf.* C. Bernard, *Recherches sur une nouvelle fonction du foie considéré comme organe producteur de matière sucrée chez l'homme et les animaux. Thèse pour le grade de docteur ès-sciences naturelles.* Paris: Martinet, 1853, 97 pp. – In spite of some simplifications and errors (for example, the omission of the fact that in the experiment with the dog on a meat diet, Bernard discovered sugar in the blood of the portal vein), this story is basically correct, especially in its emphasis on Bernard's astonishment after the unexpected results of the counter-proof experiment. The best historical presentations in English of Bernard's discovery of the glycogenic function of liver follow the text of his thesis. For example, D. Wright Wilson, "Claude Bernard," *Pop. Sci. Monthly,* 84 (1917), 567–578; F. G. Young, Claude Bernard and the Theory of the Glycogenic Function of the Liver," *Ann. Sci.,* 2 (1937), 47–83; J. M. D. Olmsted, *Claude Bernard, Physiologist* (New York: Harper, 1938, 272 pp.). In most other publications, the story is very distorted.

[10] C. Bernard, "De l'origine du sucre dans l'économie animale," *Arch. gén. Méd., 18,* 4th ser. (1848), 303–319. Published also in *Mém. Soc. Biol. 1* (1849), 121–133. An English translation ("The Origin of Sugar in the Animal Body"(is published in Kelly's *Medical Classics* (1939), III, 567–580.

[11] Claude Bernard's unpublished papers in the Collège de France, *Ms. 7b, 7c,* and others.

sugar in blood and urine. Certainly, by his long and numerous experiments he became sensitive to all the possible physiological implications of the presence or absence of sugar in various parts of the animal circulatory system.

Beginning in 1845 Bernard became interested in the clinical problems of diabetes. He observed patients[12] and formulated his first theory of the pathogenesis of this disease.[13] According to Bernard's first opinion, diabetes is "a nervous affection of the lungs." For the modern reader this theory is very surprising, but actually it was a very logical conclusion from these four premises: 1) sugar cannot be synthetized in the animal body; 2) it is normally destroyed in the lungs; 3) the principal symptom of diabetes is the presence of undestroyed sugar in the urine; and 4) the nervous system controls the breakdown of sugar in the lungs. Claude Bernard discovered that after cutting the pneumogastric nerves in rabbits the pulmonary functions are affected and glucose passes undestroyed into the urine.[14]

One important problem was whether or not the blood of diabetic patients actually contained sugar. Thomas Willis was the first to believe it. In the eighteenth century, Dobson, Cawley, and Rollo tried to extract sugar or sugar-like substances from the serum of diabetic patients. They wished to demonstrate that glycosuria is merely a sequence in glycemia. But none of these attempts produced any definite conclusion. The sweet taste of blood was not sufficient proof, and chemical analysis by alcoholic fermentation gave generally negative results. Thus P. F. Nicolas and V. Gueudeville, Soubeiran, Vauquelin, and other authorities on this subject at the beginning of the nineteenth century were not ready to accept the theory of diabetic glycemia. Their negative results can probably be explained by the fact that the analyses were performed on old blood, after glycolysis. In 1835 an Italian chemist F. Ambrosioni, was the first to give definite proof of the presence of sugar in the blood of a diabetic person. His demonstration was based on the alcoholic fermentation by yeast of blood sugar.[15]

---

[12] He worked in Rayer's and Andral's departments in the well-known hospital, La Charité, in Paris; *cf. Ms. 7b*, pp. 246 and 249–250; *Ms. 15i* and *Fasc. 25b*, f. 370.

[13] *Ms. 7b*, p. 133.

[14] *Ms. 7b*, p. 130.

[15] *Ann. univ. di med. e chir.*, 74 (1835), 160. – See introductory chapters in R. Lépine, *Le diabète sucré* (Paris: Alcan, 1909).

Even before it was definitely proved that sugar could be found in the blood of persons with diabetes, it was known that this substance could be present in the blood of healthy animals, at least in some animals under special conditions. In 1826 F. Tiedemann and L. Gmelin demonstrated the presence of fermentable glucose in the intestines and venous blood of healthy dogs after ingestion of starch.[16] In England, MacGregor (1837) confirmed the observation of Ambrosioni, and Thomson, a chemist of Glasgow, found (1845) that chicken blood normally contained a certain amount of sugar.[17]

In France, F. Magendie discovered, independently of the aforementioned authors, that sugar can be found in the blood of normal rabbits and dogs after they had been fed on starch or potatoes.[18] After Magendie's experiments, performed during his lectures at the Collège de France in 1846, the majority of physiologists and physicians agreed in supposing an alimentary origin of sugar and considering glycemia as a physiological phenomenon compatible with health, but inconstant – being a result of ingestion of special kinds of food.

Thus the presence of sugar in blood was considered to be either a pathological or an accidental fact. It was Bernard who discovered that glycemia was a normal and constant phenomenon, largely independent of alimentation.[19]

One unpublished manuscript permits us to have a real understanding of how this discovery occurred: this is Bernard's laboratory journal *Ms. 7c*, compiled from 1846 to 1848. The beginning experiments are of no interest, because, having taken a wrong turn, Bernard was unable to progress. Until May 1848 he attempted to answer a badly formulated question. Yet at this

---

[16] F. Tiedemann and L. Gmelin. *Die Verdauung nach Versuchen*, vol. I, Heidelberg and Leipzig: Gross, 1826.

[17] Lépine, *Le diabète sucré*. See also Bernard's historical sketch in *Leçons sur le diabète* (Paris: Baillière, 1877), pp. 142–161.

[18] *C. R. Acad. Sci., 23* (1846), 189.

[19] In one of his last works, at the very end of his life, Bernard states proudly: "Je montrai . . . que la glycémie est indépendante de l'alimentation; qu'elle se rencontre chez l'homme et chez les animaux nourris de viande ou soumis à l'abstinence. Je prouvai que la présence du sucre dans le sang est un fait normal coïncidant toujours avec l'état de santé et ne disparaissant que lorsque la nutrition était arretée. De sorte qu'au lieu d'admettre, comme mes prédécesseurs, que la glycémie fut un fait pathologique ou accidentel, je fis voir que la proposition contraire était vraie, et que c'était l'absence de sucre dans le sang qui constituait le véritable fait anormal"(*Leçons sur le diabète*, 1877, pp. 127–128).

time he believed that sugar must be destroyed somewhere within the organism. His main attention was evidently directed toward the lungs, and in the last week of May he observed what happened when grape sugar was exposed *in vitro* to the pulmonary tissue of freshly killed animals. After ten to twelve hours the sugar disappeared, and Bernard concluded that the lungs contained a special ferment for the destruction of glucose.[20] But following faithfully his method of experimental research, he proceeded to a counter-proof. This he did by mixing sugar with tissues of liver and other organs. He obtained positive results, and the problem became even more obscure than before he started his experiments.

On the last day of May, he injected one gram of grape sugar into the jugular vein of a dog, extracting at the same time blood from the carotid artery. This blood contained a large amount of sugar. The conclusion was evident: glucose is not destroyed in the lungs, because blood must pass by these organs in order to move from the jugular vein to the carotid artery.[21] Bernard guessed that perhaps the combustion of carbohydrates took place in the general capillaries or in the liver.[22] Numerous experiments, carefully executed by Bernard during June and July of 1848, were strongly opposed to the theory of pulmonary combustion. Grape sugar was injected into the jugular veins, or starch introduced into the stomachs of rabbits and dogs. Then either blood was taken from various parts of the animals or they were killed and blood extracted separately from different organs. Sugar was present in all samples. Bernard was unable to find a rule for its quantitative distribution.

His friend Quevenne, pharmacist at the Hôspital de la Charité, extracted and purified blood sugar from a diabetic patient, and Bernard showed that in physiological experiments there is no difference between grape sugar and the sugar of diabetics.[23]

In July 1848 Claude Bernard discovered some important facts: 1. the transformation of cane sugar into grape sugar by the action of gastric juice is not performed by gastric acid, but by some special "organic matter";[24] and

---

[20] *Ms. 7c*, p. 308.

[21] *Ms. 7c*, p. 311.

[22] He presumed that "chez un animal en digestion d'amidon, il devra y avoir du sucre dans le sang de la veine porte artériel et pas dans le sang veineux de retour" (*Ms. 7c*, p. 311; note dated May 31, 1848).

[23] *Ms. 7c*, p. 307.

[24] *Ms. 7c*, p. 312.

2. sugar is always present in the vitreous humor of the eye of a dog and also in the white of a chicken egg.[25]

Thist last finding was not immediately published, and when in March 1849 an Irish physician named Aldridge discovered this fact independently of Bernard, he claimed priority.[26] Preserved notebooks provide proof that Bernard's claim was well founded. This discovery is not without historical significance, because it invalidated the older demonstration of the presence of sugar in the blood of diabetic persons. Actually Ambrosioni and MacGregor added egg white to blood before testing its sugar content.

Bernard observed that Barreswil's copper reagent did not react well with sugar in the presence of fibrin. He imagined a new theory of the pathogenesis of diabetes. Thus sugar was supposed to be destroyed in blood, fibrin having some important function in this destruction. And diabetes was nothing more than a stopping of this destructive process probably by some chemical disorders involved in the synthesis and distribution of fibrin.[27]

This original point of view gave Bernard the possibility of foreseeing new experiments. Analyzing the blood in the vessels before and after each single organ, Bernard wished to eliminate, step by step, the ancient theory that sugar combustion is located in a particular area of the organism. The first experiments seemed to confirm his new working hypothesis. In dogs fed on a carbohydrate-rich diet, the blood from the hepatic veins and vena cava contained sugar; thus it was not destroyed in the liver. Sugar was also present in both ventricles of the heart, meaning that it had not been destroyed by the lungs.

From many laboratory notes it is clear that Bernard attained these results and was very happy that they corresponded to prediction. But as in all cases he wished to assure the results by counter-proofs. One dog was submitted to a noncarbohydrate diet, then killed by section of the spinal bulb. Blood was taken from the portal vein, from both ventricles, and from a peripheral artery. The results were completely unexpected, astonishing and puzzling. The blood of the portal system contained enormous quantities of sugar; the blood from the heart contained sugar, but in a small amount; and the arterial blood showed only traces. Chyle had no sugar whatsoever.

---

[25] *Ms. 7c*, pp. 354, 358, and 363–366.

[26] C. Bernard and Ch. Barreswil, "Du sucre dans l'oeuf," *C. R. Soc. Biol., 1* (1849), 64.

[27] *Ms. 7c*, p. 338.

It is perhaps useful to publish the exact text of Bernard's laboratory notes concerning this crucial experiment:

Rue Dauphine 32. Août 1848. Expériences sur le sucre dans le sang. Mouvements péristaltiques. Sur un chien à jeun depuis 6 jours de tout aliment solide et n'ayant bu que de l'eau, on retire du sang par la veine jugulaire; le sérum de ce sang tout frais, aussitôt après sa coagulation, donne par le liquide bleu des traces de réduction. Le lendemain il n'en donne plus. Une partie de ce même sérum traité par l'alcool, puis évaporé et repris par l'eau, mis avec la levure de bière ne donne que quelques bulles de gaz de sorte que la fermentation est à peine sensible. Il faut dire qu'il y avait fort peu de sérum, environ 15 grammes, et que la quantité de sucre devait être fort peu de chose, s'il y en avait.

Sur le même chien, dans une autre circonstance, lorsqu'il n'était à jeun que depuis 2 jours, le sérum frais donne également de la réduction par le tartrate de cuivre.

Sur le même chien remis à la nourriture de la viande et ayant mangé pendant 8 jours consécutifs uniquement des débris de viande crue pris chez le boucher; il est tué par la section du bulbe pour recueillir les sangs différents. Aussitôt le bulbe coupé, les mouvements respiratoires furent comme à l'ordinaire complètement arrêtés. L'oeil est resté sensible d'un côté et pas de l'autre. J'ouvris aussitôt le ventre, le coeur allant encore. Les chylifères étaient pleins de chyle blanc, les intestins contenus dans le ventre par la position de l'animal qui était couché sur le dos n'étaient le siège d'aucune contraction péristaltique. Alors je comprimai l'aorte dans la poitrine entre les deux doigts, et aussitôt les contractions péristaltiques éclatèrent avec impétuosité pour ne plus cesser. Seulement elles me semblaient être un peu moins violentes quand je cessais de la comprimer, pour augmenter quand je la reprenais. Du reste, cela a été de peu de durée, car bientôt les mouvements du coeur ont cessé. Ce qu'il y a eu de saillant, c'est le départ des contractions péristaltiques intestinales au moment où j'ai comprimé l'aorte thoracique.

Extraction des sangs. On a retiré à part: 1° du sang de la veine porte à son entrée dans le foie; 2° du sang du coeur dans les ventricules droit et gauche; 3° du sang provenant de la plaie faite à la nuque pour couper le bulbe.

Ces trois sangs ont été laissés en repos pour les laisser coaguler. Tous se sont coagulés au bout de quelques instants en présentant un sérum blanchâtre lactescent. (Le sang de la veine présentait également cet aspect; le chyle y avait-il pénétré ou bien était-ce un retour par le sang veineux?)

Du chyle blanc a également été extrait du canal thoracique. Il s'est coagulé au bout de quelques instants.

On a essayé avec le tartrate de cuivre les 3 sérums tout frais et le sérum de chyle également tout frais. 1° Le chyle de la veine porte donne une réduction énorme en le traîtant directement. En précipitant par le sulfate de soude sec de façon à obtenir une liqueur incolore, la réduction se fait également très abondamment. 2° Le chyle du coeur traité directement par le tartrate de cuivre donne une réduction très nette mais moins abondante que le sang de la veine porte. Traité également par le sulfate de soude, la réduction est très nette mais toujours moins abondante que dans le sang de la veine porte. 3° Le sérum du sang de la nuque traité directement par le tartrate de cuivre donne à peine des traces de réduction. Après traitement par le sulfate de soude, la réduction est toujours équivoque. 4° Le sérum du chyle traité directement par le tartrate de cuivre ne donne pas de réduction sensible.

Comment se fait-il donc qu'il y a du sucre (ou une matière qui réduit) dans le sang de la veine porte?

On recherche dans l'intestin: 1° Le liquide de l'estomac qui contenait de la viande en voie de digestion ne réduisait aucunement le tartrate de cuivre. 2° Le liquide intestinal bilieux ne réduisait pas de tout le sel de cuivre. 3° L'urine traitée préalablement par le sulfate de soude ne réduit aucunement le sel du cuivre.

Du sérum du coeur conservé jusqu'au lendemain contenait encore du sucre, c'est-à-dire réduisait le tartrate.

Cette experience est fort singulière. *C'est à n'y rien comprendre.* Il se formerait du sucre dans la veine porte. Par quel organe, par quel mécanisme?

Il faudra prendre le sang de la veine porte d'un chien à jeun et voir si l'on y trouvera cette matière qui réduit. S'il se forme du sucre dans une autre alimentation que celle de l'amidon, la question des diabétiques est singulièrement compliquée. Il faudra voir si cette matière réduisante (sucre ou autre) disparaîtra assez vite car le sang du coeur en contenait moins et le sang de la nuque d'une manière très équivoque.

Quel est donc l'organe qui formerait ce sucre ou cette matière réduisante.[28]

---

[28] *Ms. 7c*, pp. 379–382.

Where did the sugar come from in an animal without an alimentary supply of carbohydrates? Bernard wrote in his journal, as if crying in surprise: "It is absolutely incomprehensible!"

This experiment was done in the laboratory of Theophile-Jules Pelouze (1808–1867), a famous chemist and Bernard's mentor. The exact date of the experiment is not stated, but its location in the laboratory journal places it between the 10th and the 17th of August 1848, probably closer to the latter date. It is significant that in this case Bernard conducted at the same time and on the same animal two different experiments, one concerning the regulation of conditions of peristaltic movements in the intestines, and the other concerning the metabolism of sugar. It is clear enough that the second part was considered only as a routine counter-proof of previous experiments.

Bernard's notes express his astonishment. Actually, the discovered facts completely contradicted his working hypothesis and the generally accepted ideas on animal physiology. The presence of sugar in the blood of an animal without an alimentary supply of carbohydrates was such an incredible finding that Bernard, as we see from his journal, doubted the specificity of the copper reactive. This "reductive matter" – was it really sugar? He decided to repeat the experiment, using other methods of chemical analysis.

Bernard understood immediately that the presence of sugar in the portal vein of a dog without sugar in the chyle had farreaching consequences, and that it would completely change existing theories of the pathogenesis of diabetes. He decided to repeat the experiment on a starving animal, and he posed the crucial questions:

1. where and by what mechanism was sugar formed in animals?
2. which animal organ performed this "vegetable" function?

Within a few days the basic fact, namely, the presence of nonalimentary sugar in mammalian blood, was confirmed by new experiments. On August 21 Bernard obtained positive evidence of the presence of glucose in the blood of a dog fed on lard and tripe exclusively. Thus he no longer hesitated to affirm that "there is a formation of sugar at the expense of fat."[29] But the great innovation of this experiment lies in the results of chemical examination of tissues taken from various abdominal organs. I cannot resist the temptation to quote the findings in Bernard's own words:

---

[29] *Ms. 7c*, p. 387.

J'ai pris les tissues 1° de la rate, 2° des ganglions mésentériques, 3° du foie, et j'y ai recherché le sucre. Les tissus des ganglions et de la rate ne montraient pas nettement du sucre, mais le tissu du foie en contenait énormément.[30]

There was no sugar either in the spleen or in the lymphatic ganglia, but the substance appeared in *"enormous"* quantity in the liver.

What a surprising result! Many questions assailed Bernard's mind. Was the presence of sugar in liver tissues a physiological phenomenon? Was it exclusive to the liver or was it a property shared by other organs? Was it a characteristic of dog's liver only, or was it common to all animals? After a few days of feverish research, Bernard had found the answers to all these questions. Some extracts from his laboratory journal give good evidence of his investigations:

Le 22 août 1848. J'ai fait acheter chez un tripier du foie de veau et de boeuf. J'y ai trouvé énormément de sucre dans l'un et dans l'autre par le réactif et par la fermentation.

Le 23 août 1848. J'ai pris à l'Hôpital de la Charité 3 morceaux, de foie. 1° Un morceau de foie granuleux, chez un vieillard, mort très amaigri de je ne sais quoi; je n'y ai pas trouvé de sucre par le réactif. 2° Un morceau de foie très ramolli chez une femme très grasse, morte de je ne sais quoi; je n'y ai pas trouvé de sucre par le réactif. 3° Un morceau de foie d'apparence saine chez un homme empoisonné par l'acide arsenical auquel on avait donné du peroxyde de fer. J'y ai trouvé énormément de sucre par le réactif et par la fermentation.

Le 24 août. Du foie du chien de l'expérience de la page 387, mort depuis trois jours, contient encore au réactif énormément de sucre. J'avais mis le foie avec de l'eau et c'est dans cette eau à odeur forte, paludineuse, qui j'ai agi.

Le 25 août. Foie d'un albuminurique avec maladie organique du coeur, maladie chronique très longue; très infiltrée. Le foie est très congestionné; par tartrate, il y a des traces de sucre.

Sur le foie d'un homme mort de maladie du coeur il y a des traces de sucre. Il faudra doser dans les cas différents.[31]

Thus the presence of sugar in human and bovine liver was clearly demonstrated. On August 25th Bernard found sugar in the livers of a frog, a rabbit, a capon, and two veal fetuses killed in the slaughter house at Popincourt, but he was not able to find sugar in the liver of a ray or a lizard.

---

[30] *Ms. 7c*, p. 390.

These phases of Bernard's work culminated in the presenting of a note to the Academy of Science on August 28, 1848. In this communication, signed by Claude Bernard and Charles Barreswil as co-authors, it was stated that sugar extracted from the liver is glucose by chemical nature, that it cannot be found under physiological conditions in any other organ, and that its presence in the liver "is a physiological fact which is completely independent of the nature of alimentation."[32] Bernard and Barreswil presented as evidence to members of the Academy a sample of alcohol originating from the fermentation of liver sugar.

The crucial experiment quoted in this paper corresponds to the first experiment of the second series in Bernard's classical memoir on the origin of sugar in the animal body, presented on October 21, 1848, before the *Société de Biologie*.[33] But there are significant differences between the original experiment and the published text.

In August 1848 Claude Bernard was able to demonstrate only the first of the four conclusions quoted in his October memorandum. He was sure that "in the physiologic state, there exists constantly and normally the sugar of diabetes in the blood of the heart and in the liver of man and animals," but he only conjectured without any experimental proof that "the formation of this sugar takes place in the liver."

Actually, Claude Bernard was immediately led to see that the old theory about the nutritive origin of animal sugar was false, and that the liver produced sugar. But this "immediately" meant immediately after his crucial experiment in August 1848, and not immediately after the beginning of his researches concerning the metabolism of sugar.

Of course, it was easy to explain the presence of sugar in the blood of the portal vein in spite of the fact that the current of the blood should carry in opposite direction all substances found in the tissue of the liver. Bernard supposed that the blood rich in sugar had seeped back into the portal vein when, by the opening of the abdomen, the pressure on the viscera ceased.

The real demonstration of the glycogenic function of the liver was accomplished during September and October 1848 with a series of experiments characterized by ligatures of the blood vessels of living animals and determination of the sugar in differ-

---

[31] *Ms. 7c*, p. 392.

[32] C. Bernard and Ch. Barreswil, "Du presence du sucre dans le foie," *C. R. Acad. Sci.*, *27* (1848), 514–515.

ent parts of the circulatory system. Bernard showed that in properly performed experiments there is no sugar in the blood of the portal vein of an animal which is starved or fed on meat. His main argument in favor of the theory of the glycogenic function of the liver was precisely the absence of sugar in the portal vein and its presence in the suprahepatic veins and in the arterial blood.

How lucky he was to ignore some facts. First of all, there is in every case some amount of sugar in the blood of the portal vein. It was only by a special property of his chemical test that a gradual difference was transformed into an all-or-none reaction. The large amount of sugar in the blood of Bernard's dogs resulted from the manner of killing (section of the medulla oblongata) and should be interpreted as an exceptional, pathological condition. It is astonishing "how much instinctive judgement and even sheer luck contributed to a discovery which Bernard, with a good deal of justification, believed to be based upon the strictest experimental proof."[34] And how interesting it is to measure the extent to which a great scientist reconstructs his own previous thoughts to fit his later point of view.[35] The next steps in Bernard's work on the glycogenic function of the liver are from this point of view even more illuminating. In this case, as probably in the historical analysis of all other scientific discoveries, it is of invaluable help to resort to original first-hand documents. The importance of systematic conservation of this kind of document, especially of laboratory journals, can hardly be overestimated.

in: *Journal of the History of Biology 1 (1968) 141–154.*

---

[33] Quoted in note 10 above.

[34] J. M. D. Olmsted and E. Harris Olmsted, *Claude Bernard and the Experimental Method in Medicine* (New York: Schuman, 1952).

[35] Cannon's book *The Way of an Investigator,* New York, 1945, offers many excellent examples of "deductive" historically wrong approaches to the analysis of scientific discoveries. Cannon states (p. 65) that Claude Bernard "in testing the blood for its sugar content at various points after its departure from the intestine, where sugar ist absorbed ... found less in the blood of the left side of the heart and in the arteries than in the veins. He drew the erroneous conclusion that the sugar was consumed in the lungs. Then Bernard's interest in the metabolism of sugar in the body led him to examine persons suffering from diabetes, and he was struck by the evidence that the output of sugar in the urine of diabetics is greater than that represented in the food they take in. There sprang into his mind a guiding idea that sugar is produced in the organism." This is, I guess, the way in which Cannon would discover animal glycogenesis, but it has no connection with the historical reality.

The Priority Dispute between Claude Bernard and Victor Hensen about the Discovery of Glycogen

by Rüdiger Porep

I. Preliminary Comments on the Subject of Priority Disputes

If two or more authors working independently of each other simultaneously publish identical or at least very similar findings or discoveries and each author insists on having been first, we have the makings of a priority dispute. Such disputes are virtually confined to the fields of the natural sciences, medicine and technology. They are not completely unknown in the humanities and the arts but here even the jargon is different and we talk of originality or plagiarism. Priority disputes have occurred at all times but their incidence has differed widely. In the second half of the 19th century they occurred with clockwork regularity. There is hardly a volume of publications, hardly any biography of a research scientist that contains no mention of a priority dispute. The reasons why the second half of the 19th century was such a peak period for priority disputes will be briefly investigated below (cf. Mann, p. 999 [22]). Against this background, I then propose to analyse a particular type of priority dispute which to this day is periodically agitating minds and pens, namely that between Claude Bernard and Victor Hensen as to who discovered glycogen.

From 1840 onwards, the speculative, natural-philosophy orientated direction of medicine which up to then had, at least in Germany, almost wholly dominated the field was fast losing ground to the rapidly expanding scientific medicine. The physicochemical approach to medical research promised progress after decades of sensitive but stagnant speculation and fruitless systematization. Clear, reproducible observations, if at all possible supported by experiments with measurements and figures, were henceforth the order of medical research, no longer structures of ideas from old, overused building-blocks.

The natural sciences and in their wake technology now developed at breathtaking speed. Physicists offered in rapid succession new findings and new measuring devices as well as improved microscopes. In the field of chemistry, methods of analysis became more refined and permitted the ever more accurate determination of ever smaller amounts of substance. Chemists succeeded in synthesizing organic substances, they elucidated more and more chemical as well as biochemical processes. Medical scientists had only to pick up the new tools and make use of them. The results was a virtual avalanche of new discoveries and observations.

One gets the impression that the publication of discoveries in such rapid succession triggered a positive fever of success. One simply had to join in to the best of one's ability, to have a share in research, in discovery – and in fame and honour. The old custom of scientists to link outstanding achievements with the names of their authors stimulated the ambition of the medical profession. The custom was, after all, especially widespread in medicine, one stood a relatively good chance. And temptation was ever-present – a medical student's first lectures on anatomy contained countless examples of such lasting fame. We now have to discover the extent to which this era favored *parallel discoveries* and an explanation of the exceedingly violent, dogged and at times vituperous priority disputes which violated all standards of decency, destroyed friendships and caused uninvolved men to take sides.

Given the high rate of discoveries at low methodologic expenditure of the time, it is likely that coincidence played the most important part in bringing about *parallel discoveries.* At a time when, for instance, a well-trained microscopist could be almost certain that he saw what no one else had seen before providing only that he was using a microscopce of the latest construction and of a resolution that greatly exceeded anything available hitherto, conditions were favorable for duplicate discoveries.

To give just one example: Wilhelm Krause (1833–1910), an anatomist, and the physiologist Victor Hensen (1835–1924) each put a muscle fibril under his new high-resolution microscope at about the same time. Each saw that the familiar cross-bands, the anisotropic A band and the isotropic I band, were further subdivided by a narrow zone. Each promptly decided to publish, Krause in a journal, Hensen in a monograph. The publication date of the monograph was delayed by the tardiness of the engraver who was to transfer the drawing to a printing-plate. A few days before the monograph was due to go to press, Hensen picked up a copy of Krause's paper and was horrified to read of the discovery of a new cross-band in muscle. It is obvious from subsequent statements that grief and rage over the missed chance caused him to gird his loins for a priority dispute since only the laziness or illness of the engraver had prevented his monograph from appearing months earlier and thus had deprived him of the fruits of his labor. When Hensen's anger had subsided a little and he was able to read a second paper by Krause on the same subject, he found to his surprise and relief that he and Krause had in fact discovered different bands. The band described by Krause, which subsequently was named Krause's membrane but is now known as the Z band, delimits an insotropic sarcomere whilst the H band (Hensen's disk) transverses the (anisotropic) A band of a sarcomere. – Thus a priority dispute that would have arisen by chance was prevented by chance (Porep, pp. 76–77 [25]).

Coincidence is a minor factor in sponsored research, which nowadays is sometimes carried out on an industrial scale. If two scientists or groups of scientists embark on a research project on the basis of the current state of the art and with a particular objective then, given the same methods and the same rate of work, it is almost inevitable for the same results to emerge within a short space of time. The recognition of this fact has led to scientific planning. If certain conditions are observed, therefore, parallel discoveries can no longer be due to coincidence.

Not every duplicate discovery is automatically followed by a priority dispute. However, priority disputes were bound to thrive in the prevailing climate of a hectic period marked by a zest, indeed a frenzy for discovery, when in the natural sciences and technology alike progress was the spur and there was no ideal higher than fame and honor. It was a time when achievement only mattered, first of the individual, subsequently of nations. It is no exaggeration to speak of a downright ideology of achievement and success. The value of a scientist was directly proportionate to his acclaim. Such compulsive striving for success is bound to lead to excesses of which the priority dispute is an example.

Priority disputes are a human and a social problem, not one inherent in science. It is no coincidence that the most famous priority dispute of our own time, which centers on the discovery of elementary particles and the first description of transuranic elements, is being carried on between countries that cannot be regarded as being generally on the most friendly terms.

II. The Background to the Priority Dispuse about the Discovery of Glycogen

A priority dispute cannot, as a rule, be assessed in isolation from the personalities involved or without some knowledge of their field of work. The necessary background information will therefore be briefly outlined in the four sections below.

1. Biographical Notes on Claude Bernard [8, 9, 13, 19, 21, 28]

There is no lack of information in the literature about this unchallenged master of French physiology and perhaps the most important co-founder of experimental medicine. Consequently a modest sketch here may suffice.

Claude Bernard was born on July 12, 1813 in Saint-Julien-en-Beaujolais, a small place on the Rhône not far from Lyons. His father was a tenant viticulturist, i.e. he did not own his vineyard. After finishing his education at schools in Villefranche (Saône) and Thoissey (Ain), he went as apprentice to an apothecary's shop in Vaise, a suburb of Lyons. During his apprenticeship there, from 1832 to 1833, he devoted all his leisure time to the theater. He wrote several plays, including "La Rose du Rhône" and a historical drama entitled "Arthur de Bretagne". He hoped that the manuscript of the latter would secure him the sponsorship of Saint-Marc Girardin, the Professor of Poetry at the Sorbonne. Bernard wanted to become a poet.

The visit to the Professor of Literature in 1834 was decisive for Bernard's future career. The professor's advice was: Poetry for his leisure hours, medicince for a profession. The disappointed poet took this advice and without delay enrolled as a student at the École de Médecine in Paris. His clinical teacher at the Hôtel-Dieu was François Magendie (1783–1855). One of the great men of experimental medicine, Magendie was not only the Medical Director of the Hôtel-Dieu but concurrently Professor of Physiology and General Pathology at the Collège de France. He appointed Bernard as *préparateur* in his laboratories and thus made him his pupil. At the age of thirty (Paris, 1843) Bernard at last got his medical doctorate. His thesis was entitled *"Du suc gastrique et de son rôle dans la nutrition"*. After several years of trying unsuccessfully to obtain an appropriate position (despite being awarded the Prize of Experimental Medicine by the Académie des Sciences in 1845), he was at last appointed Magendie's deputy at the Collège de France. It was not until 1854 that he was offered the newly created Chair of Physiology at the Sorbonne. From then on his star was in the ascendant. In the same year he was elected a member of the Académie des Sciences (Section of Medicine and Surgery); as early as 1855 he became the successor of Magendie at the Collège de France and in 1868, after the death of the physiologist and comparative anatomist Pierre Flourens (1794–1867) he became a member of the Académie Française. In 1869 Bernard was elected President of the Académie des Sciences and in the same year the rank of senator was conferred on him for life. The last of the many honours he received was a state funeral in the cemetery of Père-Lachaise in Paris. He died on February 10, 1878.

2. *Claude Bernard's Work on Sugar Metabolism* [21, 24, 27, 30, 32]

It is impossible to do justice in a few brief lines to Bernard's monumental experimental and literary contribution. His papers cover digestion, metabolism, heat regulation, neurophysiology – especially the physiology of the autonomic nervous system – experimental pathology and (internal) medicine, anesthesia and diabetes. Some basic physiological terms were first formulated by him. In his later years he wrote on problems of basic medical research. One of these publications was *"Introduction a l'étude de la médicine expérimentale"* which was published in Paris in 1865 and is being reprinted to this day. It not only forms part of the curriculum of French medical students but is also, in the form of a primer, used in the philosophy lessons of French high school pupils [8, 9].

When *Bernard* began to investigate carbohydrate metabolism, it was known that sugar occured in the blood but only under two conditions, namely physiologically after meals rich in carbohydrates and pathologically in diabetes. It was also known that diabetics could synthesize sugar from proteins whereas under physiologic conditions, the blood sugar was regarded as representing solely the absorbed product of starch digestion by the pancreatic juice. The portal circulation was known, also the fact that sugar was excreted via the kidneys if the blood-sugar level was high.

Bernard, however, found the occurred *regularly* in the blood of experimental animals, in animals fed on a carbohydrate-free diet as well as those wholly deprived of food. He also discovered that the liver always had a high sugar content even if no carbohydrates had been fed and even if the animals had been fasted for several days. The presence of sugar in the liver, which he succeeded in demonstrating in 1848, prompted another question, namely the origin of that sugar. There were two possibilities:
1. the sugar was synthesized by means of a chemical process in the parenchyma of the liver – which seemed improbable according to accepted physiologic theory, which maintained that plants alone could synthesize substances whilst only processes of dissimilation took place in animals.
2. The liver was an *organe condensateur* i.e. it accumulated and condensed the sugar absorbed from the diet (*Mani*, p. 99 [21]). – *Bernard*, never much impressed by dogma, inclined on the basis of his experiments towards the first possibility. When dogs were fasted for some time, after which their livers were virtually free

from sugar, and then put on a diet of meat alone, their livers were once again loaded with sugar which could only have been obtained by synthesis from the muscle protein. He thus wrote in 1849: "The liver is the site and source of animal sugar" (*Bernard*, p. 131 [1]). Bernard long adhered to the theory that the sugar of the liver was formed exclusively from protein.

Ultimately, however, *Bernard* realised that the liver must have a function besides proteinogenic sugar synthesis. In his famous monograph of 1853 [2] "*Nouvelle fonction do foie considéré comme organe producteur de matière sucrée chez l'homme et les animaux*" he wrote that the sugar absorbed from the died did not increase the sugar levels in the liver or the rest of the body. Since the absorbed sugar could not after all vanish, it had to be converted into something else. This was a milky opalescent substance but its characteristics were at first entirely unknown to him.

In the winter term of 1854/55, *Bernard* said in a lecture which he had drafted in writing and was delivering at the Collège de France that the sugarlike substances which were conveyed from the intestine via the portal vein to the liver, did not pass through the latter but were converted in its parenchyma into a new substance which caused liver decoctions to have a whitish appearance and which appeared to consist of a combination of fats and proteins (*Bernard*, p. 154 [3]).

It was due to *Bernard's* indefatigable experimentation and his readiness to question beliefs that had been accepted for years that he declined to draw the tempting, almost compelling conclusion that sugar was converted in the liver into a protein and that the latter in combination with the dietary protein formed a joint and homogenous substrate for the glycogenic function of the liver. Had he believed this, he might have regarded his research as completed. Instead he found that isolated, i.e. dead, livers continued the formation of sugar for some time and that the organs lost their opalescence in the process. He drew an analogy to the plant kingdom. Plants can convert an intermediate product, starch, by enzymatic processes into sugar, so he called his sugar-forming substance *animal starch (fécule animal)*. He succeeded, in 1855, in producing a powder form of the glycogenic substance which he found to be water-soluble but insoluble in alcohol. In chemical terms, Bernard did not obtain the pure substance but he was nevertheless able to describe its most important chemical and physiologic characteristics. Glycogen had thus been discovered. Bernard invited research scientists to isolate the new substance and to elucidate it chemically (*Mani*, p. 103[21]).

In 1857 Bernard published an accurate description of the characteristics of glycogen, his *matière glycogène*. He had meanwhile produced the substance in pure form (by the standards of the time). He stated that the compound was free from nitrogen, also that it was completely converted into sugar by plant diastase as well as animal enzymes (pancreatic juice) and also by boiling with mineral acids. He also stated clearly: The synsthesis of glycogen takes place in the liver; this is a vital act. The splitting of glycogen is a chemical process the course of which is not bound to life (*Bernard*, p. 583 [5]).

In this context it has to be stressed that *Bernard*, in ten years of work of a remarkable logical consistency and fascinating lucidity of thought, discovered the key substance of carbohydrate metabolism in 1855 and accurately characterized it in 1857. His work in this field was by no means confined to the isolation and characterization of glycogen. As a result of his teachings carbohydrate metabolism was even then extensively understood and he recognised the basic mechanisms of its regulation.

3. *Biographical Notes on Victor Hensen* [25]

The name of the Kiel physiologist *Victor Hensen* is not unknown to physicians. At least candidates for the preliminary examination in medicine encounter *Hensen's* cells in the inner ear (supporting cells of the organ of Corti, or spiral organ) and, from the microscopic anatomy of striated muscle, the H band (*Hensen's* disk) in the (anisotropic) A band of a sarcomere. The terms *Hensen's* canal or duct (ductus reuniens), *Hensen's* node (primitive node), *Hensen's* stripe (a stiffening band of the membrana tectoria of the inner ear) and *Hensen's* body (a rounded body in an outer hair-cell of the spiral organ) have gone progressively out of use in the last few decades (Porep, pp. 67, 76, 90 [25]).

Victor Hensen was born in the small village of Buenge near Schleswig on 19th February 1835, when *Claude Bernard* was twenty-two years old. His father, *Hans Hensen*, was the principal of a school for deaf-mutes in Schleswig which was well-known at that time and still exists today. *Hans Hensen* was a graduate lawyer with medical and pedagogic ambitions. *Victor Hensen* studied medicine in Würzburg from the summer semester of 1854 to the summer semester of 1856, the next two semesters in Berlin and the final two semesters in Kiel. There he took his Finals in 1858. He obtained the degree of Dr. med. et. chir. in 1859 with a thesis entitled *"De urinae excretione in epilepsia"*. Shortly afterwards he was a appointed prosector in anatomy and in the same year qualified as university lecturer.

Victor Hensen, anatomist, was appointed Professor extraordinary of Physiology and Director of the Physiological Laboratory of the University of Kiel in 1864 and full professor (Ordinarius) in 1868. *Hensen* was also a member of several academies both in Germany and in other countries and many decorations, honorary titles and honorary academic degrees reflect the recognition of his achievements. His research work centered on several subjects in turn: The microsocopic anatomy of the blood, of the muscles, the eye and – especially – the inner ear, embryology, the physiologie of reproduction and – again particularly – the physiology of hearing.

Hensen's contribution to marine biology was a genuine landmark. His work marks the beginning of quantitative biological research into the fishing industry. It was he who coined the term *plankton* and he shaped the quantitative approach of planktology. *Hensen* was also the initiator and leader of several scientific marine expeditions, including the first plankton expedition in the world. He was for many years the chairman of the Prussian Commission for the exploration of the German seas.* The commission had its seat in Kiel and *Hensen* had been chiefly responsible for its inception. Hensen died on April 5, 1924 in his ninetieth year after a fulfilled scientific life.

4. Victor Hensen's Work on Carbohydrate Metabolism

In *Hensen's* early days at Würzburg, before he started clinical work, one of his teachers was *Johann Joseph Scherer* (1814–1869) Professor of Organic Chemistry (which at this time did not include the chemistry of carbohydrates and was more akin to what we now call biochemistry). *Hensen*, as a medical student, himself wrote at that time: "In consequence of the latest paper by *Bernard* on the formation of sugar in the liver, (*Compte rendu* of September 24, 1855) Prof. *Scherer* was good enough to suggest that I investigate the process of sugar formation"(Hensen, p. 219 [17]). The paper quoted by *Hensen* was the one in which Bernard [4], as mentioned above, invited other authors to isolate the new substance *(matière glycogene)* and to elucidate it chemically. *Hensen* decided to take up the challenge, in addition to the follow-up investigations suggested by Scherer. *Hensen* was given the, for a student, quite exceptional opportunity of presenting the result of his investigations at a meeting of the famous *Physico-Medica* (Physicalisch-Medicinische Gesellschaft zu Würzburg) on July 18, 1856. He confirmed *Bernard's* findings from his own investigations. In experiments on the effects of enzymes on glycogen, *Hensen* went beyond *Bernard's* communications: On the advice of the anatamist *A. v. Koelliker* (1817–1905) he exposed glycogen not only to pancreatic extract – in place of pancreatic juice which was not available to him – but he also experimented with saliva; moreover, he also used boiled liver tissue which, by contrast with fresh raw liver tissue, showed

* Preussische Kommission zur Untersuchung der deutschen Meere

no spontaneous glycolysis. The use of saliva occurred to *Hensen* because he knew of the similar behaviour of pancreatic juice and saliva on starch and starch paste. He mentioned in his talk that saliva and pancreatic extract induced the production of sugar in the boiled livers of freshly killed animals. On the whole, his talk, which was printed in the organ of the Physico-Medica, contained nothing essentially new [17]. In the discussion following Hensen's talk, *Koelliker* commented that *Hensen's* experiments promised to be of importance in elucidating the as yet mysterious function of the pancreas; on this subject Hensen had in fact expressed some incorrect though by no means implausible theories in the context of internal secretion. *Koelliker* encouraged him to continue, in particular, his investigations of the substance from which sugar was formed in the liver. This prompted Hensen to continue the work with the objective of isolating glycogen [29]. Quite soon afterwards, for the winter semester of 1856/57, Hensen, who had by now entered on the clinical part of his studies, transferred to the University of Berlin. At the same time the pathologist *Rudolf Virchow* (1821–1902) who then was already very well-known, exchanged his Chair at Würzburg for that of Berlin. It is conceivable that this was in fact what prompted *Hensen* to change his university, as immediately after his arrival in Berlin he found an active sponsor in *Virchow*. This enabled *Hensen* to continue his studies on glycogen without a break in the laboratories of the Berliner Pathologisches Institut. He had by no means forgotten *Koelliker's* suggestion.

On December 11, 1956, *Hensen* was able to present and characterize glycogen, which he had meanwhile produced, to the Berliner Naturwissenschaftlicher Verein der Studierenden. He repeated the lecture on April 1, 1857 at the Pathologisches Institut, Berlin, in the presence of Virchow and the Basle professor *J.I. Hoppe* (1811–1891). Others attending included the professors *F. Dittrich* (1815–1859) a clinician in Erlangen, J. v. Gerlach (1820–1896) physiologist in Erlangen, *A. Fick* (1829–1901) who at that time was still a physiologist in Marburg before becoming a full professor in Zürich and Würzburg, and finally the Leipzig physiologist *O. Funke* who was shortly to become Professor of Physiology in Freiburg. *Hensen* stressed that all of these gentlemen had not only watched his demonstration of the characteristics of glycogen but had expressly acknowledged it which, incidentally, none of those present ever denied (*Hensen*, p. 396 [18]).

It is surely safe to assume that *Hensen's* demonstration did not coincide by accident with the visits of all of these scientists.

Virchow almost certainly invited his student who had just passed his twenty-second birthday. To think otherwise would be to attribute to *Hensen* a blatant self-assertion that crassly contrasted with the reticence and modesty that marked his character throughout his life.

The next chapter in the history of *Hensen's* isolation of glycogen is a dramatic one. On April 12, 1857, *Virchow* read a paper by *Bernard* in the *Gazette médicale de Paris* (No. 13, dated March 28, 1857) stating that he had succeeded in isolating glycogen. Virchow grasped the consequences of this paper for the priority claims of his pupil Hensen. He passed the publication on to Hensen, suggesting that in order to preserve his priority rights he should at once write a paper on his discovery of glycogen, clearly stating the methods, the results, and the dates of his investigations. *Hensen* did not allow the alarming news to slow down his activity. On April 13, i.e. only one day later, he handed *Virchow* the paper on the isolation of glycogen and *Virchow* made it possible for it to be included in the April issue of the *Archiv für pathologische Anatomie and Physiologie und für klinische Medizin* of which *Virchow* himself was the editor.

Hensen's paper contained a description of his method of isolating glycogen. The chief difference between this method and that of *Bernard* was that Hensen removed the protein substances contained in the liver decoctions by precipitation with acetic acid without the use of heat, in accordance with the advice he had been given by Scherer as early as the fall of 1856, whereas *Bernard* destroyed the nitrogenous impurities by mixing the liver decoction with caustic alkali and boiling it. *Hensen* did not consider this method appropriate as the resultant salts and decomposition products complicated the isolation of pure glycogen [18]. It is obvious from these details and the rest of the contents of *Hensen's* paper that the author had been working very actively and for a prolonged period on the problems of the formation and metabolism of glycogen, its isolation, and finally on its physical, chemical and physiologic characteristics, and this despite the fact that his research work must have been rendered more difficult by the change of university, his limited equipment and the fact that he had no assistance.

III. The Dispute about the Discovery of Glycogen

When Bernard was told of that a student namend *Victor Hensen* had been working on glycogen and that his work had culminated in the isolation of the substance, his reaction was as violent as it was unambiguous. He maintained his views until shortly before his death, stating that "Hensen n'a jamais isolé ni montré la matière glycogène" [7] (quoted from [16]). Clearly, his pride would not allow him even to discuss the possibility that a young studend could have isolated and demonstrated glycogen. He cavalierly and irreconcilably dismissed *Hensen's* claim as fraudulent – how else can one interpret his utterance? – and that was, for him, the and of the matter.

In his paper entitled "Über Zuckerbildung in der Leber" [18] (the Formation of sugar in the liver) which *Virchow* pressed him to publish immediately after reading *Bernard's* first communication about the isolation of glycogen in the *Gazette médicale* (see above), *Hensen* wrote: "Bernard has accomplished the description of the sugar-producing substance. At the same time he outlined the mechanism by which this substance is converted into sugar . . . so *Bernard* has succeeded almost alone in discovering the essentials of this important progress from beginning to end, and I am almost afraid that my own contribution to the discovery of these latest facts will be completely lost" (*Hensen*, p. 396 [18]).

On two subsequent occasions, pupils of Hensen worked on glycogen under his tutelage but he himself was no longer actively concerned with the substance. Neither of the two papers published by his pupils contain any comments that could be taken to foreshadow a priority dispute between *Bernard* and *Hensen*. Eleven years after the isolation of glycogen, i.e. in 1868, Hensen's registrar, *C. Dähnhardt*, wrote the following lines at the beginning of his paper "Zur Glycogenbildung in der Leber" [11] (The Formation of glycogen in the liver) ". . . of the year 1857 in which *Hensen* published the discovery of glycogen which he made simultaneously with *Claude Bernard*". In 1900, twenty-two years after Bernard's death, *Ernst Harmsen*, who had studied for his doctorate under *Hensen*, began his thesis with a touch of homage to his teacher: "Since 1856 and 1857, when glycogen was disovered almost simultaneously by *Hensen* and *Claude Bernard* . . ." [23].

The personal and direct utterances listed above are, so far as I am able to discover, the only ones made by the principals involved in the priority dispute on the discovery of glycogen.

Bearing in mind the extent and violence of the usual priority disputes in the second half of the 19th century, the term dispute would hardly be applicable to the circumstances of the discovery of glycogen had not *Bernard* and *Hensen* found (unsolicited and, in the majority of cases, not very competent) partisans who conducted the dispute on their behalf. We could quote a virtually innumerable number of contributions to the controversy surrounding the discovery of glycogen, with some famous names among the protagonists, e.g. *Pflüger* and *Schiff* [cf. synopses in 24, 25 and 27]. Those favoring either *Bernard* or *Hensen* were joined by a conciliatory third party which wanted to dedicate the laurel wreath jointly to the two scientists. The best example of this last attitude is to be found in the American literature: *Lardy* compromised by describing glycogen as *Hansen-Bernard polysaccharide. Hansen* is clearly an error of transcription, due to the fact that the pronunciation of the German e is similar to that of the English a [20].

It is remarkable that most of the authors who were secondarily involved in the argument had no very profound knowledge of the whole situation. Even the well-known medical historian *Paul Diepgen* was guilty of a mistake when he wrote that: "In 1857, *Claude Bernard* discovered tissue glycogen which slightly earlier had been discovered independently by *Victor Hensen* who was then a young student" (*Diepgen*, p. 73 [12]). Not only was the glycogen mentioned in this context always understood to be hepatic glycogen – tissue glycogen as a constant constituent of muscle was not discovered until 1869 by *O. Nasse* (1839–1903, Professor of Pharmacology and Physiological Chemistry in Rostock) – but Hensen can in no way be said to have discovered glycogen independently of *Bernard*.

Of the motives of those who wanted to eulogize *Hensen*, two – both unrelated to the issue – stand out: 1. sympathy for the unknown young student who had the bad luck to get involved in a competition with France's pope of physiology, so that his defeat in a priority dispute must be a foregone conclusion, and 2. national pride which considered that France, after her defeat in 1871, could never be humiliated enough. An almost grotesque example of this attitude is supplied by *Ernst Harmsen*, mentioned above, who as a graduate student wrote his doctoral thesis on glycogen under the auspices of *Hensen*. In 1932, he put a notice in the *Münchner medizinische Wochenschrift* to commemorate the "discovery of glycogen 75 years ago" and pointedly stated that glycogen, like a fruit hanging ripe on a tree, was discovered and described simultaneously and *wholly independently* by *Victor Hensen* and *Claude Bernard*" [15]. It was a thorn in his flesh that the *Lehrbuch der Physiologie* (which is still well-known today) by *Landois* and *Rosemann* (19th edition [1929] p. 134) only mentions *Bernard* and that there is no reference to *Hensen*. He obtained little comfort from the fact that most textbooks mention the two authors side by side. Subsequently Rosemann, writing in the same journal, explained why in his opinion "Cl. Bernard's description of glycogen deserved precendence over that by *Victor Hensen*" (*Roseman*, p.1386 [26]). The entire rejoinder by *Rosemann*, which admittedly seems a shade too harsh in his attitude to *Hensen*, prompted Harmsen to a further more comprehensive article which was published in the *Medizinische Welt* in 1934 [16]. Particularly noteworthy factors in this paper are the headline "Victor Hensen, the *German* discoverer of glycogen" and the final sentence: "In any case, we now (1934!) have no longer any reason to abandon, in favor of the famous French physiologist, the just claim of one of our foremost German scientists to recognition of a discovery made when a very young man. Rather is it our bounden duty, as Germans, to restore the name of 'our' V. H. to his place beside Cl. B. as discoverer of glycogen".

IV. Conclusions

The priority dispute about the discovery of glycogen, which has sporadically flared up to this day, has a number of unusual features.

1. *Claude Bernard* and *Victor Hensen* were cast by other authors as protagonists in a priority dispute. They themselves never engaged in a priority dispute in the strict sense of the word. Neither of them so much as intervened in any of a number of controversies conducted in their life times (for instance by that specialist in priority disputes *Eduard Pflüger*, 1829–1910, Professor of Physiology in Bonn [24]).

2. It was not the *discovery* of glycogen which was in dispute, since *Bernard* knew as early as 1855 that the liver contained a substance described by him as *une espèce de fécule animale*, a kind of animal starch, which was converted to sugar by means of an enzymatic process (*Cl. Bernard*, p. 250 [3]). The question of priority concerns exclusively its *isolation*, i.e. the preparation of chemically pure glycogen.

3. The formal procedure in such disputes is that the priority is decided on the basis of the date of publication, which may be a recorded lecture at a congress or a printed paper. *Bernard's* written communication on the isolation of glycogen, which includes the preparatory procedure and the chemical and physiological characterization of the substance, has to be dated as March 28, 1857 [5, 6]. *Hensen's* paper, which refers expressly and unequivocally to the communication in the *Gazette médicale de Paris* of March 28, 1957, was not submitted for publication until April 13, 1857 (Hensen, p. 398 [18]). On formal terms, there is thus no basis for a dispute.

The fact that nevertheless a priority dispute was allowed to develop is rooted in emotional factors, some of which have been exposed above. The unequivocally false statement by Bernard that *"Hensen n'a jamais isolé ni montré la matière glycogène"* [7] was likewise the result of a solely emotional reaction, as was the concern expressed by the young student *Hensen*, born of his disappointment, that his share in the characterisation of glycogen might be completely ignored (*Hensen*, p. 396 [18]).

At a time when, by virtue of the successes and mistakes of past generation, we have gained a deeper insight into the laws of scientific research and try to base our judgment on fact unbiassed by emotion, the priority dispute over the isolation of glycogen may be concisely presented as follows: *Claude Bernard* had been working very successfully for almost eight years on the elucidation of carbohydrate metabolism when, in 1855, he discovered hepatic glycogen which he invited the research scientists of the world to isolate. A Würzburg biochemist, Scherer, who prepared *Bernard's* 1855 paper for a prestigious German publication [10], instructed his pupil, *Victor Hensen*, to reproduce *Bernard's* findings. Bearing *Bernard's* invitation in mind, *Hensen* tried to isolate glycogen from hepatic tissue. This preparatory and chemical task required neither great original thought nor chemical expenditure. In the winter of 1856/57, Bernard as well as *Hensen* were successful in their attempts to isolate and characterize glycogen. The isolation of the substance was, incidentally, very effective by contemporary methods. Later on, the impurities unavoidably associated with the methods of the time triggered controversies as to whose glycogen had been the purer and who must therefore be regarded as the true discoverer of the substance [23, 24]. The slight difference in the dates at which the discoveries were published was coincidental and without relevance. On no account can it be claimed that *Hensen* discovered glycogen *wholly independently* of *Bernard. Bernard* had a companion at the last step of the long road that led to the isolation of glycogen, namely *Hensen* who reached the same goal at the same time.

References

1. *Bernard, Claude:* Comptes rendus Soc. Biol. (mém.) 1, 121 (1849).
2. *Bernard, Claude:* Nouvelle fonction du foie considéré comme organe producteur de matière sucrée chez l'homme et les animaux. Baillière, Paris 1853.

2a. *Bernard, Claude:* Neue Funktion der Leber als zuckerbereitendes Organ des Menschen und der Tiere. Deutsch von *V. Schwarzenbach.* Würzburg 1853.

3. *Bernard, Claude:* Leçons de physiologie expérimentale appliqué à la médecine faites au Collège de France. Cours du sem. d'hiver 1854–1855. T. 1 Baillière, Paris 1855.
4. *Bernard, Claude:* Compt. rendus Acad. Sci. 41, 461 (1855).
5. *Bernard, Claude:* Sur le mécanisme physiologique de la formation du sucre dans le foie (Suite de 1855). Compt. rendus Acad. Sci. 44, 578–586 (1857). (Vortrag gehalten am 23. 3. 1857, veröffentlicht am 28. 3. 1857.)
6. *Bernard, Claude:* Nouvelles recherches expérimentales sur les phénomènes glycogéniques du foie. Gazette médicale de Paris Nr. 13, vom 28. 3. 1857, p. 201–203.
7. *Bernard, Claude:* Critique expérim. Ann. de Physiol. et Chem. VIII, 376 (1876). (Zit. nach 16.)
8. *Bernard, Claude:* Ausgewählte physiologische Schriften. Der Bauchspeichel. Das Glykogen. Die Blutgefäßnerven. Das Pfeilgift. Zusammengestellt, übersetzt und kommentiert von *Nikolaus Mani. – Hubers Klassiker der Medizin und Naturwissenschaften. Bd. VIII. Bern–Stuttgart 1966.*
9. *Bernard, Claude:* Einführung in das Studium der experimentellen Medizin (Paris 1865). Ins Deutsche übertragen von *Paul Szendrö* und biographisch eingeleitet und kommentiert von *Karl E. Rothschuh.* Mit einem Anhang: Zur Bibliographie des Schrifttums von und über Claude Bernard. Von *Rudolph Zaunick, Sudhoffs Klassiker der Medizin, Bd. 35. Leipzig 1961.*
10. Cannstatts Jahresbericht über die Fortschritte der gesamten Heilkunde in allen Ländern. – Physiologische Wissenschaften.
11. Dähnhardt, Ch.: Zur Glycogenbildung in der Leber. In: Arbeiten aus dem Kieler physiologischen Institut 1868, hrsg. von *V. Hensen.* Kiel 1869.
12. *Diepgen, P.:* Geschichte der Medizin. II. Band, 2. Hälfte. Berlin 1955.
13. *Dumesnil, R.,* und *H. Schadewaldt:* Die berühmten Ärzte. 2. Aufl. Köln (o. J.) (darin: Claude Bernard p. 218–219 und 2 Abb.).
14. *Harmsen, E.:* Beiträge zur Bestimmung des Leberglykogens. Diss. med. Kiel 1900.
15. *Harmsen, E.:* Zur Entdeckung des Glykogens vor 75 Jahren. Münch. med. Wschr. 79, 1075 (1932).
16. *Harmsen, E.:* Victor Hensen, der deutsche Entdecker des Glykogens. Med. Welt 8, 1783–1784 (1934).

17. *Hensen, V.:* Ueber die Zuckerbildung in der Leber. (Vorgetragen in der Sitzung v. 18. Juli 1856.) Verhandl. Phys.-Med. Ges. Würzburg 7, 219–222 (1857).
18. *Hensen, V.:* Über Zuckerbildung in der Leber. Virchows Arch. path. Anat. 11, 395–398 (1857).
19. *Hirsch, A.:* Biographisches Lexikon der hervorragenden Ärzte aller Zeiten und Völker, hrsg. v. *A. Hirsch.* München–Berlin[3] 1962.
20. *Lardy, H. A.* (Editor): Respiratory Enzymes. Second printing. Minneapolis 1950.
21. *Mani, G.:* Die Entdeckung des Glykogens durch Claude Bernard. Zschr. klin. Chem. 2, 97–104 (1964).
22. *Mann, G.:* Vom Streit der Ärzte. Med. Welt 39, 879–885, 995–1000 (1965).
23. *Pflüger, E.:* Über die Darstellung des Glykogens nach Viktor Hensen. Pflügers Arch. Physiol. 95, 17–18 (1903).
24. *Pflüger, E.:* Das Glykogen und seine Beziehungen zur Zuckerkrankheit. Bonn[2] 1905.
25. *Porep, R.:* Der Physiologe und Planktonforscher Victor Hensen (1835–1924). Sein Leben und sein Werk. Kieler Beiträge zur Geschichte der Medizin und Pharmazie. Hrsg. v. *Robert Herrlinger †, Fridolf Kudlien* und *Georg E. Dann.* H. 9. Neumünster 1970.
26. *Rosemann, R.:* Zur Entdeckung des Glykogens vor 75 Jahren. Eine Berichtigung. Münch. med. Wschr. 79,1367–1368 (1932).
27. *Schuth, W.:* Die Entdeckung der Glykogenbildung in der Leber. Ein geschichtlicher Beitrag. Med. Diss. Freiburg/Br. 1962.
28. *Sigerist, H. E.:* Große Ärzte, Eine Geschichte der Heilkunde in Lebensbildern. München[5], 1965.
29. Verhandlungen der Physicalisch-Medicinischen Gesellschaft in Würzburg 1857. (Darin: Sitzungsberichte für das Gesellschaftsjahr 1856. Sechzehnte Sitzung am 18. Juli 1856, p. XLIX.)
30. *Wolff, G.:* Der Zuckerstoffwechsel – eine biographische Studie. Med. Mschr. 12, 766–774, 838–846 (1958).
31. *Wolff, G.:* Beiträge berühmter Studenten zur Erforschung des Zuckerstoffwechsels. Münch. med. Wschr. 102, 1203–1208 (1960).
32. *Young, F. G.:* Claude Bernard and the Discovery of Glycogen. A century of retrospect. Brit. Med. Journ. 1957, p. 1431–1437.

in: *Medizinische Monatsschrift 25 (1971) 314–321.*

Paul Langerhans – of Islets and Islands

by GÜNTHER WOLFF

Thomas Carlyle (1795–1881), British historian and author of biographies ranging from Oliver Cromwell to Frederick the Great of Prussia, said in the mid-19th century that "the history of the world consisted of the biographies of great men". In my view, this exemplarly statement applies not only to the history of the world but equally to the history of medicine.

The names of many great physicians and surgeons are for ever linked with a disease they discovered, with a symptom or sign, an important instrument, a specific operation or a diagnostic procedure.

Now, we have all heard of the islets of Langerhans- in a pathologic, histologic and, in connection with diabetes, also in a clinical context. Some of us may even know that these particular cell formations in the pancreas were first described by a student, Paul Langerhans, in his doctoral thesis of 1869. He was then 22 years old.

Biographical data, however, have so far been very few. Born 25th June 1847 in Berlin, the son of a physician, died 20th Juli 1988 – only occasionally with the addition: on the island of Madeira.

The data – such as there are – always center on the thesis "Contributions on the Microscopic Anatomy of the Pancreas" – to which we shall revert below and which, when the importance of its contents was recognised, was to usher in a new era in diabetology.

Wheter I am compiling my own family history or attempting a contribution to the history of medicine, I always try to reach beyond figures and dates. What I was looking for here – as in genealogy – was rather the man with all his strengths and weaknesses that were concealed behind the bare facts.

Who was the man behind the name of Paul Langerhans? What were his scientific interests after his thesis, what work did he do, how and where did he live, how did he die? Specific searches produced no progress until as Nietzsche once aptly expressed it – I "got tired of seeking and discovered finding". I intended to go on holiday to Madeira in 1975 but before I left a friend, Hans Schadewaldt, Director of the Institute of Medical History of the University of Duesseldorf, encouraged me to resume my research on Hans Langerhans.

At this point the direction of our research was changed by a battery of the proverbial strokes of luck. The first one occurred in the Department of the Cultural Attaché of the German Embassy in Lisbon and led us via the Honorary German Consul in Funchal and the local museum of the British cemetery. Then Professor Jahnke, of Wuppertal, actually put us in touch with a surviving niece of Langerhans. This led to a meeting with other members of the family who had not known each other previously. The Honorary German Consul (Frau Elisabeth Gesche) knew the name of a German physician in Erlangen whose forebears were said to have been acquainted with Langerhans. And there had indeed been a meaningful and extremely frequent exchange of letters between the grandfather of Dr. Hoffmann of Erlangen and Paul Langerhans. Furthermore, despite the problems of World War II, some of the correspondence had survived. The owner kindly allowed me to look through the letters which became the source of additions to the history of medicine via the discoverer of the islet cells. At the same time, they reflected the personality of the man. Goethe for example – in the 19th century, when people still communicated in writing – stressed the importance of the contents of letters for biographical research when he said that letters were so valuable because they preserved the essential core of existence.

Another mirror of the personality is represented by a portrait which according to Leonardo da Vinci was "worth more than a thousand words". And this brings us to something else that is curious about the biographical data of Paul Langerhans hitherto:

Most of the portraits shown in our medical textbooks are, quite simply, not of Langerhans. An error had occurred which was then perpetuated unchecked and uncritically from one book to the next. As recently as the Deutsche Diabeteskongress in 1977, the Belgian scientist Gepts, who was awarded the Paul-Langerhans Plaque, presented a portrait which did not represent Paul Langerhans but Hans Strasser, a fellow registrar at the Pathological Institute, Freiburg.

The error was rectified by Professor Schadewaldt – who has been working in Freiburg for many years – after his attention had been drawn to the mistake by a member of the Strasser family. Who then was guilty of this historical prank?

The Freiburg picture does indeed bear the name of "Paul Langerhans". However, the initial letters "s.lb." ([To] his dear) had been omitted (the name of the dedicator is missing).

Other books contain pictures which are details taken from family groups. However, we now have other, previously unpublished photographs which were kindly made available to me by a member of the Langerhans family. We cannot tell whether the previously unpublished and undated photograph of Langerhans as a young man was taken when he was a student of Rudolf Virchow. On the other hand, we know his *doctoral thesis* which was reprinted in facimile a few years ago. For a better evaluation, it seems useful to touch on at least a few fragments illustrating the state of knowledge about diabetes at that time. Diabetes mellitus, described as "honey diuresis" or "the mysterious disease", was known to the Ancient Greek, Roman and Egyptian physicians.

The symptoms of diabetes were described as early as 1550 B.C. in the Ebers papyrus. An early "test strip" for sugar in the urine consisted of . . . ants, which, attracted by the sweetness of the sugar, were drawn to the urine. By 1674, the physician Thomas Willis no longer relied on the sweet tooth of ants but detected the sweetness by tasting the urine himself. This was the principal sign of the disease in which the sugar ran through the body – diabainein – and which since the time of Aretaeus and Galen about the 2nd century A.D. has been known as diabetes.

Morgagni, the founder of modern morbid anatomy, had to admit as late as 1761 that diabetes was a *"morbus in sede inceta locus"* – a disease the site of which in the body was quite unknown.

From the middle of the 17th century onwards, Johann Conrad Brunner had pioneered further discoveries which were ultimately to lead to modern diabetology. Brunner came very close to discovering the site of diabetes which was still unknown at the time of Morgagni.

He found that the partial removal of the pancreas of an animal was followed by the typical symptoms of diabetes, i.e. severe thirst and polyuria. However, these effects disappeared soon after the operation. The reason was that Brunner, as mentioned above, did not remove the entire pancreas and – as we now know – left part of the gland with its islets of Langerhans.

And this brings us back to the key term – islets of Langerhans.

There can be little doubt that Virchow, a friend of the Langerhans familiy – a brother of Paul also became his graduate student and subsequently his registrar – suggested the pancreas to Langerhans for his doctoral thesis. Some years previously, the famous French physiologist Claude Bernard had made major contributions to endocrine secretion, with his "milieu interne" and with his now well-known *piqûre* or puncture diabetes – diabetes provoked by puncture of the floor of the fourth ventricle – demonstrated a neurogenic triggering of glycosuria.

The thesis, which is dedicated to "Professor Virchow in admiration and gratitude", is a thin volume of only 31 pages. Which shows once again that in scientific papers, it is not so much the size as the content that matters!

The findings in the thesis are presented with the utmost modesty – a human attribute which in science as elsewhere is becoming ever rarer. I am quoting a few major passages:

"In the summer of 1867, I began work at the Berliner Pathologisches Institut, to which I was admitted by the kindness of Professor Virchow, and carried out a series of investigations into the fine structure of the pancreas."

He apologized for "the slight contents" and then modestly continued . . .

"I am unfortuntely obliged to start my communications with the statement that I am by no means in a position to present the finished results of a successful study but can at most contribute a few isolated observations which suggest that the organ investigated has an infinitely more complex structure than was assumed hitherto."

"I must apologize in case these lines fall into the hands of an experienced microscopist and he finds a little too much of what is known and much too little of what is new . . ."

He then described, by means of his simple "teased" preparations, the peculiar clusters of cells that he was the first to observe; unfortunately no sketches of these are attached to the paper. He concluded with a statement hinting at an endocrine secretion.

". . . that in the pancreas, we have no direct transition of the secretory elements into the epithelia of the ducts."

The importance of the findings in Langerhans's thesis was not recognised in his lifetime. It was sometime after his death, that the Frenchman Édouard Laguesse (1893) described the cell clusters as "îlots de Langerhans" – the islets of Langerhans – the scientific term by which they are known today throughout the world. And as early as 1909, Jean de Meyer used the term *"insulin"*, to describe the contents of the islets of Langerhans, i.e. even before Banting and Best, in 1921, isolated the secretion of the beta granules in the B cells.

In this context, I refer to recurrent comments in the literature that the discoverer of the islet cells was no longer concerned with questions of carbohydrate metabolism. I believe, however, that such sweeping statements should not be made rashly as there are indications in his letters that Paul Langerhans at least retained an interest in the questions first raised in his thesis.

For instance, the two friends exchanged views across thousands of kilometers – Hoffmann had meanwhile become a professor at the German University in Tartu – about carbohydrate metabolism and in particular the glycogen findings of Claude Bernard, about the relationship of carbohydrates and the creation of energy, about the provocation of experimental neurogenic diabetes, etc.

Hoffmann reproduced Claude Bernard's diabetic puncture and the description he dispatched to Madeira included a blood-sugar curve, plotted in his own hand.

As the surviving letters of Langerhans were chiefly written in 1877, we cannot tell whether, when he died in 1888, he had heard of the experiment carried out by v. Mering and Minkowski in 1886. The experiment involved the use of phloridzin to induce a transient experimental diabetes which, it was soon discovered, was due to poisoning of certain areas of the pancreas with involvement of the cell structures discovered by Langerhans. The paper by v. Mering and Minkowski on the provocation of "Diabetes mellitus after extirpation of the pancreas" was not published until one year after Langerhans's death.

At this point I cannot resist the inclusion of a curious sequence of events not previously known which I only discovered from the correspondence. It was another little story communicated by Hoffmann to his friend in Madeira and shows once again how often accident plays a part in great discoveries.

When an assistant in Berlin, v. Mering had "made improper suggestions" to nurses and was removed from his post. He was taken on by Minkowski in Strassburg who was at that time interested in excretory pancreatic enzymes – i.e. not at all in diabetes. Mering assisted him in ligating a pancreatic duct and went on holiday.

The credit for discovering pancreatic diabetes should really go to the laboratory servant who noticed the constant thirst and frequent urination of the operated dog as typical symptoms of diabetes.

In the jargon of the modern gutter press, the discovery of pancreatic diabetes would no doubt read: "Professor Disciplined for Sex Orgies with Nurses Makes Discovery of Global Importance".

However, back to Langerhans. When he had finished his thesis and taken his Finals in 1870, he travelled in Egypt, Syria and, for purposes of exploration, in the region west of the Jordan. These travels, which may be described as "educational journeys", differed from subsequent ones after he contracted tuberculosis and which via several places including Silvaplana, Capri and Badenweiler, finally took him to Madeira. The latter journeys combined scientific interest with the probably primary objective of alleviating his tuberculosis.

He returned from his educational travels to find his country at war with France. He immediately joined the army and took part in most of the campaign. Papers of the Langerhans family, unlikely to have been previously used for a biography of Langerhans, show that the young army surgeon very rapidly gained the respect of his colleagues and that he was often consulted as an authority even by older officers of the medical corps. The Franco-Prussian war of 1870/71 is, incidentally, itself of interest in the context of the history of medicine as, although the International Red Cross was founded by Henry Dunant in 1859 after the battle of Solferino, this was the first time that its humanitarian activities were given any real scope. Now, 100 years later, we can only reflect how far we have moved back from the statement: "In the battle of Solferino the conscience of the world remembered the duty of compassion" (commemorative stone in Vienna, Ministry of War).

The friends discussed field hospitals and especially the progress that Lister's antisepsis meant for war surgery, but also "the scandalous conditions of patronage" and the "Social Question" which was a burning topic of the day. "We cannot", Hoffmann wrote to Langerhans in a letter dated 7th July 1877, "make it go away, so we have to see if it is possible to solve it".

And an observation that is no less topical today: "If only one could get a majority of them to the point where they thought more deeply and were less inclined to pick the man who promises most as their Messiah, an advance in reason that is urgently needed and not only by the working-class".

Bismarck took a sceptical view of Hoffmann. In his own opinion, the "Iron Chancellor" had nothing to fear even from the *Fortschrittpartei* (progress party) founded jointly by Virchow and the father of Paul Langerhans, a Berlin physician and city counsellor.

When peace was restored in 1871, Langerhans first went to Leipzig and then accepted an appointment as prosector in Freiburg where some years later he became an associate professor. In 1874 he contracted tuberculosis – whether he caught the infection from autopsy material can only be conjecture, the more so in view of his mother's early death from the disease.

Langerhans was forced to give up his promising career, though at first he hoped only temporarily, in the interest of his health. He retired – which a legacy enabled him to do – to Madeira. Why he chose this particular island will become clear in a reference to the pathography below.

It is very clear from the correspondence, in which the two friends dealt in detail with the *situation in the German universities,* the power of the *scientific press*, and with the political and sociomedical problems of the time, that even in his "island exile" Langerhans never abandoned hope of recovering from his tuberculosis and resuming his place in the world of medical science in Germany. However, this wish was subordinate to the long "cure" he had prescribed for himself – and recommended to other patients – in the hope of ultimate recovery.

The *description of German university life* in the correspondence – from which I can only include extracts – would fit the motto of preacher Solomon from the Old Testament: "What is it then that one has done . . . there's nothing new under the sun". The "faculty gossip" in connection with the appointment of professors, for instance, has quite a contemporary ring. Lacking in respect but not in vigour, the friends were agreed that any professorships falling vacant were being filled by incompetent successors.

To quote one passage: "I have no idea who is going to Leipzig. I expect they will ofter it to Kussmaul" (remembered by Kussmaul's respiration) "but whether he'll go is in the lap of the gods. And who'll be offerd the chair if he turns it down, perhaps not even the gods know".

The „faculty gossip" reached its peak with caustic remarks such as (L. to H. 2nd March 1877): "Things are getting more and more uncomfortable in Freiburg, from what I hear Heinrich Funke, malicious lout that he is, is progressively dominating the scence. The Devil take him! and with that sentiment, I am yours ...". Or in another letter (of 16th January 1877, L. to H.): "So Czerny's position is to go to ..." (illegible). "I do not consider it a very fortunate choice either but who else is there? There are not many shining lights among the young surgeons ... The fact is that much of research is a matter of words and weaker successors often inherit the fruits of their predecessors' labor".

On another occasion, (12th February 1877) L. wrote to H.: "I have not heard any scandals, except the one about Ebstein in Göttingen. Nice faculty they seem to make themselves there".

And his friend's reply (H. to L.) ". . . perhaps they could have got someone better in Göttingen. Possibly E. is a comfortable and safe personality and old Henle" (of Henle's loop) "may think: why sould Imake a rod for my own back?" And a few lines further down: "We have had no scandals here of late nor is one in prospect in the near future; the main eruption will be at the election of the next rector".

Their exchange of views on the *German scientific press* and the *publication of papers* might easily have been written at the present time.

The two friends exchanged their views on research projects and papers across the considerable distance of 5000 kilometers. Langerhans was, however, clearly depressed by his scientific isolation when he wrote: ". . . but where would I get the books to look it up? Books are the problem. Couldn't you send me down the college library for a little while?"

Other comments that could have been written today were those made by H. in a letter to L. in which he criticised the craving for acclaim of some scientists who founded new "private periodicals" – as he contemptously called them – solely to publicise their own names. He emphasized that a fee should be paid for every paper submitted, otherwise such publications should never "become more than rags . . ." He also pilloried the ostentation of medical societies which by no means always met an urgent need.

And yet another contemporary-sounding comment from Tartu (1st April 1877): "But it is dreadful to emerge from one's tranquil study in a laboratory into this world of affected tattle, the unsubstantially of the literature, the mountains of little results each of which is made to support a large theory, the many words and little sense".

Criticism of the medical press and the ever increasing new journals recurs continually in the correspondence. We are even now in the midst of a luxuriant proliferation of scientific organs. These numbered about 100 around 1800; according to modern estimates, they will have increased to one million by the fast-approaching year 2000.

A comment on the splitting of one publication, the *Zentralblatt für Chirurgie,* into one for surgery and one for gynaecology, touches on the commercial element in scientific journals and then continues: "I dare say the 'Gynäkologe' will also make its profit. It is just the same as in the world of commerce – you don't produce to meet a demand, you produce to create a demand. The many new journals are not being founded because there are so many authors yearning for publication, but many papers are written because there are so many journals. The multitude of journals means that the medical profession may not be able to meet the demand, but if the publishers are competing with each other they can be squeezed. As everywhere in the world though, the rich have all in their favour, the professors and the poor practitioner have to pay with their sweat and allow themselves to be exploited by the public and the publishers. Here too, we have only a fight for survival and no moral philosophy of life . . .". This was written in 1877 and how apt it is for our own day.

It is obvious from Langerhans's early educational travels that his interests included besides medicine all aspects of *natural science*. It is likely that his teacher Virchow, to whom he remained close across the distance, had stimulated his interest in this particular field.

He was commissioned by the *Königliche Akademie der Wissenschaften* in Berlin to study the maritime worm fauna. This resulted in the discovery of a large number of previously unknown species of worms. In addition, the maritime environment stimulated his interest in fishes and in fact in the entire fauna of his "island exile". His studies included work on a newt *(Triturus)* which he had used in the experiments for his thesis. He augmented these studies by a stay on the island of Tenerife with its rich vegetation in the Orotava valley and its thousand-year old dragon trees. As author he continued to sign himself – still hoping for a return to Germany: Doctor Hans Langerhans, Professor in Freiburg, currently physician on Madeira.

He was interested in Darwinism and encouraged his friend to read about such matters which could only be useful to him. The Madeira studies also established new links with papers written in Freiburg which concerned the nervous system. This shows that Langerhans was by no means inactive in his "island exile" where, as he wrote, he studied "island zoology".

Before Langerhans went to Madeira, he was one of the first Germans to work for a time at the Naples Zoological Institute which was founded in 1872 by Anton Dohrn (1840–1909). Unfortunately we do not know whether he visited Ischia from there.

He did not omit to publish his findings. Here his close association with Virchow was obviously very useful to him. We can also gather from his reports that he turned to his old teacher for financial assistance and, worried about the latter's agreement, wrote to his friend: "My old chap is taking an unconscionably long time in settling our financial transaction. He is always dawdles about business matters but I cannot very well put anyone else in his place and in any case he is the only friend I have got left in Berlin". The end of the story comes in another letter: "My old chap (Virchow) has written to say that the Academy has granted me the sum requested. So I am once again beholden to my old benefactor – and glad to be so. "He may have expressed his gratitude to his old teacher, benefactor and friend of his family by giving his name to a newly discovered species of annelid *"Accularia virchowii"*.

Langerhans wrote a handbook on Madeira. His style was one of scientific precision but wholly comprehensible to the general public. The book is a mine of information, not only of the historical, geographical and geological characteristics of his "island exile" but also of the countryside, the people and the record of this Atlantic isle.

In writing about the expatriate colony and the tourists, or those who came to Madeira in search of health, he commented characteristically on his compatriots: "As is inevitable in view of the close relationship of the nations, we Germans share in full and undivided measure the dislike and envy". This statement too is reminiscent of the present day.

Other chapters of the book contain useful information for tourists and the sick, on the few doctors on the island, on pharmacies, nurses and hospitals but also on ways to obtain books and periodicals to combat bordeom during their "cure" on the island. He also advised them to fill up their time by attending English language courses.

The guidebook includes a sketch of the island and a plan of the town of Funchal and its immediate environs. The letter, Langerhans wrote in his foreword of April 1884, was "the work of a German officer who did not want his name to be mentioned".

Langerhans dealt in particular detail with the *climatic conditions* of the island with special reference to their therapeutic value for consumptives. This section offers an interesting insight into contemporary phthisiology. As for the question that everyone reading these lines must be wanting to ask, why did he pick on Madeira as his health resort, his considered answers are given in Chapters 10 and 11 of the Madeira Handbook. He recommended the dust-free air and the humid climate especially for patients with tuberculosis of the larynx from which he himself was suffering.

In his Madeira book as well as in his scientific papers, he wrote, no doubt prompted by his own condition, on the epidemiology of tuberculosis on Madeira where, incidentally, in the church of Monte above Funchal, is the tomb of an Austrian Emperor, Charles, who also died of a tubercular condition.

His letters turned into a case history when he described the changing signs and symptoms of his disease and in keeping with contemporary views, he kept returning to the importance of the elastic fibers in the sputum. "The elastics are still in bloom" he wrote in one letter, perhaps a simile with the flowering splendour of the island.

His larynx had to be painted with lapis (silver nitrate) and his voice, he wrote, "was coarser than that of any riffraff". There were also repeated mentions of hemoptysis. His medical advice to his consumptive patient was very modern in that, even at that time, his counselling included general health education and he recommended exercise, diet, an outdoor life and skin care as the best treatment for diseases lungs. However, he also attached particular importance to the treatment of each patient as an individual. He described a regard for the invidualty of the patient as the greater part of a physician's care. And how modern he strikes us when he writes: "We do not treat diseases but patients" and in conclusion appeals: "People only get well if they have the will".

The final stage of Langerhans' tuberculosis with renal involvement and uremia is known from a letter by his wife, Margarethe, whom Langerhans married after her husband had died of pulmonary disease in Madeira. The heart-rending letter is a record both of human grief and accurate medical observation.

This harrowing document and a two-page case note in English by a Dr. Hicks on his colleague Langerhans, also found among Hoffmann's papers, are reproduced verbatim in our paper published in "Medizin. Welt", Nos 1 and 2, 1977.

Langerhans was a good and popular physician in Madeira. I was told this by the Honorary German Consul whose father had actually known Langerhans.

Langerhans's last resting place in his island exile is the English cemetery. He had described its tranquility and lush southern vegetation in his book on Madeira, concluding with the words: "It is a still, secluded place where one may rest in peace".

The Odyssey of Langerhans ended on the island of Madeira and it was from the fourth song of the Odyssey that he chose the inscription for his grave: "Weeping I sat in the sand, wanting to live no longer and look on Helios's rays".

The Deutsche Diabetesgesellschaft responded to a suggestion by my friend Schadewaldt and myself to mark the grave of the discoverer of the islets with a commemorative plaque.

I should like to conclude this talk with a question and answer and at the same time give a brief outline of the current state of diabetology.

The question is: Has the discovery of Paul Langerhans still any relevance today, more than a hundred years later?

My I refer you to my "Biographical Calendar".

In 1869, Paul Langerhans discovered the special clusters of cells that make up about 1 to 2 percent of the pancreas and are scattered throughout the organ.

A quarter of a century later when their importance was realised, Laguesse gave these structures the name of their discoverer.

In 1901, which happened to be the year in which Henry Dunant was awarded the Nobel Peace Prize for his humanitarian idea to create the Red Cross, Lane distinguished two different cell forms, the A and B cells, within the islets of Langerhans. The B cells make up 60 to 70 percent.

Twenty years later, Banting and Best actually succeeded in isolating the active principle, till then the object of repeated hypotheses and assumptions, from the islets of Langerhans by ligation of the pancreatic duct. The substance yielded by the islets was called insulin. But cells other than the two known forms were to be discovered.

In 1931, Blume discovered that the islets contained yet another type of cell, the D cells, of which there are 1.5 to 2.5

millions in the human pancreas. The number is reduced in diabetics. The total weight of the islets is only 1 to 2 g, and the diameter of an islet is 75 to 500 μ (1 μ = one-millionths mm). The diameter of a single B cell is 12 to 15 μ. A B cell is thus about twice the size of a red blood cell.

There are however still more cells in a small islet. This brings us to the discovery of the V cells. Each cell form secretes a different hormone.

I shall follow up this morphologic outline with a brief review of the pathogenesis of diabetes.

After the discovery of "pancreatic diabetes" by v. Mering and Minkowski, the theories obviously centered on the pancreas and its islets. Then came the advocates of the so-called counter-regulatory diabetes, while others favored pituitary or neurogenic diabetes. At the same time it became increasingly obvious that the disorder was not confined to carbohydrate metabolism but also involved fat metabolism so that the popular term "sugar diabetes" seems an incorrect description of this multifactorial condition.

Despite the changes in the pathogenesis of diabetes, the islets have withstood the onslaught of scientific opinions.

In the age of organ transplants, there have obviously been attemps to replace the pancreas of a diabetic or one extirpated because of carcinoma with a donor organ. However, of 32 such transplants carried out in the USA, only two patients survived. The rejektion response was too great.

After the failure of pancreas transplants, attempts were made in animals, but also in man, to inject or infuse isolated islets or isolated B cells into different parts of the body, the liver having proved the most successful. With the concurrent administration of immunosuppressants, the highly purified cells were successfully implanted and functioning. Nevertheless, it proved very difficult to achieve metabolic stabilisation with such cell implants.

Hopes then centered on an "artificial pancreas", a "pancreatic prosthesis" or "artificial islet cells".

We all know that it is the instability of his metabolism that constitutes the chief risk to a diabetic. The greater the fluctuations in blood-sugar, the more severe are the various complications. A "pancreas machine" has in fact been developed. A computer continuously monitors the blood-sugar, the level of which – again via a computer – governs the dispensing of the required levels of insulin or glucose by means of an indwelling cannula and a pump. This method ensures a stable blood-sugar profile by contrast with the instability that occurs even if insulin is injected in two daily doses.

The artificial B cell is used in comatose or pregnant diabetics, in extreme instability of carbohydrate metabolism, before and during operations on diabetics and in severe complications.

Whilst at the present time such "machines" require special premises, some diabetologists are looking forward to the development, on the lines of the kidney machine and home dialysis, of an artificial "domestic pancreas" (Pfeiffer).

A further objective is to reduce these machines to the size of a cardiac pacemaker. And yet, despite all the magnitude of these technical inventions they leave me with an uneasy feeling. As I was writing down these thoughts, I kept thinking of the French physician and materialist philosopher La Mettrie who in his work "L'homme machine" dating from the middle of the 18th century saw man as a machine.

Should we in this increasingly dehumanized, meterialistic and "high-tech" age of ours allow ourselves to be reduced to the level of "machines"? Should we not despite all the technical and medical advances, which should of course be exploited, remain human and not be degraded to the level of a machine? Admittedly, remaining human involves the acceptance of disease, suffering and death.

A lucky break, especially the discovery of an exchange of letters, enabled me to put some flesh on the bare bones of what was so far known of the life of Paul Langerhans. The biography of this exceptional man was thus brought to life. But only the pathography shows his true greatness.

After his death, the cell structures he discovered were to become known as the "islets of Langerhans" and to carry his name to all corners of the world. The isolation of the secretion of the B cells of the islets – insulin – saved the lives of millions of diabetics. They owe thanks to Langerhans and to the other workers who built their work on his islets and created scientific "dry land".

This is why Paul Langerhans must never be forgotten. In the beautiful words of the German poet v. Zedlitz (Joseph Christoph Freiherr v. Z., 1790–1862) dating from the middle of last century "He's only dead who is forgotten".

The Discovery of Pancreatic Diabetes

The role of Oscar Minkowski

by Bernardo Alberto Houssay

In 1889 von Mering and Minkowski reported that total pancreatectomy in dogs was followed by severe diabetes. This was a discovery of historic importance. It demonstrated that diabetes occurs in the absence of the pancreas; and this finding furnished the starting point for research which proved that this organ produces an internal secretion, thus leading to the discovery of insulin and its application to the treatment of patients suffering from diabetes. Studies on carbohydrate metabolism were considerably extended, and it became possible to demonstrate the role of the liver in this metabolism and the regulatory functions of hormones secreted by several endocrine glands in normal conditions and in diabetes. This work was done in the laboratory of the Medical Clinic at the University of Strassburg, under the direction of Professor B. Naunyn, who in his book "Erinnerungen, Gedanken und Meinungen" refers to it in a statement which can be translated as follows:

"The discovery of pancreatic diabetes by von Mering and Minkowski gave a powerful impetus to out experimental research in diabetes. They had had a conversation about the extirpation of the pancreas. Next day Minkowski recounted that von Mering had upheld the dogma, accepted since Claude Bernard, that animals did not survive total pancreatectomy. He, Minkowski, had maintained that in dogs survival was possible; what did I think about it? I said: 'Since you have been able to remove the liver, you will also be able to carry out the removal of the pancreas, and if geese survive the liver operation, dogs will come through this one with even greater ease.' The next day Minkowski performed the first pancreatectomy in my laboratory; Mering assisted and then left on a trip. When Minkowski returned to the laboratory, 24 hours later, he could already report that the dog had severe diabetes with 5 per cent sugar. Incidentally, as long as he was in Strassburg, Mering did not perform pancreatectomy on his own, nor did he attempt to, and took little interest in following up the discovery."

When Naunyn's book was published, Thierfelder, a pupil of von Mering, wrote the following letter to Minkowski on May 5, 1926:

"You will be surprised to receive a letter from me. In fact, a special circumstance makes me write to you. It has to do with the description of the discovery of pancreatic diabetes given by Naunyn on page 457 of his 'Erinnerungen' (Memoirs). That description is undoubtedly mistaken, or at least incomplete. It not only minimizes Mering's contribution to this discovery, it completely suppresses it. This cannot remain unanswered, because it is already becoming current in medical literature. Thus, in the book written to commemorate the sixtieth birthday of Ludolf Brauer (reprint from the *Zentralblatt für Herz- und Gefässkrankheiten,* 1925, p. 2), Büdingen says: 'According to Naunyn, his great teacher, this discovery of genius should be attributed solely to Minkowski; von Mering only helped him in the operation'. Because of my friendship with von Mering while he lived, you will understand that it appears to me to be my duty to defend his interests also after his death. Would you not wish to make use of the occasion to correct Naunyn's version in some appropriate place?"

I asked Minowski's wife, who is now living in Buenos Aires, for information about the discovery of pancreatic diabetes and she gave me a copy of the letter written by Minkowski in answer to Thierfelder. This letter, written from Breslau and dated May 8, 1926, says:

"You are not fair to Naunyn if you imagine that in his account of the discovery of pancreatic diabetes he has unjustly belittled von Mering's contribution. Naunyn, as director of the Institute where the work was carried out, and as editor of the *Archiv für experimentelle Pathologia und Pharmakologie* in which it was published, kept in touch with the development of this research and guided the authors of the manuscript. Thus all that he wrote in his memoirs in his desire to be 'truthful even to harshness', was very familiar to him.

"Nothing is further from my mind than the wish to detract from von Mering's memory. I never quarreled with him; I was friendly with him until his death and I always felt grateful to him for having suggested the operation of pancreatectomy to me in a conversation we had. I do not think he had any grounds for complaint of my behavior, at any rate he never expressed any, either on his visit to me in Cologne shortly before his death or when I returned his visit in Halle. There were, however, good reasons (and he agreed with them) why all the communications on pancreatic diabetes, such as those to the Medical and Natural Science Society of Strassburg, the First International Congress of Physiology at Basel, the Assembly of Natural Science Research Workers at Heidelberg and the Congress of Internal Medicine at Leipzig, should be presented by myself alone, and also why our joint work in the *Archiv für experimentelle Pathologie und Pharmakologie* should have been written by me only. The same reasons explain why further work on diabetes should be conducted by me while von Mering, as far as I know, did no further experimental work on the problem.

"I am sorry I did not publish a detailed history of the discovery of pancreatic diabetes while von Mering was still alive, as he could only have confirmed my statements. It is not very pleasant for me to do so after his death because my account of the affair can easily be misinterpreted. Personalities seem to me to be of no importance compared with the value of positive results. However, your prejudice against Naunyn's statements forces me to describe exactly what happened as it has remained engraved in my memory.

"You know I worked in the laboratory of the Medical Clinic at Strassburg while von Mering was working at Hoppe-Seyler's Institute when you were an assistant there. One day in April 1889 I went over to your Institute to consult some chemical periodicals in your library, which were not available in our Clinic, and there I met von Mering, who shortly before had recommended 'Lipanin,' an oil with 6 per cent free fatty acids, as a substitute for cod liver oil in the belief that its favorable therapeutic effects might be due to its free fatty acid content.

"'Do you use Lipanin frequently in your clinic?' von Mering asked me."

"'Oh, no,' I answered. 'We give our patients only good fresh butter, not rancid oil."'

"'Don't scoff,' he replied. 'Healthymen must split fats before absorbing them. If, however, the pancreas does not function properly, fats already split must be given.'

"'Have you proved this experimentally?' I asked."

"'That is not so easy,' he answered, 'since pancreatic lipolytic enzymes pass into the gut even if one ties the pancreatic duct."'

"'Well, then,' I said, 'remove the whole pancreas!"'

"'That is an impossible operation,' he replied."

"As I did not know that Claude Bernard had stated that animals could not be kept alive after total pancreatectomy, and my youth led me to presumptuous overestimation of the results I had already obtained in my surgical experiments, I exclaimed: 'Bah! there are no impossible operations; pancreatectomy cannot be more difficult than hepatectomy; give me a dog and I will remove its pancreas today."

"'Good, I have dog which I can let you have now. So try it."'

"That same afternoon in Naunyn's laboratory, with von Mering's help, I took out his dog's pancreas. Perhaps, as a lucky coincidence, that particular animal possessed especially favorable anatomical conditions; they vary considerably in different animals. The whole gland was removed and the abdominal wall sutured; the animal remained alive and apparently well for nearly four weeks. I intended to return it to von Mering for his experiments on the utilization of fats, so I did not bother much about it; but because there was no suitable cage available it was kept tied up in one part of the laboratory. The day after the operation, von Mering had to go to Colmar urgently because his father-in-law was seriously ill with pneumonia. He had to stay there over a week. Meanwhile the dog, which was house-trained, very often micturated in the laboratory. I scolded the servant for not letting it out frequently enough, but he said: 'I do, but the animal is queer; as soon as it comes back it passes water again even if it has just done so outside."

"This observation induced me to collect some of the urine in a pipette and do a Trommer's test. Finding the urine reduced strongly, I made a 10 per cent solution with 1.5 cc. I still had in the pipette and found it contained 12 per cent sugar.

"I thought at first that the glycosuria might be due to the fact that von Mering had treated his dog for a long time with phloridzin. So I immediately pancreatectomized three more dogs with no sugar in their urine previous to the operation. The second and third animals died two days later of necrosis of the duodenum, but both had glycosuria before they died. The fourth animal survived and from the second day after pancreatectomy had a persistent diabetes just like the first animals.

"It was then von Mering returned, but did not come at once to the laboratory. I met him again on the first of May, the Anniversary of the foundation of Strassburg University at the festival celebration in the auditorium. Purely by chance, I was sitting behind him and I said over his shoulder, 'Do you know, von Mering, that all pancreatectomized dogs become diabetic?"

"'That's interesting,' he replied, 'we must follow up this question.'

"I then operated on a whole series of dogs, assisted sometimes, but not always, by von Mering. Once he tried to operate, but the animal died of hemorrhage on the operating table so he gave up trying.

"He took part in some of the work, in particular the glycogen determinations with which he was familiar. He was prevented by other circumstances from coming regularly to the laboratory of the medical clinic and he left me to finish the work alone. At the end of the semester I proposed to von Mering we should publish the results of our research together and that I would carry on the further conduct of the work alone. He agreed and also left me to prepare the manuscript of our work. When it was finished and ready for the press, von Mering was away on vacation and as I did not wish to delay its publication, I was unable to let him see it. Naunyn had no scruples about publishing the manuscript I had prepared in his *Archives,* so von Mering read the paper for the first time in proof and praised its make-up. Because I had written it, I put his name first, out of courtesy and also because von Mering was somewhat older than I and his name came before mine in alphabetical order. It is curious that because of that order, 'von Mering and Minkowski,' some have inferred that von Mering's contribution was necessarily greater than mine.

"Naunyn who was in a position to judge, considered I had shared too much with von Mering in not keeping the work on diabetes for myself and leaving him to follow up the further work on fat absorption. In knew, however, that I owed the discovery of diabetes to a lucky accident, and that I had not, any more than von Mering, imagined until then the importance the pancreas had in carbohydrate metabolism. Moreover, perhaps I would never have tried the extirpation of the pancreas if that conversation with von Mering had not taken place. I thought it only decent to invite him to collaborate in the work on diabetes, and I have never omitted to place his name together with mine even in recent times, as for example in my report on insulin in the Kissingen Congress of 1924."

"You must remember that in work done over many years I alone defended the doctrine of pancreatic diabetes and the internal secretion of the pancreas against many attacks, in particular against those of Edward Pflüger; also that I have contributed new proof of my ideas by experiments with transplants, doudenal extirpation, etc. In all these discussions von Mering took no part or interest. It is also peculiar, perhaps because he did not master the technique of pancreatectomy, or because he had no further interest in the problem, that he did not resume the work on fat absorption after pancreatectomy. With his consent, I suggested that Mr. Abelman in the laboratory of Naunyn's clinic should examine fat absorption after pancreatectomy. Later Burkhardt and Lombroso in my clinic in Greifswald busied themselves with this question which even today merits further research.

"I do not intend to publish this information. I shall, however, leave a copy of this letter in a suitable place, for at some future time a student of the history of diabetes may be interested in the true facts. Only if you or anybody else were to take a definite attitude against Naunyn's account, would I consider myself obliged to take action to clarify the circumstances."

It is not worth while to report or discuss the innumerable versions of the story of the discovery of pancreatic diabetes, some of which have been published while others have passed into the oral tradition of laboratories.

Professor E. Frank, now of Istanbul, and himself a pupil of Minkowski, is in possession of a copy of this letter and quotes its contents in his book written in 1949. The letter was deposited by Minkowski in the Medical Section of the "Schlesische Gesellschaft für Vaterländische Kultur" in Breslau. When Hitler came to power in 1933, the General Secretary of this section, Professor Rosenfeld (the same who coined the slogan, "The fats are burnt in the fire of the carbohydrates") and Professor Frank were asked to resign from membership. Professor Rosenfeld abstracted this document and, being an elderly man, gave it to Professor Frank.

Oscar Minkowski was born in Alexoten (Kowno, Russia) on January 13th, 1858, and in 1872 became a naturalized Prussian. He studied in the Gymnasium at Kowno from 1867 to 1872 and in the old Gymnasium of Königsberg. His inaugural thesis for the doctorate in medicine was accepted in 1881.

He was an assistant to Professor Naunyn in the Medical Clinic at Strassburg and later became Professor of Internal Medicine at Greifswald and afterwards at Breslau. He died in Fürstenberg (Mecklenburg) on June 18, 1931. Naunyn refers to Minkowski in his Memoirs in the following terms:

"In Minkowski I found a force of the greatest magnitude. When a student, he went back from Freiburg to his home in Königsberg, before taking the State Examination, and he asked me for a subject for his thesis. I proposed the following: Changes in the excitability of the psycho-motor cortex of the brain caused by experimental variations in the blood circulation. Perhaps the subject was the reason that no important results were obtained. In the course of this work, however, I came to appreciate Minkowski so much that when Stadelmann left I gave him the latter's position. This was a great acquisition for us, because Minkowski was a man of rare intelligence. The agility, clarity and universality of his mind, and the quickness and accuracy of his observations and opinions, endowed him with powers for exact judgment and for research in natural science. In his experimental work his great manual dexterity was very useful to him. It was surprising how easily he adapted himself to different circumstances. His elder brother, a business man of great ability, recounted to me how Oscar (my friend), when a student, frequently did his homework in his father's shop. Thus he sometimes saw samples of wheat which were passed from hand to hand. Not long after, his advice used to be asked and he would give his verdict with as much assurance and sometimes more accuracy than the experts. The removal of the liver and the removal of the pancreas were surgical achievements of the first quality, and several years passed after he had taught them before they were performed in other laboratories than my own. He had never done microscopic work; however, when we worked together on polycholic jaundice he prepared the slides and from the beginning he made them perfectly; I have never seen better sections. Already at that time we found the 'Kupfer cells,' before they were given Kupfer's name. When he was in Strassburg, a gentleman came to see me in whom I found a small polyp placed exactly on the anterior commissure of the larynx. It is very difficult to see these small tumors in this place and even more difficult to operate on them. As at that time there was nobody in Strassburg who cared to operate on this case, I asked Minkowski to do so. Minkowski, who had never even thought of operating on the larynx, laughed and would not do it. Finally, he made up his mind and practiced during a few days. About fifteen days later he told me he had 'removed the polyp completely and cleanly in one session.' 'It is not easy, but it can be done.' He was never interested in surgery; however, he was fascinated by problems. When a problem was suggested to him, with astounding acuteness he saw the decisive aspects and knew how to cope with them. Even today I 'dip my flag' to the powerful intelligence which endowed Minkowski for all this, but at times I overestimated his capacity. That spirit which pushes us into research and tortures us, and is only appeased by work done in its service, was not always alive in him and sometimes it was neccesary to stimulate it. When it awoke, Minkowski worked powerfully; otherwise, my friend could also live without an absorbing task. Ambition and the wish for official places were foreign to him. Minkowski arrived too late at a position which gave him independence and free reign to his genius. Even today I feel indignant when I think he was almost fifty years old when he obtained his first appointment. When eventually he went to Greifswald he was again passed by for many years, while places that were right for him were occupied by others. I was so annoyed by this that I decided to take a very unusual step. I sent a personal memorandum to the Prussian Minister of Education, in which I drew attention to the importance of Minkowski and to the fact that, in my opinion, this man of great worth was continually being passed over for incomprehensible reasons. I have cause to believe my request was given due attention in Berlin. In the meantime my friend found in Breslau a position worthy of him and a place where his genius could develop, but I still bear a grudge against the faculties of medicine who overlooked him for so long; my whole school suffered because its most outstanding member was forgotten. I was always having to exert my influence in favor of Minkowski to the detriment of others."

The discovery of pancreatic diabetes is usually considered as the result of chance; but luck favors those who deserve it, that is to say, those who are prepared to make use of it. The discovery was made in Naunyn's clinic, where diabetes was the main subject of study and where experimental work on problems of pathology and pharmacology was being done. A factor in this discovery was the boldness which youth sometimes brings to research, as was the case with Minkowski in 1889 and Banting in 1921. Minkowski's surgical ability and his previous training in experimental work made his achievement possible. The discovery was correctly understood from the beginning, and through many years Minkowski gave further proof of his interpretation of it by means of patient and cleverly performed experiments. He was not only an able man, he was also fair to von Mering and associated him in the publication of the results as was his due. Later both discoverers had distinguished scientific and medical careers. Undoubtedly, however, the discovery of pancreatic diabetes was due to Minkowski's determination and technical dexterity; it was he who removed the pancreas from a dog and found sugar in its urine. This experiment opened a new and fruitful era in the study of diabetes and its treatment, in metabolic research and in endocrinology.

Von Mering carried out a very distinguished scientific career; he discovered phloridzin diabetes and, in collaboration with Emil Fischer, he developed veronal. The true fact is that von Mering did not discover pancreatic diabetes nor did he do research in this field after his first publication with Minkowski.

Bibliography

Frank, E.: Pathologie des Kohlehydratstoffwechsels. Benno Schwabe, Basel, 1949.

Von Mering, J., and Minkowski, O.: Diabetes mellitus nach Pankreas extirpation. Arch f. exper. Path. u. Pharmakol. *26*:371, 1889.

Minkowski, O.: Weitere Mitteilungen über den Diabetes mellitus nach extirpation des Pankreas. Arch f. exper. Path. u. Pharmakol. *31*:85, 1893.

Minkowski, O.: Untersuchungen über den Diabetes mellitus nach extirpation des Pankreas. Berl. Klin. Woch. 90, 1892.

Minkowski, O.: Störungen des Pankreas als Krankheitsursache. Lubarsch. Osterag's Ergebnisse der allgemeinen Aetiologie. *I*:78, 1896.

Minkowski, O.: Bemerkungen über den Pankreasdiabetes. Arch f. exper. Path. u. Pharmakol. *53*:331, 1905.

Minkowski, O.: Ueber die Zuckerbildung im Organismus beim Pankreasdiabetes. Arch f. d. ges. Physiol. 11:13, 1906.

Minkowski, O.: Die Totalextirpation des Duodenums. Arch. f. exper. Path. u. Pharmakol. 58:271, 1908.

Minkowski, O.: Zur Kenntniss der Funktion des Pankreas beim Zuckerverbrauch. Arch exper. f. Path. u. Pharmakol. Suppl. *59*:395, 1908.

Minkowski, O.: Totalextirpation des Duodenums. Deutsche med. Wchnschr. 45, 1908.

Minkowski, O.: Discussion of paper of Michaud. Verhandl. d. Kong. f. inn. Med. 564, 1911.

Naunyn, B.: Erinnerungen, Gedanken und Meinungen. J.F.Bergmann, München, 1925.

in: *Diabetes 1 (1952) 112–116.*

Apollinaire Bouchardat 1806–1886

by Elliott P. Joslin

Bouchardat's life and soul were wrapped up in the problems of diabetes and diabetics. Until his buoyant and enthusiastic entrace upon the stage, diabetes was universally considered a fatal, a deadly, hopeless disease. Over and over again, Bouchardat emphasized this fact and then went on to say that it was his purpose to show the contrary and to proclaim that, barring serious complications, diabetics could live as long as most people, the strict hygienic regime which they were obliged to follow counterbalancing the handicap of the disease. Above all else, Bouchardat was the apostle of hope in a diabetic world of despair.

Bouchardat grasped the fundamental point that glycosuria had its origin in the sugar of the blood, which in turn came chiefly from carbohydrate in the diet, from bread and cereals – although he recognized, as his contemporary Claude Bernard was then demonstrating in his laboratory in Paris, that it could be derived from protein. Bouchardat urged his patients to make their own analysis of the sugar-producing content of a food by eating it and then testing their own urine. In this way Bouchardat introduced into diabetic therapy the personal responsibility of the patient in his own treatment. This was one of his cardinal contributions. At first his patients made their tests for glucose with unslaked lime. Later he employed a copper reagent anticipating Fehling's test. Fortunately, he was able to make quantitative tests of the glucose excreted in a given period by taking advantage of Biot's discovery of the polariscope and thus compute carbohydrate intake and outgo.

No disease, according to Bouchardat, was more apt to relapse than diabetes. He cites the example of a man who became free from diabetes for ten years until at the age of eighty it reappeared, thus illustrating the insidious onset and sly return of the malady.

Although Bouchardat devised all sorts of measures to make the forbidding, nauseating, rancid meat-fat diet of Rollo palatable, he never lost sight of the fact that the aim of treatment was to keep the urine sugar free. Primarily he lowered the carbohydrate in the diet by his limitation of bread and the exclusion of milk. He introduced the use of gluten bread, but he had no illusion regarding it. He did not want to be called a "gluten bread doctor." He advocated moderation in its use as well as of all foods in treatment. *"Mangez le moins possible."* He noted the favorable effect of undernutrition during the Siege of Paris. He occasionally fasted a patient. He emphasized green vegetables and even washed them to lower the carbohydrate.

Bouchardt was the first to utilize exercise to control the glycosuria. He pushed this to the limit in season and out of season. He taught his patients to exercise particularly the muscles of the arms and chest, because thereby he hoped to improve the strength of respiration. He explained in many ways to his patients the good effect of exercise, and in support of it he cited the high incidence of diabetes among the professional classes in contrast to that among manual workers.

He recognized that the mental capacity of the patients was retained long after the loss of muscular and nervous power, though he admits that the memories of his patients suffered. He observed the diminution and occasional regain of sexual activity both in males and females, although he stated in his first edition in 1875 and again in the second in 1883: *"1. Les femmes atteintes de vrai diabète sucré deviennent très-rarement enceintes. 2. Dans le nombre ṣi considérable de diabétiques qui sont venus me consulter, je n'ai pas mémoire d'avoir vu une seule femme enceinte."*

Apollinaire Bouchardat was Professor of Hygiene in the University of Paris. He was a friend of Claude Bernard, who over and over again in his *Leçons sur le Diabète* calls attention to Bouchardat's activities in the experimental field and his conceptions of the etiology of diabetes, although he does not mention his clinical activities. This is not strange, because Claude Bernard's work was confined to the laboratory. He was concerned with his discoveries of

1. curare glycosuria,
2. the glycosuria following the puncture of the 4th ventricle,
3. the invention of a method to estimate the sugar in the blood,
4. the changes that followed in the sugar content of the blood in the right heart upon the exclusive feeding of protein to dogs,
5. the discovery of glycogen in the liver and its glycogenic function and the disappearance of glycogen after death, as a

result of a diastatic enzyme. Claude Bernard held the liver as the organ primarily concerned with diabetes. He does not appear to have been interested in the treatment of the diabetic and actually contributed nothing directly to it.

Bouchardat suspected the pancreas as the cause of diabetes. He was the first to attempt to prove this by its removal, but sugery then was too crude. Bouchardat was a good chemist. He noted the difference in action between glucose and levulose and tried to make use of the latter's peculiar behavior as well as that of its precursor, insulin, in the control of the disease. He recognized inosite and various other carbohydrates. Both clinically and chemically he observed acetone in the breath and urine of his patients with severe diabetes, but did not clearly associate it with diabetic coma although recognizing coma could be pricipatet in such cases and for them he prescribed relaxation. He determined the intake and excretion of carbon dioxide and pointed out the advantages of potassium in the low carbohydrate vegetables.

Although he knew alcohol was not directly sugar producing, more and more as he grew older he restricted its use.

Bouchardat examined the blood for sugar, even though to carry out the test it required 300 cubic centimeters. He explained why it was that glycosuria could be high and glycemia low, because in one the percentage found in the urine represented the quantity secreted by the kidney during an average period of several hours but with the other it was the analysis of the existing sugar in the blood for the moment. In emphasizing the frequency and ready detection of diabetes he related how even a hotel bell-boy had diagnosed the disease in an old man by observing the white spots on his pants which would not brush off or disappear with benzine, but would wash off with water.

It is a great pleasure to have the photograph of Bouchardat (from which the cover drawing was made) which came to me through the friendly intervention of Mrs. William B. Bell and Mr. Maurice Paz, Président de L'Association Française de Diabétiques through the assistance of Professor and Mrs. Boulin, who succeeded Professor Labbé, in charge of the Hopital de la Pitié in Paris. It appears that Apollinaire Bouchardat's granddaughter married Professor Francis Rathery, whose *Diabète Sucré, Leçons Cliniques* in 1934 and 1935 I received from him and prized. It was eventually through their son, Dr. Michel Rathery at the Hopital Bichat that the picture was obtained.

When anyone attempts to write an account of an historical period or phase in diabetes, he invariably becomes indebted to Dr. Frederick M. Allen, whose detailed compilation of the story first appeared in 1919 in the Rockefeller Monograph, entitled *Total Dietary Regulation in the Treatment of Diabetes* by Allen, Stillman and Fitz. This monograph is now out of print. What a contribution to the world it would be if Dr. Allen would amplify it and publish it so that the material, which he so painstakingly gathered years ago, could be available to us all. I hope this year at the annual meeting of the American Diabetes Association action can be taken to encourage Dr. Allen to fulfill this task. No one else in the world could do it as well.

Bouchardat wrote simply and clearly. His French is therefore easy to read. I wish that space permitted quoting some of the sentences which constantly are in my mind. It is most unfortunate that his monograph was not translated immediately into English, because thereby in this country we failed to benefit from it for almost two generations.

Apollinaire Bouchardat was born in 1806 and died in 1886. He was buried in Paris in Père Lachaise cemetery. Would that his spirit might know the gratitude of millions of diabetics whose lives he prolonged and made endurable and to whom he gave, and still gives, courage and hope.

in: *Diabetes 1 (1952) 490–491.*

The First Case of Diabetic Retinopathy
(Eduard von Jaeger, Vienna 1853)

by Franz Fischer

We have before us the plates and documentation of a case of retinitis (retinopathy) in diabetes mellitus, the first of its kind. It derives from the *Beiträge zur Pathologie des Auges* by Eduard von Jaeger for the year 1855. That it was the first such case we have the best guarantor, Theodor Leber. In 1875, he collected the cases from the literature – there were 19 in all, of which Jaeger's case was the first – and coined the term *retinitis diabetica.* So characterized, Jaeger's case wanders through the literature. After Leber he found no-one more appreciative. We thought it stimulating as well as conducive to the continuity of research to exhibit this case.

It is no accident that the observation was made in Vienna, and made by Eduard von Jaeger. In the second half of the 18th century and subsequently, Vienna was very fruitful medical soil, a place where the new seed of ophthalmology could flourish. We see Joseph Barth, the gifted individualist, Georg Joseph Beer (first professor, 1818), the first teacher and founder of scientific ophthalmology, Friedrich Jaeger, Ritter von Jaxtthal (Eduard's father), Professor at the military medical Joseph's Academy (Josephinum), the most sought-out eye-surgeon in Europe. In the so-called II Vienna Medical School, Eduard von Jaeger with Ferdinand von Arlt and K. Stellwag von Carion was an outstanding champion of the specialty. As the son of Friedrich von Jaeger and grandson of the great Joseph Beer, Eduard von Jaeger had glittering prospects. Nevertheless, and with all his personal accomplishment, he was denied what he felt to be his heart's desire: only at the age of 65 did he become Professor at the II Ophthalmic Clinic, Vienna, not long before his death (5 July, 1884). His main creative work lay in ophthalmoscopy. The best witnesses on his account are two competent ophthalmologists: Ludwig Mauthner (in the obituary): "Eduard von Jaeger's career is inextricably bound up with the history of the ophthalmoscope. He was one of the first who turned Helmholtz's discovery to practical use. He also produced an improved form of Helmholtz's instrument very soon for everyday practice. Eduard von Jaeger was the greatest ophthalmologist the world had yet seen." Then Maximilian Salzmann (in the preface to the reworked Atlas of 1890): "The time has its expectations, which Eduard von Jaeger, linked with the appearance of his *Atlas* has satisfied in full measure. His work is recognized as the most important in the field of ophthalmoscopy and has become a foundation on the basis of which numerous young doctors have been introduced into this important oculists' discipline."

So much for the environment and personality of our author. And now for the case. Te description begins as follows:

"The gardener Wilhelm W., then 22 years old, of slender physique and medium height, had always been healthy and strong in childhood and adolescence. However, 4 years previously, through catching cold, he developed a disorder which repeatedly kept him in bed with slight fever and swelling of the right foot, loss of strength and appearance. As this continued, the *phenomenon of a diabetes* emerged, coupled with marked anorexia, dry throat, frequent vomiting after eating and feelings of great decline and weakness. For a short time the patient had also complained of frequent cough with much sputum and feelings of oppression and pressure in the chest."

We now shorten this account. 5 weeks before he had experienced a disturbance of vision: transient seeing of flashes and "slight clouding of the outer half of the visual field in the left eye". The clouding had spread to the other eye and was increasing. The sight in the left eye had temporarily improved. The disorder had steadily increased. It is stated: "The patient presently appears very ill and low, is thin and has a sallow complexion." Then a "disturbance of the visual field in the middle" with reduction of visual acuity is described. Passing to the ophthalmoscopic findings: The media had appeared quite transparent and normal. The peripheral parts of the fundus were free from lesions.

On the other hand, the site and vicinity of the transverse section of the optic nerve (in the extent of the extravasate illustrated in the picture) is dull in color, less translucent, more blood-red, and the optic nerve cross-section is so completely covered by the aforesaid color change as to be no longer perceived and can only be recognized by the union of the retinal vessels.

"Anomalous redness of the optic fundus" and "radiate spreading of the optic fibers in the vicinity of the optic nerve" were reported. Then it states:

"In the region of this anomalous coloring of the optic fundus there are to be perceived a considerable number of apparently uniformly distributed blood-red flecks, some punctate, some striate or otherwise shaped, of the most various size, which seem to lie in the plane of the retinal vessels, i.e., deep to the retina, are predominantly elongated, and whose arrangement and orientation correspond partly to the optic expansion and partly to the paths of the retinal vessels, particularly the veins. Between the flecks, at some distance from the optic disc, there also appear numerous irregular, rounded, light-yellow spots whose brightness makes them very obvious."

It then states that the retinal vessels in the region of the optic disc were hazy. The arteries showed an especially brilliant media. The diameters of the arteries and veins were significantly increased above normal.

The description ends as follows: "The left eye exhibits objectively and subjectively exactly teh same appearances, though to a lesser degree and the patient is still capable with its aid of getting about in the street and even doing some work as a gardener."

We note that plate and text are quite consistent. The text, based on the author's principle, is descriptive, not explanatory. The illustration is quite true to life and free from any exaggeration. The lithography and color printing, carried out by the Imperial and Royal Court and State Press in Vienna is an emazing technical achievement for a hundred years ago.

What was Eduard von Jaeger describing? At the fundus: an edema of the optic disc and adjacent retina, streaked and radially arranged hemorrhages at some distance from the disc, light-yellow spots, to be explained later, as essential features. The question whether this complied with the concept of diabetic retinitis (retinopathy), then and now, may be answered as follows. Th. Leber (1875) remarked of Jaeger's case that it resembled the retinitis occurring in albuminuria. Later, the edema (with the star figure in the macula) were counted as characteristics of albuminuric (nephritic, angiospastic) retinitis as against diabetic retinitis. What can we say today? Diabetic retinopathy embraces a whole range of retinal lesions: "blood-spots (anatomically: capillary aneurysms) at the outset, hemorrhages and white degenerative foci subsequently, and finally vascular and connective tissue proliferation, vitreous hemorrhage, retinal shrinkage, etc. (retinitis proliferans), though these stages are not always observed. As always with retinopathy, the edema is not part of the fundus picture. It is the view of not a few workers today that, when an edema appears, the case is one of nephritic and not diabetic retinopathy. We believe, however, that diabetic retinopathy can, exceptionally, imitate nephritic retinopathy. Edema formation is shown especially by young diabetics, as confirmed by R. Thiels and our own observations. Frankly, we cannot share Thiels' view (1956) that this depends on the special nephropathic forms of diabetes, the Kimmelstiel-Wilson glomeruloscleroses. The fact that most Kimmelstiel-Wilson cases are heralded by retinopathy *without* edema formation is an argument against. Therefore nothing prevents us from acknowledging Jaeger's case as one of true diabetic retinopathy, despite any similarity with albuminuric retinitis. Jaeger's case admits of another interpretation. The indistinct disc, the numerous radially arranged hemorrhages, the markedly reduced visual acuity – all are very suggestive of a thrombosis of the central vein of the retina. This is not at all an uncommon event in older diabetics (with advanced arteriosclerosis), in any case commoner than in non-diabetics; in young diabetics it was unknown. Now, J. Dietzel and P. White have recently observed a central vein thrombosis in a young diabetic, followed by a retinitis proliferans in the other eye. This demonstrates that the angiopathy specific to diabetes (and not just the usual arteriosclerosis) is capable of producing such a picture. Jaeger's case in a 22-year-old diabetic could be interpreted in this sense; but, frankly, the fundus picture is not at all consistent and the appearance in both eyes arouses doubts. The possibility exists.

Now for the "rounded light-yellow spots" in our fundus picture. That this referred to the usual retinal degenerative foci we believe can be dismissed without more ado. K. vom Hofe was the first (1938) to point out the frequency of such a finding in diabetic retinopathy, and we confirm this from our own experience. It only surprises us how little awareness of this there was until now. Vom Hofe interpreted the picture as lipid infiltration of the deep retinal layers or choroid and proved correct. For the picture certainly is not related to "choroiditis in diabetic retinopathy" as we have recently described it. How accurate, then, were Jaeger's observations!

If we leave the fundus picture: the patient's age of 22 years leads to the following remarks. Until some 10 years ago, diabetic retinopathy below 40 years of age was an absolute rarity. Thus we find in a world-famous textbook of ophthalmology of 1935 that only a single case is quoted from the literature. A marked change has occurred here. The number of young diabetics is large and steadily increasing, due to insulin and other modern treatment. The young diabetic is becoming older and now experiences its vascular complications, notably nephropathy and retinopathy; at the age of 30 or 40, he is confronted with a gloomy fate. For us, this is the main problem of diabetes mellitus today. On the other hand, the practicality of oral treatment of diabetes is fading. And now back to Jaeger's case. At that time, and for one of his age, he was certainly a rarity. And it should be considered that in the pre-insulin era young diabetics died off very quickly without exception from coma; young diabetics did not live to experience vascular complications.

As for the duration of the diabetes – in our case barely longer than 5 years – the following may be noted. As far back as 1858, Albrecht von Graefe was struck by the fact that the ocular disorders in diabetes mellitus belonged to "an advanced stage of the general disease". It required intensive research up to our own time to reveal the role of the duration of the diabetes in the development of retinopathy. Today, many workers, notably Dolger (USA) adopt the standpoint that every diabetic will experience the "vascular complications" of nephropathy, retinopathy, etc., if he lives long enough, for 20 years or more. On the other hand, Joslin's school in the USA advances the view that the vascular complications can be prevented or at least postponed by precise management of the diabetes from the outset without interruption, with proper treatment and surveillance. The advocates of the "free diet" (which actually is not a free diet) for diabetic children and adolescents rather incline to Dolger's view. We ourselves acknowledged Joslin's requirements in various articles though, like other authors, we were well aware that in by no means a few cases, and despite the best monitoring of the diabetes, a retinopathy (and nephropathy) develops after quite a short duration of the diabetes, while others remain unaffected despite continuously poor monitoring and overlong duration of the disease (30 or more years). We sought to explain the "bad" cases by a special penetrating power of the diabetes on an unherited basis. We are further of the opinion that, not only the diabetes as such, but also the associated vascular constition are inherited, and in a decisive manner. On this, the findings have yet to be made known. Jaeger's case, with its relatively short duration of diabetes, therefore also falls outside the rule in this respect and requires a special explanation, as given above.

What does the case tell us otherwise? We may pass over the classical diabetes symptoms. Nothing is said relating to albuminuria or nephritis. Th. Leber felt this as a defect in the completion of his task. Thanks to the exact illustration, we can say with fair certainty that a nephropathy did exist, indeed in the uremic end-stage. This is not surprising, since we know how much alike are diabetic retinopathy and nephropathy, both clinically and pathologically; and it is just in young diabetics that nephropathy, as Kimmelstiel-Wilson's glomerulosclerosis, runs a deleterious course. That the report contains nothing about the blood-pressure only evokes the late development of blood-pressure measurement. A hypertension would not be surprising; according to our findings, it is associated just like the nephropathy with the retinopathy of young diabetics. The disease was ushered in by an infection, as we know well today. We amplify: the course of the diabetes was also unfavorably influenced by infection. Unfortunately, the eradication of focal sepsis has been pushed into the background in modern diabetes treatment. The description even suggests pulmonary tuberculosis. Over and again, this disease plays a noteworthy yet too little noted role in juvenile diabetes, being the second cause of death after uremia.

We may conclude: The case reported by Eduard von Jaeger in 1855 is unusual as regards age, duration of diabetes and fundus findings. It withstands any check by current standards. We are right to see in it the first observation of diabetic retinopathy. The strictly scientific approach of the author has saved the case from oblivion. Yet it is quite remarkable that our acquaintance with diabetic retinopathy should have begun in such an unusual way. And what is even stranger is that in Jaeger's case we encounter the problem case of diabetes mellitus today.

Eduard von Jaeger published this case in his *Beiträgen zur Pathologie des Auges* (1855-1856). Just listen, in conclusion, to what our historian, J. Hirschberg, writes on this: "No sacrifice for science was too heavy for him. For his wonderful *Contributions to the Pathology of the Eye* he plunged into a debt of 20,000 gulden, which he gradually paid off from his earnings." Such was Eduard von Jaeger. May he be a model to all young ophthalmologists!

Summary

The priority of the case is certified by Th. Leber (1875). That the observation was made in Vienna and by Eduard von Jaeger (1855) is not a matter of chance. Though this case of diabetic retinopathy is unusual in many respects, the diagnosis is beyond doubt and satisfies any check. The author's comprehensive and very factual approach gives us cause, even today, for valuable inferences and reflections, and not only as regars the fundus appearances. The spirit of a true natural scientist reveals itself.

References

F. Fischer: Probleme der diabetischen Retinopathie. Klin. Mbl. f. Augenheilkunde 125 (1954): 666 – Einst und jetzt. Die historische Entwicklung der Retinopathia diabetica. Münchner med. Wschr. 44 (1954)1287. – Die Retinopathie des jungen Diabetikers (unter 40 Jahren). Graefes Arch. 1957. – *J. Hirschberg:* Geschichte der Augenheilkunde. In Handbuch Graefe-Saemisch, Bd. XV, 1916. – *Eduard von Jaeger:* Beiträge zur Pathologie des Auges. 2. Lieferung, S. 33, Tafel XII. K. K. Hof- und Staatsdruckerei, Wien 1855. – *Th. Leber:* Über die Erkrankungen des Auges bei Diabetes mellitus. Arch. f. Ophthalm. 21, 3 Abtlg. (1875): 206 – Die Krankheiten der Netzhaut. In Handbuch Graefe-Saemisch, Bd. VII/2 (1914): 969. –*I. Mauthner: Eduard von Jaeger.* Wiener Med. Wschr. 28 (1884): 878 – *Th. Puschmann:* Die Medizin in Wien während der letzten 100 Jahre. M. Perles, 1884. – *M. Salzmann:* Ophthalmoskopischer Handatlas von *Eduard von Jaeger,* neubearbeitet und vergrößert. F. Deutike, Leipzig und Wien 1890. – *L. Schönbauer: Das Medizinische Wien. Geschichte, Werden, Würdigung.* Urban & Schwarzenberg Berlin und Wien 1944.

in: *Wiener Medizinische Wochenschrift 107 (1957) 969–972.*

The History of Traumatic Diabetes

by VIGGO THOMSEN

Traumatic diabetes constitutes an interesting and special chapter in the history of diabetes. Already at the end of the eighteenth century *Pouteau* and *Malaval* described cases of coincidence of trauma and diabetes, and in the beginning of the nineteenth century several such cases were published, for instance, by *Larrey*. In contradistinction to the former the diagnosis in these latter cases was substantiated by the detection of glycosuria. However, at that time nobody thought of a causal relationship between trauma and diabetes. It was *Cl. Bernard's* (1) detection of the diabetic puncture which gave rise to the notion of the morbid picture of traumatic diabetes. By means of the diabetic puncture it was possible to provoke experimental glycosuria; the influence of the nervous system on the regulation of the sugar metabolism was demonstrated, the consequence naturally being the publication of reports, in which endeavours were made to show the importance of certain cerebral affections for the etiology of diabetes, whence the question of the importance of head traumatism naturally acquired actuality. In 1854 *Goolden* in the "Lancet" published the first report of diabetes witnessed in sequel to head traumatism, and *Cl. Bernard* (2) himself utilized his experimental experience by applying it to man. Thus in the lectures he delivered in 1855 he mentioned a quarry-man who had become "diabetic" after a fall and recovered when the wound in his head was healed.

Griesinger was the first who in 1859 in his "Studien über Diabetes" took up the question of traumatic diabetes and made it the subject of discussion on the ground of 20 cases of diabetes observed in sequel to trauma, which he had collected. Since then traumatic diabetes has constantly been the subject of discussion, and the literature contains numerous reports of such cases.

In the course of time the different authors have set forth divergent opinions with regards to the etiological importance of traumatism, evidently in some degree on account of the varying ideas of the pathogenesis of diabets. According to the opinion prevailing at different times, I think we may speak of three periods, namely, the first up to the turn of the century, the second up to the world-war, and the third from that time up to the present.

The literature comprises numerous casuistic reports besides compilation works, and particularly on the ground of the latter I shall in the following endeavour to give an account of the history of traumatic diabetes.

As was mentioned before, the first compilation work is due to *Griesinger* who had come across such a case and, on reviewing the literature, was surprised to find so many cases in which a trauma must be suspected of having given rise to diabetes. When he studied these cases he was struck by the fact that many of them, for instance his own case, presented no cerebral lesion at all but merely a general concussion of the body or an injury of parts of the body, which could not be attributed to any direct connection with a nerve-centre; consequently he did not either detect any cerebral symptoms during the development of the disease. In four cases only were rather severe cerebral symptoms detected, and three of these patients recovered entirely. Accordingly *Griesinger* concluded that cerebral traumatism rarely gives rise to chronic diabetes and that there often is a question of transitory melituria with a favourable prognosis. He expresses his opinion of the importance of trauma in the following manner:

"Dagegen können Verletzungen, Contusionen, heftige Zerrungen der allerverschiedensten Theile des Körpers zur Ursache, oder vielmehr zu einem der mitwirkenden Momente bei der Entstehung ebensowohl eines vorübergehenden, als eines chronischen Diabetes werden. Dies lässt sich wohl für jetzt nicht weiter erklären, die Experimente mit der "Piqure" passen nicht darauf; aber es ist die Wahrheit."

In 1862 a great French paper was published by *P. Fischer* who had collected 21 cases of "traumatic diabetes" incurred after head traumata and 22 after various other lesions. He divides the cases into the following groups: "Polyurie simple sans Glykosurie"., "Polyurie avec Glykosurie légère", "Glykosurie passagère", and "Glykosurie permanente, Diabète confirmé", which he considers simple varieties of the same disease, namely, of diabetes.

The first three groups are characterized by their rapid occurrence after the trauma and their tendency of being transitory, i.e. of from about 1 week to 2–3 months' duration. They differ from one another by their presenting various degrees of, or no, glycosuria. The first group presents very pronounced polyuria, the patients being reported to consume up to 30 liters of fluid and the specific gravity of the urine amounting to 1.001–1.007, whereas, in the third group, the specific gravity of the urine sometimes attains the high figure of 1.052. The latter group, namely, of diabetes, only comprises 6 of the 21 cases. About these the author reports that the onset is somewhat obscure, whence it is impossible to ascertain whether the disease manifests itself immediately after the trauma or after a shorter or longer lapse of time. However, everything tends to suggest that the glycosuria observed in these cases does not appear so soon after the trauma as in case of transitory diabetes. The symptoms appear from 2 to 18 months or more after the trauma. The author indeed mentions that there is a break in the observation, and that it may justly be objected that, in these cases, he has not furnished any conclusive proof of the causal relationship.

In 16 of the 22 cases of other than head lesions there was a question of diabetes, in 3 of them of temporary diabetes, and in the remaining 3 cases of simple polyuria *Fischer* divides these 22 cases into two groups, namely, commotio of the medulla and the nerves of the spinal marrow, and commotio of the abdominal ganglion plexus. He expresses his conclusion derived from the clinical observations of diabetes after traumata in the following terms: "On doit toutefois considérer comme acquises à la science ces conclusions déduites des observations cliniques, que des traumatismes du cerveau, de la moelle, des nerfs rachidiens, et du grand sympathique, sont suivis de diabète tout aussi bien que dans les expériences physiologiques par lesquelles ces mêmes organes ont été lésés."

Frerichs likewise acknowledges the importance of head traumata; this author moreover emphasizes the importance of psychic trauma in the form of sudden or more protracted agitation. Quite a similar point of view is later advocated by *Seegen*.

An important work is due to *Brouardel & Richardière* who in 1888 endeavoured to set up the clinical picture of traumatic diabetes on the ground of 33 cases. The existence of traumatic diabetes is by them considered certain. In the discussion of the importance of predisposition they admit its causative concurrence though they attribute no more than secondary importance to this question, since the trauma is the decisive factor for the appearance of the disease and it is in many cases impossible to detect such a disposition. They think that traumatic diabetes is most frequently met with in men of middle-age, who are more exposed to injuries than women and other age-classes. The lesions are of extremely different nature, the majority of them being head traumata – 17 out of 33 cases – and, in the second place, lesions of the columna. They emphasize, however, that it must be considered reliably proved that a peripheral trauma, however slight it may be, is sufficient to give rise to traumatic diabetes. It is not necessary at all that the lesioned spot should topographically correspond to a region with nervous centers. Diabetes can occur from a couple of days to many months after the trauma. If several years, for instance more than 5 or 6 years, elapse before the diabetes becomes manifest, they consider the causal relation doubtful and claim that the patients in the interim present certain symptoms or complications suggestive of diabetes and, moreover, severe and permanent nervous disturbances. If such were absent, anybody might attribute his disease to some indifferent trauma or other incurred during childhood or a later period of life. As to the symptoms and complications of traumatic diabetes it holds that they are identical with those met with in ordinary diabetes. However, among the complications of traumatic diabetes are emphasized those nervous symptoms which, on account of their frequency and particular nature, often characterize this form of diabetes. They are disturbances of sensibility, hyper- or anesthesias, and neuralgias which, after having been located to the injured spot, may subsequently involve the whole body. They may be conjoined with giddiness and tremor. The patients frequently are affected with hypochondria, their trauma forming an object of their constant anxiety. Some patients presented pareses, particularly of the eye muscles. The authors attribute great importance to these symptoms, as they show that the trauma has given rise to functional or organic disturbances in the central nervous system and, thus, may be directly responsible for a diabetes of nervous origin.

After the difference in the course of the disease *Brouardel & Richardière* distinguished between two forms of diabetes, which they termed "Diabète traumatique précoce ou aigu" and "Diabète traumatique retardé ou chronique", and although this division in that form subsequently proved inadequate, it has long been in general use, and the terms of "Diabète précoce" and "Diabète retardé" may still be met with in modern literature.

The former sets in suddenly a day or two after the accident, with polydipsia, polyuria and glycosuria. The symptoms are conjoined with other diabetic phenomena, but they gradually disappear, and the patient may be considered to be cured after the lapse of 2–3 months. One of the symptoms, polyuria, may however be seen to persist some time after the disappearance of the others. In case of diabète retardé the disease runs quite a different course, the symptoms, to begin with very faint, gradually becoming so marked that they reveal it at last. This form of the disease usually has a fatal issue though reliable cases of recovery are on record also. *B. & R.* assert that diabète retardé in reality runs quite the same course as classical diabetes, and they think that the causative factor in this form of the disease probably is an organic lesion, whereas in case of diabète précoce there is a question of disturbances of a more functional nature. From a medico-legal point of view diabète précoce owing to its favourable prognosis plays no great part. As regars diabète retardé it is difficult to determine whether there is a causal relation between it and the preceding trauma. Here they emphasize the nervous disturbances as being suggestive of traumatic diabetes. In referring to *Frerichs* they likewise emphasize the importance of the patient's having experienced fear or great excitement, mentioning that it must be examined whether the excitement does not play the part of chief causal agent of traumatic diabetes.

In 1894 appeared a great German work the author of which, *Asher*, just as *Brouardel & Richardière*, proceeded particularly from a forensic point of view. Asher's work comprises 124 cases from the literature. With regard to onset, symptomatology and prognosis of traumatic diabetes *Asher* agrees with *Brouardel & Richardière*. With regard to the etiology the former emphasizes more strongly than the latter two the importance of head traumata though he, too, finds that diabetes does not infrequently occur after other traumata. This is evidenced by his distribution of the material according to causes: Head trauma in 58 cases, non-head trauma in 62, and uncertain trauma in 9 cases. He denies *Griesinger's* presumption that diabetes after head traumata should afford a favourable prognosis. He decidedly disagrees with *Brouardel & Richardière*'s assertion that the two forms of Diabète précoce and retardé should be of importance for the prognosis. He acknowledges that forms with an acute and an insidious inception should be discriminated between, but both these groups comprise cases running a chronic course or rapidly leading to recovery. With regard to the prognosis of the cases running a chronic course he agrees with *B. & R.*, as was mentioned before, and declares that they may end fatally in the course of 1–5 years. The prognosis of traumatic diabetes is particularly serious in predisposed subjects. After a discussion of the physiological and pathologo-anatomical facts, which latter may be summarized by the statement that the floor of the fourth ventricle was normal in the cases submitted to autopsy, he concludes as follows: "Gegenwärtig ist es uns nicht vergönnt, durch die Erfahrungen und Forschungen der pathologischen Anatomie und der Physiologie den ursächlichen Zusammenhang zwischen Trauma und Diabetes zu begründen. Es existieren nur Tatsachen, welche ihn wahrscheinlich machen".

W. Ebstein (1) in *1892* reports a case of traumatic diabetes which is not revealed till 6 years after the trauma. The reason why he puts the diabetes into causal relation with the trauma is that the patient immediately after its occurrence developed traumatic neurosis, which by *Ebstein* is considered the predisposing factor in this tardy case of diabetes. In a comprehensive work issued in 1895 he (2) again treats this subject and reports a new case, where a comparatively slight trauma gives rise to traumatic neurosis and diabetes is detected 6 months later. This work moreover contains a synopsis of 50 cases of traumatic diabetes. On that ground *E.* emphasizes the importance of disposition, since only a minority of the victims incurs diabetes. With regard to diabetes in sequel to traumatic neurosis he is of opinion that, on the ground of his own cases and those recorded in the literature, he is justified in concluding that, just as there is a causal relation between trauma and subsequent functional disturbances in the nervous system on the one hand and between trauma and diabetes on the other hand, there must be a correlation between neurosis and diabetes. He emphasizes, however, that the traumatic diabetes in the majority of cases seems to occur independently of a traumatic neurosis, and that the fact that diabetes not only occurs after, but often simultaneously with, traumatic neurosis, justifies the assumption that this form of traumatic diabetes need not to be a consequence of the neurosis but that both it and the neurosis may be the direct consequence of the trauma. Similar cases of diabetes after traumatic neurosis were during the same period reported by *Heimann* and by *Asher* etc. The etiological importance of traumatic neurosis was substantiated by a series of investigations of alimentary glycosuria after administration of glycose to patients suffering from traumatic neurosis published by *v. Jaksch, Strauss* (1), *Geelvink, v. Strümpell, van Ordt, Arndt* and others. *Arndt* who collated *Strauss', Geelvink's* and *von Oordt's* investigations with his own, obtained positive results of the test in 32.6 per cent of the cases of traumatic neurosis, whereas, in case of other neuroses, such as neurasthenia, hypochondria and hysteria, alimentary glycosuria was detected in 14.4 per cent of the cases only.

Those important works issued prior to the turn of the century, which I have recorded in the preceding pages, have each afforded a contribution to the precision of the picture of the picture of traumatic diabetes as it presented itself at that time. I shall finally quote *v. Noorden*'s (1) point of view set forth in 1898 with regard to the discernment of the cases that came under medical estimation. This author asserts that the traumatic origin of diabetes must *certainly* be diagnosed, if the patient until a twelvemonth period prior to the trauma has not been found to suffer from glycosuria and this has been detected within a twelvemonth subsequent to the trauma. He likewise admits the traumatic origin without preceding urine test, if a previously healthy subject incurs diabetic symptoms and discharge of sugar in the urine within the first weeks after a trauma. Although the urine is not tested during the first months or even years after the trauma, the occurrence of diabetic symptoms is considered sufficiently convincing. He admits the *possibility* of traumatic origin, if persons who have not previously presented any signs of diabetes, incur this disease in the course of 1–2 years after a trauma without the symptoms appearing in immediate sequel to the accident. However, such a causal relationship is probable only in case of intracranial lesions, concussion of the brain or traumatic neurosis supervening to a trauma of another kind. Lesions of another kind than those mentioned are too rarely followed by diabetes to permit of attaching importance to them as causal agents in such dubious cases.

On casting a retrospective glance upon this first epoch it must at once be emphasized that all the authors consider the existence of traumatic diabetes a fact. They consider it a neurogenous diabetes due to a change in the central nervous system brought about by the trauma. It is interesting to follow up the evolution of what is considered a necessary trauma. From the cranial trauma, which may naturally be assumed to give rise to lesions proper of the central nervous system, it is on the ground of clinical observations extended to comprise purely psychic traumata, and later the traumatic neurosis is pointed out as an intermediate link imparting importance to traumata insignificant in themselves. Particularly *Ebstein* (2) draws attention to this circumstance, emphasizing however that *Brouardel & Richar-*

dière in their discussion of the nervous symptoms attending traumatic diabetes in reality have supplied an excellent description of the traumatic neurosis.

Whereas the authors thus are generous as to what may be considered a trauma of the central nervous system, the majority of them despite clinical observations are very cautious in attaching importance to the peripheral traumata. Already *Griesinger* emphasized the frequency of diabetes after peripheral traumata even at the cost of the head traumata, and *Brouardel & Richardière* likewise emphasize that even a slight peripheral trauma may be followed by diabetes. *Fischer* in two equal groups of patients detects a good many more cases of diabetes in the group of peripheral traumata than in the group of head traumata, and *Asher,* who attaches special importance to the head trauma, only finds 58 such traumata against 71 not involving the head.

Even though *v. Noorden* from the works at issue thus derives the logical conclusion, he cannot be considered quite justified in declaring that other traumata than those affecting the central nervous system too seldom give rise to diabetes to permit of attaching importance to them. Even if the various authors, such as for instance *Asher*, admit that neither physiology nor pathological anatomy affords any explanation of the cases of diabetes, their objection to the importance of peripheral traumata must certainly be explained by their respect to the fact of *Cl. Bernard's* diabetic puncture.

On glancing at the cases described as traumatic diabetes it is evident that several of them are characterized by lacking limitation of the notion of diabetes. Thus there are no doubt many cases of diabetes insipidus. Of greater interest is the stress laid upon a transitory form of diabetes which is for the first time made the subject of special discussion by *Brouardel & Richardière.* Finally it is of interest that, at that time already, more or less stress is laid upon the diabetic disposition as being of importance for the occurrence of the disease, this fact affording the most adequate explanation of the small number of traumata being followed by diabetes.

With the second period a somewhat severer criticism of traumatic diabetes begins to assert itself.

This criticism is for the first time met with in the work issued in 1900 by *Stern* (1). In accounting for the theory concerning traumatic diabetes he just as some of the authors of the first period assumes a sceptical standpoint with regard to its appearing after peripheral traumata. He writes for instance with regard to the theory that a trauma giving rise to diabetes, as far as we know, affects the nervous system. It is true that it is possible that a severe injury of the pancreas or of the liver may cause diabetes, but convincing facts in that direction are not known from human pathology. A trauma may be thought to give rise to permanent, partly anatomically detectable and partly functional changes in the central nervous system, by which a permanent state of irritation may be thought to have arisen, which affects the carbohydrate metabolism. As the changes in the nervous system may develop slowly there is also a possibility of unterstanding that a diabetes does not become manifest before the lapse of weeks or months, in contradistinction to the rapidly passing glycosurias which are observed after diabetic puncture and also in sequel to head traumata in man. For the cases in which the diabetes shall have occurred after a lesion not involving the central nervous system the causal relationship is not known. The hypothesis that a peripheral lesion should exert such a reflectory influence on the central nervous system that the result would be a permanent disturbance of metabolism lacks all foundation. In his opinion the clinical observations also give rise to doubts, as diabetes appearing after peripheral traumata usually do not differ from diabetes. In his considerations of the clinical observations of diabetes following a head trauma he directs his attention especially to those cases running a rapid course to recovery, i.e. such cases as by *Brouardel & Richardière* are designated as diabète précoce. For these he thinks that the trauma may certainly be made responsible. In the cases running a chronic course the possibility cannot be excluded that the disease has existed perior to the trauma, and in contradistinction to the transitory cases these do not present any signs by which they may be distinguished from ordinary diabetes. However, in case of other severe lesions not involving the head he admits the possibility of an influence on the central nervous system, if the whole body has been exposed to severe commotio. As to the importance of traumatic neurosis for the appearance of traumatic diabetes he does not consider the cases at issue numerous enough to exclude a fortuitous coincidence.

It is evident that, as to physical traumata, he entirely disregards peripheral ones, and as to diabetes following a head trauma he has his doubts with regard to any others but those which are cured.

Kausch' criticism is still more severe, for he asserts that the objection may be raised against all the reported cases that the disease existed beforehand! He only found two cases in the literature where the urine had previously been examined and found to be free from sugar; in neither of the cases, however, were the circumstances under which the urine test had been performed accounted for. There may have been a question of slighter diabetes, in other cases, where the urine portions need not all contain sugar. In other cases, where the examination was not performed, there may have been a question of "diabetes decipiens", i.e. the only symptom of which is glycosuria – a disease which is not diagnosed unless the urine is accidentally examined. In many cases he thinks that the diabetes might have been detected long before the trauma if the patient had consulted a physician or the physician had tested the urine. In some cases the patient may have been aware of his disease and purposely tries to put it into causal relation with the trauma. In many of the reported cases he thinks that the diabetes has appeared after the trauma though independently of it; this holds for instance for those cases, where the first symptoms appear several years after the trauma. Finally there is the difficulty of determining the moment of inception of the diabetes. The only reliable symptom is glycosuria; but it would, of course, be a mistake to assert that the disease commenced on the day where the urine test revealed sugar for the first time. The other symptoms, such as thirst, polyuria, hunger, tiredness etc., must likewise be taken into account though with some reservation. However, with regard to these non-objective symptoms we depend of the information afforded by the patients who, as we know by experience, are inclined to attribute their complaint to some external cause or other. In his work *Kausch* gives a survey of many of the cases of traumatic diabetes and glycosuria recorded in the literature and of a series of his own cases of glycosuria. He divides the cases into two groups, namely, direct and indirect diabetes and glycosuria, indirect diabetes meaning that an affection due to the trauma has been its intermediate cause. There may, for instance, be a question of meningitis, traumatic neurosis, pancreatitis, etc. This is a point of view which *Stern* likewise advocates though he opines that, strictly speaking, the latter cannot be considered traumatic diabetes. According to the degree of the glycosuria *Kausch* divides the cases into 4 groups:

1. genuine diabetes,
2. diabetes or glycosuria which is cured,

3. ephemeral, spontaneous glycosuria, and
4. alimentary glycosuria.

As to the cases of genuine diabetes he emphasizes that they present absolute irregularity. There are all the transitions between immediate inception and after the lapse of many years. Now they are slight, now severe cases, now leading to death or not. The kind of trauma seems to be without influence on either inception or course of the disease. Nor does an acute or an insidious inception influence the course. As to the next group, i.e. the cases of diabetes followed by recovery, he makes the same observation as *Stern* (1), namely, that they are chiefly due to head traumata, in contradistinction to the cases of permanent diabetes, which frequently are caused by other traumata even though the head traumata predominate here too. These cases are characterized by the prompt appearance of glycosuria, frequently during the first days subsequent to the trauma; the glycosuria is often preceded by polyuria or, more frequently, the polyuria persists for a long time after the cessation of the glycosuria. Finally the glycosuria often is strikingly small as compared to the polyuria. On account of all these properties he just as *Stern* (1) considers these cases which, in a much higher degree form a unity, analogues to the diabetic puncture, where it is likewise possible by puncture at different heights to provoke polyuria + glycosuria or polyuria alone, respectively. However, *Kausch* is sceptical in regard to the thought that diabetes should be curable. In that case the diabetes either became latent, or there was no question of chronic diabetes but of transitory glycosuria. In his opinion there is merely a quantitative difference between a diabetes that is cured and transitory glycosuria, whence he prefers the latter term for the cases discussed.

Finally, the third group comprising the cases of ephemeral traumatic glycosuria is characterized by the sudden occurrence of glycosuria, which only lasts 8–10 days, the small quantity of sugar and the absence of other diabetic symptoms. *Kausch* is surprised that such cases, apart from *Redard*'s cases, have not been reported before.

As regards the fourth group, i.e. alimentary glycosuria, he reports that he detected it in 6 out of 12 cases submitted to the test.

He is of opinion that the slightest forms of glycosuria, namely alimentary and ephemeral glycosuria, occur particularly after slight fractures, whereas the transitory form is especially observed after head traumata. As was mentioned before, he thinks that genuine diabetes is a very rare direct sequel of the trauma. On the other hand he does not deny that it may indirectly be caused by a trauma though very seldom also. Conclusively he admits that he cannot produce proofs of genuine diabetes actually being so rare or failing to appear as he asserts.

In 1911 *Hoeniger* submitted to a critical estimation all the previously reported cases of diabetes following a trauma, collecting all those which presented one or several components of the diabetic symptom complex. According to the symptoms he sets up a probability diagnosis and, thus, thinks he is able to show that only very few cases represent genuine diabetes, whereas the majority of the cases should represent diabetes insipidus or various forms of transitory glycosuria. This seems, however, to be exaggerated, for on counting the 206 cases reported it becomes evident that he has diagnosed diabetes or diabetes ? in 115 cases. In his conclusion he in concert with *Kausch* assumes that traumatic glycosuria may well exist but no traumatic diabetes.

However, this epoch does not lack advocates of the existence of traumatic diabetes, among whom are two of the most prominent investigators of diabetes, *Lepine* and *Naunyn.*

Lepine thinks that, even after a critical estimation, the trauma must in 5 per cent of all the cases of diabetes be considered the cause, though not always the only cause, as there is a question of hereditary predisposition in various cases. He attaches great importance to the head trauma, referring to a work of his disciple *Jodry* who found head traumata in 72 out of 145 cases. He cautions against assuming, as does *Kausch,* that a pre-existing diabetes is the general rule. If the influence of the trauma is contested, what then is the explanation of the not infrequent cases where the diabetes is cured after a few months' duration, and how shall it be explained that head traumata are more diabetogenic than other traumata? Diabetes occurring after a fall is by him accounted for, for instance, by the probability of commotio cerebri even in cases where the head has not been struck.

In his book issued in 1906 *Naunyn* submits the whole question to thorough examination, and he amongst other cases includes 8 of his own presenting diabetes after head traumata as well as after non-cerebral traumata and traumatic neurosis. With regard to the latter he refers to v. *Jaksch, Strümpell* and *Strauss* who, like himself, have observed that alimentary glycosuria in case of traumatic neurosis is strikingly frequent after administration of 100 g. of glycose. He emphasizes that cases of transitory nervous glycosuria cannot be distinguished as differing essentially from diabetes, but that there are all kinds of transitions between them. He absolutely contests *Kausch'* judgment of the etiological importance of the trauma. In his opinion *Kausch'* demand that it must be proved that the patient has not previously had diabetes is too rigorous, for it would render continual observation with administration of glycose necessary, while the absence of symptoms or of glycosuria in a single urine test would be no proof, as is also asserted by *Kausch.* What is of practical importance is whether the patient has previously been *afflicted* with diabetes, but *Kausch* goes further and claims the detection of a morbid disposition. Even though such a disposition existed it would not be equivalent to the disease, nor does *Naunyn* think that it need become so. He thinks that, in the majority of cases of traumatic diabetes, such a disposition plays a part, whence it must be taken into account except in cases of severe head traumata. Whether it is justifiable, in cases of diabetes after a trauma, to declare that the disease has arisen under the influence of the trauma on an eventually or probably existing disposition, or there is a question of a decidedly deleterious action exerted by the trauma on a possibly or certainly nascent disease, must be decided in each individual case. His standpoint is clearly expressed in the following words: "Im allgemeinen muß in der Praxis mit aller Bestimmtheit dafür eingetreten werden, daß dem Trauma im weitesten Sinne (körperliches Trauma + psychischem Choc), dem Unfall, eine hervorragende Stellung unter den Ursachen des Diabetes mellitus zukommt." He winds up his deliberations by emphasizing *Pape* and *Navarres'* demonstration of the fact that, amongst the "Unfallsmännern par excellence", i.e. engine-drivers, twice as many die of diabetes as in other professions, and that there are seven times as many cases of diabetes amongst the engine-drivers as amongst the other railwaymen of the same railway company. In examining how a disturbance in the central nervous system may lead to diabetes he mentions that disturbances in the carbohydrate metabolism may be due to changes in the regulating influence of the nervous system on liver, pancreas, muscles, etc., but that it must much more frequently be assumed that, simultaneously with the morbid condition in the central nervous system, functional disturbances develop in the organs which are of importance for the carbohydrate metabolism, namely, in pancreas and liver. He draws a parallel with the motor system, where an affection of the motor neuron gives rise to an affection of the muscle. Thus, he thinks, a "secretory neuron" may be imagined forming a unit together with its terminal organ. The secretory organ cell, in which a disease gives rise to diabetes, is affected simultaneously with the nervous system, together with which it forms an entirety.

Welz (1) in his work issued in 1915 comes to the conclusion that genuine diabetes can be caused by a trauma but that neither the location of the trauma, definite clinical symptoms nor the course of the disease afford reliable criteria for the etiological relationship. He emphasizes that the probability of relationship decreases with the duration of the symptom-free interval, setting the limit at 2–3 years at the highest. He is very sceptical with regard to the importance of traumatic neurosis, which he considers an artificially constructed intermediate link between diabetes and a trauma which is not acknowledged as direct cause.

Thiem agrees with *Welz'* views.

Finally I shall mention *v. Noorden* (1) who in 1912 emphasizes that there certainly are cases of acute neuropathogenous glycosuria but that it must be deemed dubious, and probably impossible, that a genuine chronic diabetes can persist on account of a nervous disturbance without the pancreas being affected. What is decisive is that diabetes must now be considered a complaint which is due to a strictly located organic disease.

Thus this epoch is characterized by very conflicting views, which are most strongly advocated by *Kausch* who denies, and by *Naunyn* who highly emphasizes, the etiological importance of the trauma. Whereas the authors acknowledging its etiological importance continue adhering to the possibility of neurogenous diabetes, *v. Noorden* (1) almost absolutely denies its existence and emphasizes that diabetes is a localized pancreas affection.

This standpoint forms the transition to the third period the commencement of which coincides with the beginning of the world war.

In 1916 *v. Noorden* (2) calls the world war with its enormous tax to the nervous system a mighty and terrible physical experiment, which must clear up the question whether we shall henceforth reckon with the notion of chronic neurogenous diabetes and so-called traumatic diabetes. He is decidedly of opinion that the physical and psychical claims of the war, with the inclusion of the lesions, act as an irritant on an existing disposition though without being able, if the disposition is absent, alone to provoke the appearance of diabetes. Those soldiers who incur diabetes during the war, have taken the field as masked diabetics, whose disease as a rule is merely accelerated. He emphasizes that, as regards the etiology, he does not deny neurogenous influences as provocative factors, but attaches importance to such only if they strike an inefficient pancreas. As a hypothetical explanation he assumes that the neurogenous irritants continually set the production of sugar going again via the central nervous system, the sympathicus, the adrenals, the blood and the liver. Consequently the pancreas must continually act as a suppressing agent, and the increased hormone production will gradually exhaust this previously inefficient organ.

A similar point of view, namely, that the various war influences cannot give rise to diabetes but merely to its manifestation in case of existing disposition for the disease, is advocated by *Albu, Gottstein* and *Umber* as well as by *Hermann Strauss* (2).

On the ground of some interesting statistics *Gottstein* and *Umber* endeavour to elucidate the question. During the war they counted up the diabetics among the civil population of Charlottenburg and found 2.3 per mille, which they considered a maximal value, as there was a question of a fairly well-to-do population. For Berlin itself they report a value of 1.2–1.3 per mille. For the sake of comparison they quote the figure from *Umber*'s military infirmary, where 11 out of 2232 soldiers, i.e. 4.9 per mille, had diabetes. However, several of these had just been sent to that infirmary because of their diabetes. In another military infirmary they found 1.2 per mille of diabetics, i.e. a much smaller rate per mille than in the population of Charlottenburg.

Hermann Strauss (2) likewise emphasizes that diabetes was not more frequent among the soldiers than among the civil population. Thus, up to the autumn of 1916, there were found 1525 cases of diabetes only in 279 military infirmaries, and Strauss reports that the number of diabetics in the military hospitals amounted to no more than 0.5 per mille as compared to the home infirmaries, where it was 0.8 per mille. Although *Strauss* does not either consider the war influences the cause of diabetes but merely as an activating factor in case of existing disposition, he emphasizes that they are able to aggravate an existing diabetes and of importance for the severe course which the disease often runs. Hence he is of opinion that a diabetes detected during the war must in the majority of cases be considered an injury received in the discharge of official duties.

For the sake of comparison with these observations on the part of the Germans it deserves mention that diabetes according to *Hurst*'s reports seems to be less frequent among English soldiers, and *Joslin* by examining 40,000 front soldiers found two cases of diabetes only.

In opposition to these authors *Lenné* (1, 2) thinks it justifiable to assume that there actually are "war diabetics", i.e. patients whose diabetes *is due* to physical strain. On the other hand he admits that injuries and diseases apparently have not had any essential influence on the appearance and the character of the disease. He refers to a material of 258 diabetics, mentioning, amongst other things, as a proof of the afore-mentioned influences promoting the appearance of diabetes, that the number of diabetics among soldiers of 20–30 years of age amounted to 24 per cent, whereas, in the corresponding age-class in *Gottstein* and *Umber*'s report concerning a civil population, it only amounted to little more than 2 per cent of the total number of diabetics. *Lenné* thus created the new picture of "war diabetes" which, to judge from the post-war literature, has played no small part in Germany, where such cases frequently came to be judged as injuries received in the discharge of official duties. Perhaps, this is one of the causes of the great attention which, after the war, was paid to traumatic diabetes in Germany, while very few reports of it are met with in the literature of other countries.

On reviewing the post-war literature it becomes evident that the war has not afforded the elucidation of the question prophesied by *v. Noorden* (2) in 1916.

In a paper published in 1919 *Magnus-Levy* thus admits both head traumata, psychic shock, severe general commotio of the body, and blows against pancreas and liver as causal factors. *Now Hermann Strauss'* (3) further commentary (1922) upon the afore-mentioned material of 1525 cases of diabetes among combatants is of interest, as he treats it according to the etiological factors. However, applicable reports have been available in 200 cases only. Among these he rejects about 30 cases in which as causes are mentioned cold, physical hardship, exhaustion and the like, besides two small groups with thyreotoxicosis and gas poisoning. The remaining cases are divided into three groups: I. Physical influences: 70 cases; II. Preceding infectious diseases: 45 cases; III. Shock: 10 cases.

It is interesting to see that group I only contains 7 cases of head trauma, whereas the remaining 90 per cent of the cases present lesions of the trunk, abdomen, or extremities, i.e. lesions which, as he points out, do not always imply commotio of the central nervous system. In two cases there was a question of a gunshot-wound and a contusion of the pancreas, respectively.

Stauss concludes that one must be somewhat more liberal with regard to the acknowledgment of traumata as diabetogenic factors and that, at any rate, it is not warrantable to acknowledge such cases only, in which the brain has been struck directly or indirectly. On the other hand, it is somewhat puzzling that he with regard to the cases of shock, in group III, declares that they are quite easy to understand, merely substantiating our experience of near relationship between psychic trauma and appearance of diabetes. However, he immediately afterwards emphasizes that there were strikingly few such cases.

The authors who, above all, have imparted to the conception of traumatic diabetes its special stamp after the war, are *Umber* and *v. Noorden*, and particularly the former has treated the subject over and over again. His standpoint was dictated by his conception of diabetes as being, pathogenetically, exclusively dependent of a pancreas affection, i.e. a hereditary hypofunction of the islands of Langerhans. His conception is clearly formulated in the following sentence found in his work from 1927 (1): "Es gibt keinen einwandfreien experimentellen oder klinischen Beweis dafür, daß durch eine Verletzung des Gehirns oder des Kopfes, des Rumpfes und der Gliedmassen ein echter Diabetes entstehen kann. Hingegen ist die Entstehung des Diabetes durch Unterfunktion des Pankreas-Inselapparates gesichert, und die Beseitigung aller diabetischen Störungen durch das Insulin hat den letzten noch ausstehenden Beweis dafür gebracht, daß lediglich eine anatomische oder funktionelle Erkrankung des Pankreas einen Diabetes hervorbringen kann". In support of his repudiation of a traumatic origin of diabetes he takes the war experiences into account also.

Over and over again (1, 2, 3, 4,) he accounts for the points of view which he applies in deciding whether there is a relationship between a trauma and a diabetes appearing after such a trauma. In case of post-traumatic glycosuria it must above all be determined whether there is a question of extra-insular irritative glycosuria ("Reizglykosurie") or of genuine insular diabetes. As prototype of extra-insular irritative glycosuria he mentions *Cl. Bernard's* diabetic puncture, which is a sympathicogenous glycosuria. Amongst such irritative glycosurias he mentions as being known, partly, constitutional spontaneous cases running a chronic course, and, partly, cases of a transitory nature witnessed after agitation, traumata, particularly head, traumata, and intoxications. He thinks that it is such cases which, in the older literature, were termed diabète précoce. Still, he mentions bulletins of chronic extra-insular glycosurias, which were detected after traumata and in which he is inclined to acknowledge a causal relationship. However, such a complaint is no progressional affection liable to compensation but should sooner be termed an innocent anomaly.

True traumatic diabetes cannot be thought to occur unless the very pancreas is injured, and in that case the lesions must be very severe, for experiments have shown that at least 4/5 of the pancreas must be removed before diabetes appears. However, such severe traumata will as a rule lead to death; nor are, according to *Umber,* reliable examples of such an origin of diabetes on record in the literature. In this connection he moreover mentions the possibility of the insular apparatus being indirectly injured via acute pancreatitis and severe necrosis of the organ.

Whereas he denies that other physical or psychic traumata are able to give rise to diabetes, he admits that, in rare cases, they may aggravate an existing diabetes and, hence, render a latent diabetes, prediabetes, manifest. By such a prediabetes he means a condition, in which the insular apparatus is already affected and somewhat inefficient but, as yet, not so severely as to give rise to glycosuria or other diabetic symptoms, if the individual lives on an ordinary diet. Just as in case of manifest diabetes there may in such cases arise an impairment of tolerance which makes the previously latent diabetes manifest. Diabetes would at any rate have appeared, and he does not reckon with the possibility of a trauma being able to accelerate its appearance by more than weeks or months. In such cases the trauma just as in case of existing diabetes plays an aggravating part only. Later (5) he has made a restriction with regard to the kind of traumata, declaring that such induction or aggravation is only probable if a trauma has directly struck the pancreas region or has given rise to severe inflammation or general infection with ensuing impairment of tolerance. In regard to the aggravation of diabetes he writes that, as a rule, it is negligible and can in the majority of cases be suppressed by an adequate treatment; nor does it give rise to any persistent change of the future course.

Amongst a very great number of diabetics he has experienced this twice only. In the one case an abdominal trauma gave rise to bilious colic with secondary pancreatitis followed by diabetes. In the other case a shell-shot in the arm had given rise to constantly recidivating osteomyelitis which, at each attack, caused transitory impairment of tolerance which finally became permanent. In these cases the diabetes was not previously recognized, but

Umber is of opinion that the pancreas in both cases has been inefficient. Evidently in these cases the aggravation is not due to the trauma as such, but to an affection caused by the trauma as intermediate link.

If we summarize *Umber's* standpoint, it will be as follows: Traumatic diabetes is only conceivable if the trauma has given rise to a severe injury of the pancreas itself. Other physical and psychic traumata cannot give rise to true diabetes; at the highest they may acquire importance as activating or aggravating factors, respectively, in cases of latent or manifest diabetes, respectively.

Finally it deserves mention that *Umber* in the course of time emphasizes more and more strongly that diabetes is a heredofamilial disease. He draws attention to the works of his disciple *Finke* who amongst 1500 diabetics detected a heredofamilial disposition in 26.4 per cent of the cases, a figure which corresponds to the findings of other authors. This is very interesting, as *Danforth* has calculated that, in case of recessive heredity of diabetes and a frequency of 2.5‰ of the total population, 72 per cent of the diabetics need not have any diabetic relations during three generations comprising siblings, parents and their siblings, and grandparents. Hence, it will almost never be possible to exclude with certainty the existence of diabetic genes.

In 1934 *Umber* (6) on the ground of the detection of diabetes in three pairs of enzygotic twins comes to the conclusion that diabetes is a recessive property dependent of the hereditary disposition and on which external factors may produce an inducing or an inhibitory effect but never give rise to the disease. He considers this the final proof that it is justifiable to deny traumatic diabetes in practice.

On the ground of his conception of diabetes as a pure pancreas affection *Umber's* standpoint is by *v. Noorden* (1) agreed to, who as early as 1923 writes about neurogenous diabetes: "Einen neurogenen Diabetes gibt es überhaupt nicht, die Kriegserfahrungen haben ihn vollends zu Grabe getragen". On the other hand he also recognizes neurogenous glycosurias to which he applies the common term of chromaffinogenous glycosurias.

In 1933 he (3) published a detailed study of the question of the importance of the trauma as provoking factor. He assert that, if diabetes is detected shortly after a trauma, the patient has nearly always had a previously unrecognized diabetes, or the chromaffinogenous glycosuria provoked by the trauma has for the first time given rise to its manifestation. He emphasizes that there has been a question of diabetes and not of a disposition to diabetes. If there were a disposition to diabetes, a causal relationship must certainly be acknowledged. He declares that diabetes does not originate from the moment of detection of sugar in the urine or of discharge of sugar, but that it frequently must have been preceded by a protracted development of disturbances of the pancreas function and of metabolism. He draws a parallel between diabetes and the first attack of podagra, which is not the inception of, but a long prepared sequel to, the uratic arthritis.

As a contrast to the views set forth by these authors may be mentioned *Hijmanns van den Bergh's* standpoint. If there is no clue to the patient previously having had diabetes, he is inclined, if the patient after the trauma incurs symptoms resembling neurasthenia which are later followed by special diabetic symptoms, to acknowledge the probability of traumatic diabetes, even though the glycosuria has not been detected till long after the incurrence of the trauma. Against *v. Noorden's* assertion that diabetes is due to a pancreas affection only, he raises the objection that the function of the pancreas is so highly influenced by other systems, such as for instance endocrine glands, central nervous system and sympathicus, that the assumption of a possible causal relationship between trauma and diabetes is quite justifiable. Whether, in case of diabetes occurring after a trauma, there has been a question of predisposition may be very interesting from a scientific point of view but is quite indifferent from a social point of view. He concludes by emphasizing that, for the sake of a transitory theory, one should not wrong the patients by taking no notice of the possibility of a relationship between trauma and diabetes where it can really exist.

These points of view are more or less unanimously espoused by the other authors of that time. Thus, *Rosenberg, Kaufmann, Klieneberger, Wiechmann, Bahn, Steinthal, Landé, Krone, Stursberg, Broglie, Behrendt, Sellner, Weber,* and others agree with *v. Noorden-Umber.*

Joslin entirely agrees with *Umber.* Thus in the latest edition of his book (1935) in the discussion of the etiological importance of the trauma he contents himself with an ample quotation of *Umber's* works. *Matz* who has examined 300 former soldiers with diabetes, also deems it unlikely that a neurogenous or a traumatic factor is of importance for the occurrence of diabetes.

Jacobi and *Meythaler* in a great work fairly agree with *Umber* and *v. Noorden* though, with regard to organic lesions of the central nervous system and psychic traumata, they make greater allowances than those authors. However, in advocating the view that cranial traumata, encephalitis, meningitis and severest psychic traumata fail to give rise to but are able to provoke or aggravate diabetes, this is done from a purely legal point of view, as they do not think it can be proved scientifically. However, they consider such a standpoint justifiable as long as the psycho-physical connection between the brain and the insular apparatus, which probably priceeds through the autonomic nervous system, is not reliably established. They add, however, that the factors mentioned as activating the diabetes must only be acknowledged after the most rigorous criticism.

Isaac (1) advocates a practical standpoint, for, presuming a constitutional disposition, he acknowledges a causal relationship if the diabetes manifests itself within 4 weeks after the trauma. A further presumption is, however, that there must be a question of severe trauma, such as for instance a cranial lesion or a trauma conjoined with shock. A similar standpoint is advocated by *Grote* who likewise asserts that an interim of more than 4 weeks between trauma and diabetes renders a causal relationship unlikely, whence he thinks that an eventual indemnification must depend on the temporal interval.

Liebig who has published 9 cases of traumatic diabetes, in which he has been very liberal with regard to the acknowledgment of causal relationship, advocates nearly the same standpoint as *van den Bergh* though with the reservation set forth by *Umber* and *v. Noorden* that an existing disposition must be considered a necessary intermediate link. *Krause* and *Schur* hold similar views, the latter particularly stressing that we are totally ignorant as to whether a latent diabetes would become manifest at all or, at any rate, much later than *Umber* thinks, if the patient did not incur the trauma.

As experienced an author as *Stern* (2) in his manual of the traumatic origin of internal diseases formulates his conditions for acknowledging the traumatic origin of diabetes in the following axioms: A causal relationship must be deemed probable, if (1) there are no indications with regard to the existence of the disease prior to the accident; (2) if the accident has caused a lesion of the pancreas or of the central nervous system, particularly of the head, or if the patient has experienced a severe general commotio or a violent emotion; (3) if the diabetes has developed during the first weeks after the accident. To these axioms he adds that, even though other etiological factors should be detected which, from a scientific point of view, might alter the aspect of the disease, this fact should not detract from the patient's right of indemnification; moreover, the appearance of diabetic symptoms should be parallelled with the detection of glycosuria in cases, where this was detected later. This shows that he agrees entirely with *van den Bergh*. *Lichtwitz*, *Grafe* (1) and *Thannhauser* hold similar views. With regard to the war experiences *Stern* (2) and *Grafe* (1) are of opinion that *v. Noorden* and *Umber* attach too much importance to them. *Grafe* (1) thus writes that it is not correct to apply to the total population observations made with regard to the health of the pick of it, and he thinks that neurogenous activation of latent diabetes is not only possible but even probable.

A special view is held by *Veil* who in 1930 very sharply contests *v. Noorden-Umber*'s standpoint. He calls their attempt at explaining cases of diabetes after trauma by the presumption of the previous existence of latent diabetes a construction and a phantastic hypothesis. He asserts that the explanation of traumatic diabetes does not at all require the renewal of the theory of neurogenous diabetes. He himself is of opinion that it is not difficult to imagine the occurrence of a functional impairment of the pancreas – an organic neurosis.

Even though the afore-mentioned authors disagree with regard to the estimation of the etiological importance of the trauma, very few of them will probably consider a pure, neurogenous diabetes probable, at any rate scientifically speaking. However, the continual investigations of the importance of the interbrain for the regulation of the carbohydrate metabolism have maintained the idea that this regulation mechanism likewise plays a part in clinical pathology, and thus kept up the notion of neurogenous diabets. Thus, *Leschke* for instance goes as far as declaring that typical diabetes mellitus according to its entire character and course must be considered a central – vegetative disturbance of the regulation of the carbohydrate metabolism.

On the ground of isolated cases, in which not only severe cerebral disturbances but also diabetes occurred in sequel to a trauma, *Arneth*, *Woll* and *Curschmann* in those cases are inclined to assume a neurotraumatic basis of the disease. *Curschmann* moreover reports 2 cases of diabetes after carbon oxid poisoning, and since this poisoning tends to give rise to changes in the interbrain, he deems it possible that really centrally conditioned, genuine diabetes may arise in that manner. On the whole he recommends a less offhandish attitude in regard to the neurotraumatic origin of diabetes.

Falta who, on the ground of his own and collaborators' works on insulin resistance in case of genuine diabetes, so strongly emphasizes that diabetes in many cases involves an extrainsular component, and suggests the theoretical possibility of all transitions form pure insular to pure extrainsular diabetes, naturally is one of those authors who discuss the possibility of neurogenous traumatic diabetes. He admits that its existence has not been proved, but the knowledge of the regulating influence of the central nervous system on the carbohydrate metabolism, and the fact that reports of changes in the central nervous system of persons having died of diabetes continue to appear, and finally that many cases do not present any changes in the pancreas, are the reason why such a form of diabetes cannot be excluded. Just as *Naunyn* he suggests the possibility of trophic disturbances in the insular apparatus.

Whereas *Woll* and *Arneth* in the afore-mentioned papers reported cases of diabetes the course of which did not differ from that of ordinary diabetes, *Gebhardt* in 1934 reported a case of glycosuria and ketonuria with normal blood sugar after a cranial trauma. The alimentary blood sugar curve was approximately normal and unaffected by the insulin. *Gebhardt* is inclined to consider this case a particular form of renal diabetes due to lesion of a center which regulates the filtration power of the kidney.

Finally *Kretschmer* in 1935 reported three cases of diabetes after cranial lesion characterized by being refractory to insulin, which in a certain degree holds for *Curschmann's* previously discussed case also. However, *Kretschmer*'s cases are so briefly recorded that it is impossible to judge them correctly.

However, despite the small number of observations he sets up the following rules for a causal relationship with a trauma:

1. There must be a severe cranial trauma with clinical signs of commotion;
2. it must have been proved that the patient has not had diabetes prior to the trauma:
3. besides the diabetic disturbance of metabolism the patient must present other cerebral symptoms or cerebral nerve symptoms;
4. glycosuria and blood sugar level must prove refractory to insulin. To this latter symptom is attached special importance.

Before I terminate the exposition of the views held during the last epoch I shall refer to one of the latest works treating of the subject published by *W. v. Drigalski,* whose views concerning several decisive points are opposed to those held by the chief authors.

In the first place he raises objections against the idea that, if a case of diabetes shall be considered traumatic, the trauma must have been "appropriate", i.e. it must have struck the skull or the pancreas, as appears also from the preceding.

Emphasizing the frequently observed temporal relationship between purely psychic traumata and diabetes, he asserts that it is practically never possible to decide whether a trauma has had a psychic or a physical effect, whence it cannot either be proved whether the sequels must be attributed to the one factor or to the other. Therefore, in his opinion any other mechanical traumata besides those mentioned may give rise to diabetes: "Worauf es beim Trauma ankommt, ist nicht der Ort und die Art der Einwirkung, sondern im wesentlichen die Schwere der Erschütterung der psychophysischen Gesamtsituation".

In the second place he raises objections against the common distinction between the importance of the trauma as "giving rise" to a disease and that of the trauma as merely "activating" a latent disease. He claims that, in each single case, it must be determined whether there is any reason to assume the existence of an endogenous morbid disposition. If this is the case, the estimation of the importance of the trauma as causal factor will require the determination of how great a probability there is that the disease would also have been incurred without the trauma. If there is no clue to disposition, which in his opinion is very rare in case of traumatic diabetes, the disposition must be considered an unknown factor and, hence, left out of consideration in judging the case at issue; then only the trauma can be incriminated as cause of the disease. It is evident that *v. Drigalski* thus will be able to acknowledge practically any case of diabetes witnessed after a trauma, if only the temporal relationship is in order.

If we review this last epoch our attention is arrested by the fact that the different authors are far from agreeing in their estimation of traumatic diabetes. In the preceding pages I have endeavoured to convey an idea of the various points of view prevailing with regard to traumatic diabetes, and I think it possible to distinguish between four. The clearest standpoint is that set up by *v. Noorden* and *Umber*, who only consider a traumatic origin of diabetes possible, if the very pancreas has been injured. However, their further definition comprises more indefinite factors, if they, though with the greatest reservation, acknowledge that a trauma can activate diabetes in case of existing latent diabetes, prediabetes or diabetic disposition. This renders the estimation unreliable; for, firstly, the different authors may be of different opinion in regard to the meaning of latent diabetes or of the other terms applied to an abstraction which we are not accustomed to deal with and which is characterized by lack of symptoms. Secondly, when shall we assume the existence of such a condition? Even if we are informed that some members of the patient's family suffer from diabetes, the investigations carried out for instance by *Pincus* and *White* and, in Denmark, by *Secher*, show that there need not be any detectable disturbances of the carbohydrate metabolism in all the members of the family. On the other hand, the circumstance that the patient's nearest relations are not diabetic does not exclude that he may have a diabetic disposition. Finally the rules of inheritance can scarcely be said to have been cleared up entirely, even though the results of the investigations tend to suggest that there is a question of recessive inheritance.

As to what traumata may be assumed to have an activating effect there is ample scope between *Umber's* essential acknowledgment of traumata striking the pancreas region and other authors' acknowledgment of other slighter or severer physical and psychic traumata.

According to what I have termed *van den Bergh-Stern*'s standpoint the causal relationship between traumata and diabetes is acknowledged, if there is a question of pancreas traumata, trauma of the central nervous system, or psychic traumata. Scientifically speaking the existence of predisposing factors in a certain degree tends to reduce the importance of the trauma, though it is at the same time emphasized that such factors must not be taken into account for the estimation, particularly in regard to insurance.

The third standpoint is that advocated by *Veil* who acknowledges traumatic diabetes, thinking that it is dependent upon pancreas neurosis.

The fourth standpoint, which is advocated by *Kretschmer* and which may likewise be termed clear, implies a special form of diabetes depending of an organic lesion of the central nervous system, which is no pancreas diabetes but its contrast, a diabetes refractory to insulin.

Thus, even though it is possible and justifiable to set up a series of chief points of view, this fact alone reveals the uncertainty prevailing in regard to the whole question. The various, more or less liberal interpretation of the principles held by the chief authors may lead to extremely varying estimation of the etiological importance of the trauma, which is evidenced by the above recorded, more or less divergent standpoints held by numerous authors. As a marked example in this respect I need only refer to *W. v. Drigalski.*

Of the two main standpoints that held by *v. Noorden-Umber* may be termed scientifically most reliable, whereas that held by *van den Bergh-Stern* is of a more social character, permitting of acknowledgment of a relationship between factors where we so not scientifically know any such intermediate link and which afford verdicts that can easily be made to accord with generally prevailing popular and forensic notions of right. In Germany *v. Noorden-Umber*'s standpoint has the preponderance now, for the German Reichsversicherungsamt pronounces its verdicts according to it, as is evidenced by the following verdicts, the first of which, dated October 7th, 1928, is worded as follows: "Die Erfahrungen auf dem Gebiet der Zuckerkrankheit in den letzten Jahrzehnten haben gelehrt, daß die Krankheit nur ganz ausnahmsweise Unfallfolge sein kann, und zwar nur dann, wenn der Unfall zu einer Verletzung der Bauchspeicheldrüse geführt hat. Es muß sich also um einen schweren Unfall handeln, durch den die Bauchspeicheldrüse unmittelbar verletzt worden ist". The wording of the second verdict, dated June 9th, 1934, is as follows: "Zuckerkrankheit Unfallfolge nur bei Zerstörung von neun Zehnteln der Bauchspeicheldrüse. Verschlimmerung des Leidens durch Unfall nur wahrscheinlich, wenn unmittelbarer zeitlicher Zusammenhang und mittelbare Gewalteinwirkung auf die Pancreasgegend oder schwere Eiterung, bzw. Allgemein-Infektion".

Before I terminate this historical account, I shall quote a couple of verdicts from recent years which show the standpoint that asserts itself in Denmark.

Danish investigations of the problem are not on record in the literature; only *Holger Strandgaard* (1913) in a work on diabetes and surgery mentions the question of traumatic diabetes though without accounting for his standpoint in regard to it.

A verdict of the *working men's insurance council* (Arbejderforsikringsraadet) pronounced in 1924 with regard to a case of diabetes incurred two months after a peripheral trauma has the following wording: In order to be able to acknowledge the existence of traumatic diabetes, which is so rare a disease, it is necessary, for the sake of complete reliability in accordance with general medical experience, to know, firstly, that the urine has not contained sugar prior to the accident and that it has contained sugar immediately or shortly after the accident; secondly, it must generally be demanded that it is proved that the trauma has involved the head or, by its violence, has been able to give rise to changes in the brain or in the central nervous system.

The verdict of the *medicolegal council* (Retslaegeraadet), dated March 11th, 1932, refers to a case of diabetes detected in a woman, aged 51 years, on admission to hospital after a cranial trauma. The wording of the conclusion is as follows: According to the information it must be assumed that Mrs. H. F. *can* have incurred the diabetes detected immediately after the accident on account of the accident.

According to this verdict it may be assumed that the medicolegal council agrees with the working men's insurance council, and a comparison with the two repeatedly quoted chief standpoints shows that both the medicolegal council and the working men's insurance council are of quite the same opinion as *van den Bergh-Stern.*

in: *Viggo Thomsen: Studies of trauma and carbohydrate metabolism with special reference to the existence of traumatic diabetes, Kopenhagen 1938, S. 9–36.*

Insulin Precursors – a Historical Sketch

The First Attempts at Treating Diabetes with Pancreatic Extracts

by Karl Heinz Leickert

Sir Frederick Grant Banting was just 30 years old when, together with the 22 year old medical student Charles Herbert Best, he administered pancreatic extracts to pancreatectomized dogs in 1921. This was made possible by the skill of the biochemist J. B. Collip who, by means of acids, alcohol and cold, had produced a purified and concentrated extract which was also very active in man. A dog without a pancreas survived for 70 days on this bovine pancreatic extract. These results were first published in 1922 by Banting, Best, Collip, Campbell and Fletcher; they called the insulin[1] "isletin" [2, 33].

For this discovery, F. G. Banting and his chief John J. R. Macleod were awarded the Nobel Prize for medicine in 1923, whereas Best and Collip went empty-handed. Later, Banting demonstratively shared his prize with Best and nothing was left to Macleod but to act similarly towards Collip.

But were these Canadian investigations actually the first researches that finally led to the preparation of insulin?

Even in 1892, Capparelli was using an extract obtained by trituration of fresh pancreas in 0.76% NaCl solution. He injected this mixture "into the abdominal cavity of a dog made diabetic by extirpation of the pancreas; 36 hours later the sugar in the urine had already begun to fall and in most cases disappeared completely soon afterwards" [5]. According to Pflüger, it was of course only a partial extirpation of the pancreas that was involved in these experiments [28].

In 1893, Comby [6] informed the convention of the "Hospital Medical Society" in Paris that he had obtained no effect in a patient aged 25 with severe diabetes by the "hypodermatic" injection of guinea-pig's pancreatic juice – which was well-tolerated – over 5 days.

---

[1] After Zuelzer had previously contacted other drug firms.

In Turin, in 1893, Battistini checked this published result in two patients, using glycerin solutions and fresh calf pancreas in a NaCl solution for the treatment of diabetes. The amount of sugar excreted certainly fell, but Battistini also noted pyrexia and abscess-formation [3].

In the same year, Wood [37] reported a fall in urinary sugar after injections of pancreatic juice in one case, Hale-White found the same in one case [10] with 2 ounces of fresh pancreas daily and injections of two drops of pancreatic juice morning and evening, while Knowsley Sibley had good results with boiled pancreas in one case [16].

In 1894, Vanni described a reduction of glycosuria in pancreatictomized animals after the injection of pancreatic extract [36]. In 1895, Ausset observed that the glycosuria of pancreatectomized dogs subsided after the administration of lightly cooked pancreas, and he also gave cooked pancreas to patients. He describes a patient of "diabetic type" who excreted 38 g of glucose daily, suffered from cachexia and "excreted more than double the normal amounts of chloride and phosphate". By the second day after medication, Ausset found only 2 g of glucose and at the 9th day sugar was no longer demonstrable in this diabetic. This state lasted for a month. The question arises as to why Ansset did not pursue his favorable observations. On the other hand, and this may well have been the reason, other clinicians could not confirm these results with the same medication [1, 20].

In 1898, Blumenstein treated the juice expressed from the pancreas with alcohol, thereby destroying – quite unconsciously – the proteolytic trypsin. He wrote an optimistic essay on his experiment, but abandoned his researches soon afterwards [4]. All the communications mentioned above were single case reports.

As Reuter reports, at about the same time other authors, also unsuccessfully, tried administering pancreatic extracts in enemas [29, 30]. In 1902, Hess undertook serotherapy, but also without significant results [11].

In 1903, Zuelzer began his first studies with pancreatic extracts and adrenal juice. In his clinic in Berlin-Hasenheide he then used rabbits as experimental animals, in which he first established that the injection of at least 1 ccm of adrenalin regularly produced hyperglycemia and glycosuria. Later, Zuelzer [41] added the simultaneous subcutaneous administration of pancreatic extract and arrived at the following result:

3.3 kg rabbit
19. 9. 1903 = 1 ccm adrenal juice (right)
19. 9. 1903 = 2 ccm pancreatic extract (injected left)
19. 9. 1903 very little urine, sugar 0

4.3 kg rabbit
20. 9. 1903 similar injection
21. 9. 1903 no sugar in urine

He repeated these experiments innumerable times in the most varied combinations. Sugar excretion regularly failed to appear. It is true that Zueler had misinterpreted the mechanism of action of the pancreatic extract in the sense of a theory of adrenalin/insulin antagonism. However, the methodology of this experiments was reasonable. At that time, Zuelzer was still not describing a specific method of extraction of his pancreas preparations. He merely mentioned that "in order to obtain a not too toxic pancreatic secretion, all the proteins of the pancreas must be removed"! [38–45].

Numerous authors (Reuter [29, 30], Kenez [13], Lausch [19], Holscher [12], etc.) attribute these first experiments to the year 1907; actually in the paper published by Zuelzer in 1907 [41] there appears the footnote: "These short communications were submitted to the editors about 3 years ago. Publication was postponed at the author's request in the hope, not as yet fulfilled, that he would be successful in obtaining practical results from the theoretic investigations."

In the meantime, Zuelzer had further endeavored to prepare an extract which could be tolerated by humans without side-effects. The pancreatic glands of horses, sheep, pigs and other animals were processed as follows: they were first pounded with sand in mortars, then the gland pulp was mixed with kieselguhr and pressed through fabric. This fluid extract was treated with alcohol to precipitate the proteins. Results that were to some extent satisfactory as regards activity against the glycosuria were obtained, but side-effects such as rigor and fever developed. It was not only animals that were treated with this first pancreatic extract, as described in the literature (Kenez [13]), but also humans.

In 1908, Zuelzer gave his pancreatic extract the name "Acomatol". At that time he in no way believed in the possibility of a continuous treatment of diabetes, only, as the name indicates, the control of diabetic coma [22].

In 1909, on Minkowski's advice, Forschbach repeated Zuelzer's experiments at his Breslau clinic and noted side-effects in 2 patients as well in animal experiments. It is true that the glycosuria also decreased. Because of these side-effects, Forschbach discontinued his experiments, stating the symtoms as tachycardia, high fever, vomiting and, in one of the two patients, inflammation of the oral mucosa. Finally, however, he endorsed Zuelzer "as having been the first to produce successfully from the pancreas a preparation that eliminates sugar excretion in a shorter or longer period by i.v. administration, even in cases in which nutrient supply remains unaltered". Yet Minkowski finally notified Zuelzer that his preparation was unusable because of side-effects [7]. "I reproach myself that we did not then endeavor to follow up the causes of the side-effects, in view of the undoubted effects on sugar excretion, and contented ourselves with establishing the unsuitability of the preparation for the treatment of human beings." (see Mallinghof, jun [21]).

In 1909–1912, Ott and Scott had positive results with pancreatic extract in dogs, but not in cats. They also reported febrile side-effects [26, 32].

In 1914, Mohr and Vahlen [23], using a very complicated technique (the pancreas was boiled with dilute sulfuric acid, then heated at 140° with zinc chloride, and lactic acid later added), obtained a substance which reduced sugar excretion in pancreatectomized dogs. It would certainly now have been interesting to determine whether the blood-sugar was similarly reduced in the same way by this substance.

In 1914, Rose [31] published, in a preliminary report, amazing results obtained by the administration of an alkaline pancreatic extract, according to which 4 patients had lost their sugar for months!

In 1913–1914, the collaboration flourished between the clinican Zuelzer at Berlin-Hasenheide and the firm of Hoffmann La Roche[1], who sent their then laboratory director, Camille Reuter, to Berlin. This collaboration prospered so much that Reuter at Grenzach was able to process up to 114 kg of pancreatic glands in copper vessels. With this Grenzach preparation, Zuelzer now noted particularly convulsions in dogs which had never been seen previously in laboratory experiments on rabbits [29, 30].

As the preparation techniques for large-scale production had been altered (probably at the instigation of M. Guggenheim,

---

1 After Zuelzer had previously contacted other drug firms.

Karl Petrén. A Leader in Pre-Insulin Dietary Therapy of Diabetes

by Russell M. Wilder

One of the most distinguished medical teachers and clinical investigators of his time was Karl Petrén. Some of his biographers have called him the most distinguished in Sweden. We know him in America principally because of his studies of diabetes and his advocacy in the very early nineteen twenties of a diet very high in fat. He was even more renowned, however, in neurology, and participated actively in Swedish public health affairs, notably in programs for the control of tuberculosis.

Born in 1868 of a line of clergymen on his mother's side, one of five brothers all of whom became outstanding, his medical training in Lund was followed by a year of study under the guidance of Dejerine, in Charcot's former clinic, the Salpétrière, in Paris. An equally lengthy sojourn was with Naunyn in Strassburg, then in Germany. He was called in 1902 to the professorship of internal medicine at Upsala, and in 1910 to the chair of medicine in his alma mater, the University of Lund.

It was not until he took the professorship at Lund that Petrén's scientific interest was drawn to diabetes. Thereafter this became a major concern to him, largely because of dissatisfaction with the then current treatment by starvation. Extensive facilities and many patients with diabetes of severity, whom he could maintain for months and years under continuous supervision, enabled him to conduct extensive clinical and laboratory observations, employing various dietary procedures and ultimately arriving at conclusions of significance.

It is true that others, before Petrén, among them especially Weintraud, also a pupil of Naunyn, had found protein restriction to be beneficial in diabetes; but Petrén's studies went much further in revealing, as they did, that an increase of the nitrogen exchange would aggravate pre-existing acidosis, and that, with a rigidly restricted protein intake, even in patients with diabetes of severity, fat possessed a nitrogen sparing effect not much inferior to that possessed by carbohydrates in the normal. Thus the Petrén diet, as finally developed, became sufficiently high in fat to provide the calories required to maintain near normal body weight and this diet, to the surprise of everyone, could be tolerated without augmenting acidosis. Petrén's diets also were restricted in their carbohydrate content to that contained in leafy vegetables, and almost always, by these means, blood sugar levels, in chronic cases of severity, could be held near normal.

Because of the war (1914–1918) Petrén's early work on diabetes came to our attention late. The procedure, developed independently by Newburgh and Marsh [1], closely resembled that which he was recommending; also, without knowledge at the time of Petrén's observations, I conducted a metabolic study with Boothby and Beeler [2], and our findings were in support of his conclusions. His high fat diets were opposed, nevertheless, in many quarters and controversy raged until the discovery of insulin, in 1922, which soon permitted liberal diabetic diets and put an end to further need for such procedure. However, certain facts, brought to light by Petrén's studies and those of the others to whom I have referred, ought not to be forgotten: that fat like carbohydrate spares protein and that uncompensated acidosis, even when diabetes is severe, does not follow fat combustion if the nitrogen exchange is low and a minimal amount of carbohydrate is tolerated.

Petrén traveled widely and became an intimate of many of the foremost internists and neurologists in Germany, France, England and Scandinavia. He visited the United States and Canada before his death and left most pleasant memories of him here. Those who went to see him and his gracious wife, in their friendly home in Lund, found a generous and charming host. He was a gourmet nonpareil. He loved good food and vintage wines, which explains perhaps his indignation at the starvation of the diabetic patients of the period.

Petrén was said by those who studied under him to have been a forceful teacher. I can well believe it, recalling as I do an apt analogy he drew between the defenses of the body and those of a European state, in danger always of sudden invasion by a foreign power. The buffers of the blood, bicarbonates and phosphates, are like the standing army of the state, ready for battle at a moment's notice; the ammonia mechanism, whereby the fixed bases of the blood are preserved in long-standing ketogenic acidosis, like the army of reserves, takes time to mobilize. Also, just as the country's army of reserves, its national army when mobilized, takes over and permits the standing army to be brought back to former strength, so too the carbon dioxide combining power of the blood, though depleted in the early combat with accumulating keto-acids, again may be restored to normal levels when the rate of mobilization of ammonia has been sufficiently increased.

Petrén was a fervent advocate of international cooperation, especially in the world of science. Following World War I he labored mightily to bring together, as promptly as might be, the colleagues from the opposing sides in that dreadful conflict. He nevertheless was a nationalist at heart, the civilized type of nationalist. I well recall his enthusiastic pleasure at the rolling landscapes of southeastern Minnesota. "Just like Sweden," he would say. "I have seen nothing so lovely since I left my home."

Petrén's magnum opus, his "Diabetes-studier," a volume of 1000 pages, published in Copenhagen in 1923, with his assistants, Smith, Otterström, Odin and Malmros, with a foreword by B. Naunyn, stands as a landmark, as Naunyn expressed it there, between two eras of research on diabetes.

References

1. Newburgh, I. H., and Marsh, P. L.: The use of a high fat diet in the treatment of diabetes mellitus. Arch. Int. Med. 26:647–62, Dec. 1920.
2. Wilder, R. M., Boothby, W. M., and Beeler, Carol: Studies of the metabolism of diabetes. Jour. Biol. Chem. 51:311–57, April 1922.

in: *Diabetes 4 (1955) 159–160.*

Discovery of Insulin

On the History of the Discovery of Insulin

by JOSEPH H. PRATT

FREDERICH G. BANTING, a young surgeon, and CHARLES H. BEST, a medical student still in his preclinical years, worked in the summer and autumn of 1921 in the physiological laboratory of Professor J. J. R. MACLEOD at the University of Toronto in Canada. They worked together night and day. The task they had set themselves was to reveal the internal secretion of the pancreatic gland. They proceeded on the false assumption "that extracts of the pancreas usually contained powerful protein-splitting enzymes which split or destroy the products of an internal secretion that are simultaneously present". (1) This idea was shared by MACLEOD. They were unaware that HEIDENHAIN (2) had already, in 1875, demonstrated that extracts of the fresh pancreas possessed no proteolytic capacities. "The cells of the living pancreas," wrote Heidenhain, "contain no protein enzyme, but on the other hand a substance from which this may be formed under certain conditions (zymogen)".HEIDENHAIN had removed the pancreatic gland of an experimental animal immediately after sacrifice and divided it into two parts. One half was at once finely minced and a glycerin extract made from the tissue. The other half of the organ was left at room temperature for 24 hours before the glycerin extract was prepared. The first extract was absolutely inactive in a 1.2% solution of sodium bicarbonate, the second extraordinarily active as regards protein digestion. BAYLISS and STARLING (3) mention that HEIDENHAIN's experiments had been confirmed by LANGLEY (3): "Langley demonstrated that the proteolytic enzyme is present in the fresh gland, but not as an active enzyme, but as a precursor, trypsinogen". These authors further referred to investigations made by DELEZENNE and FROUIN (4) at the Pasteur Institute: pancreatic juice obtained via a cannula from the pancreatic duct, thus avoiding any contact with the small portion of mucous membrane forming the floor of the fistula, was completely trypsinfree. In Pawlow's experiment, however, where the pancreatic juice from the opening of the pancreatic duct runs over the mucosa, trypsin is formed from trypsinogen. According to Northrop,[1] the trypsinogen is gradually converted into trypsin in the pancreas. This happens through traces of trypsin which are present in the gland. This fact explains the positive result in HEIDENHAIN's experiments when the pancreas had been kept at room temperature for 24 hours.

On the wall of the laboratory in which BANTING and BEST had carried out their experiment is a plaque with the following inscription: On 30 October 1920, FREDERICK GRANT BANTING advanced the hypothesis that the inability to isolate the internal secretion of the pancreas was due to the fact that, during the extraction process, enzymes were liberated that destroyed the internal secretion (now known as insulin). In May 1921, BANTING and CHARLES HERBERT BEST, both members of the University of Toronto, performed in this room the experiment which ended in the isolation of insulin.

This inscription was reproduced without special comment in the pamphlet published by ELI LILLY & Co., the producers of insulin, in 1947 on the 25th anniversary of the discovery of insulin. Its text also appears in Dr. LLOYD STEVENSON's (5) authoritative biography, Sir FREDERICK BANTING, in 1946. His knowledge of the facts and respect for the truth compelled STEVENSON, despite his admiration for BANTING, to print under the reproduction of the plaque inscription the following sentence: The hypothesis mentioned was not confirmed by more exact investigation. STEVENSON then refers to a footnote he had made on another page: "The lytic enzymes of the pancreas must be activated in the intestine before they exert their destructive power." In another footnote, he states: "It has been shown since that even the islets, though to a lesser degree, undergo the same degenerative processes as occur in the rest of the gland, and that a gland whose excretory duct has been ligated actually contains fewer islets than a normal gland." Even MACLEOD, in his last article on insulin, published in 1929, refers to the extremely strong enzymes of the intact pancreas." (6) Textbooks of physiology, pathology and medicine still support BANTING's view that closure of the excretory ducts of the pancreas leads to destruction of the acini, but leaves the islets of LANGERHANS intact. In the 8th edition of the leading American textbook of medicine (7), published in 1951, there can be found, for example, the remark that "BANTING and BEST prepared an extract from the islet tissue of the pancreas

[1] Crystalline Enzymes. New York 1939, S. 80

after bringing about degeneration of that part of the gland which produces the tryptic enzyme by ligature of the pancreatic ducts. This extract eliminates all disturbances of carbohydrate metabolism in both pancreatectomized dogs and human diabetes". It is obvious that the magnitude of the discovery made in Toronto so dazzled the judgment of scientists that they accepted BANTING's premise without quibble. Had they tested it more exactly, they would have found that the two most careful studies of atrophy of the pancreas after ligature of the ducts clearly demonstrated that, after the performance of this procedure, on the one hand there developed a more or less severe destruction of the islets and, on the other hand, a considerable number of acini were preserved (MILNE and PETERS [8], F. M. ALLEN [9]). In a still older study (10), the author of these lines reported that after ligature of the pancreatic ducts in 4 dogs, no islets were to be found in the atrophic pancreas, but that, on the other hand, acini could very easily be demonstrated. These observations were checked and confirmed by Dr. FRANK B. MALLORY, the great authority on pathologic histology.

The only author to express in writing that BANTING's hypothesis was not confirmed is his co-worker, CHARLES H. BEST. In the BEAUMONT LECTURES (11), published in 1948, BEST asserted "that a success with the chemical and physiologic methods we then used could have been guaranteed, since active trypsin is not present in simple pancreatic extracts made by the methods originally used. That this is the case can very easily be demonstrated." BANTING died without it ever having been said to him publicly that he had tried in his experiments to destroy something that did not exist, namely, an active proteolytic enzyme in the fresh pancreas.

The inscription on the plaque in the Physiological Institute in Toronto contains yet another error. BANTING was not the first to advance the hypothesis that the internal secretion of the pancreas could be obtained after ligation of the excretory ducts, because the ligation produces degeneration of the acini of the gland and the chemical products of the islets were preserved unmixed with digestive enzymes. Even in 1902, SSOBOLEW wrote (12): "Now, however, we have in ligation of the excretory duct a means of isolating the islets from the anatomic paths and of studying the chemistry of these separated structures with exclusion of the digestive enzymes. However, this anatomic isolation of the islets also allows us to try out an organotherapy for diabetes in a rational manner."

LYDIA DE WITT at ANN ARBOR, in 1906, advanced the same hypothesis as BANTING 15 years later. On the idea that stimulated her to carry out her investigations, *Morphology and Physiology of Areas of Langerhans in some Vertebrates,* she writes: "As the experiments of SCHULZE and SSOBOLEW and other authors showed that ligature of the excretory duct and prevention of outflow of the pancreatic secretion produced complete atrophy of the acini of the gland, whereas the LANGERHANS' islets were isolated in large parts of the pancreas and the physiologic effect of its extract could be determined, our experiments were undertaken." E. L. SCOTT (14) started from similar ideas in 1912, when he began a series of experiments in CARLSON's laboratory in Chicago aimed at producing an active pancreatic extract. He expected that the atrophy of the gland which developed after complete ligature of the ducts would elevate the formation of the digestive enzymes. But after numerous experiments on dogs, which, as far as complete atrophy of the gland was concerned, proved unsuccessful, this method was abandoned as impractical. The Toronto researchers were aware of SCOTT's work. They regarded the fact that SCOTT had extracted the pancreas with alcohol as extraordinarily important as, in their view, the alcohol destroyed the action of the proteolytic enzymes.

One must do MACLEOD justice, and acknowledge that other important American physiologists were also wrongly convinced that active proteolytic enzymes are present in the normal fresh pancreas. SCOTT, and also his chief CARLSON, shared this belief. SCOTT writes that "these enzymes are immediately rendered ineffective by high per cent alcohol." Professor JOHN R. MURLIN (15), of the University of Rochester, was also of the opinion that the action of the enzymes must be excluded. He and his coworkers extracted the pancreas with strong hydrochloric acid "with the idea of destroying the trypsin."

A number of researchers have demonstrated that simple ligation of the pancreatic ducts does not lead to permanent digestive disorders or to atrophy of the gland. PRATT, LAMSON and MARKS (16) demonstrated that the negative results have their source in the activation of the pancreatic juice by the necrotic tissue in the vicinity of the ligatures. The activated pancreatic juice digests the adjacent tissue and a new connexion is formed between the pancreas and the intestine. This connexion permits the re-entry of the pancreatic juice into the intestine. If this process were prevented, by permanently displacing a section of omentum between pancreas and intestine, marked weight-loss of the experimental animals developed and bulky stools were produced, whose cause was the poor absorption of fat and protein. A dog sacrificed two months after exclusion of the pancreatic juice from the bowel had a pancreas which "was converted into a small, shrunken, very hard, nodular, almost horny mass." The mid-section of the gland and the uncinate process consisted of a mass of tissue 3 cm long, 2 cm wide and 1.5 cm thick, embedded and fused with the duodenum. Surely, very little tissue juice could be obtained from such an atrophic pancreas, at most 1–2 ccm. When BANTING and BEST claim to have extracted 125 cm of tissue juice from the pancreas of a dog whose excretory ducts had been ligated for 10 weeks, they were providing a convincing proof that they were not working with an atrophied gland. It must actually be assumed that, essentially, BANTING and BEST were extracting normal tissue. It would therefore be expected that an extract of the fresh normal pancreas would produce as marked a fall in the blood-sugar as an extract from one of their "atrophic" glands. That this is the case can be shown from the figures published by BANTING and BEST themselves. The following review has been compiled from their own tables (17):

It emerges very significantly from these figures that the extract from the normal gland had just as much effect on the blood-

Pancreatectomized dog

	Blood-sugar	Blood-sugar-reduction mg %	Intravenous injection of
15 August			
noon	300	70	10 ccm extract from degenerated pancreas
1 p.m.	230		
16. August			
10 a.m.	300	120	10 ccm extract from degenerated pancreas in 0,1 % solution HCl
11 a.m.	180		
17 August			
6 p.m.	300	130	10 ccm extract from normal gland
7 p.m.	170		
18 August			
midnight	220	70	10 ccm extract from normal gland in 0,1 % solution HCl
4 a.m.	150		

sugar as did the extract from the so-called "degenerated" gland. How BANTING could consider his own figures and then conclude "that it is obvious from the table that the extract from the normal gland is much weaker than that from the atrophied gland" is altogether puzzling. Already in December 1922, ROBERTS (18), of the Physiology Department of Cambridge University, pointed out in a letter to the Editor of the *British Medical Journal* that the only reasonable conclusions that could be drawn from BANTING's tables were the following: 1) the normal gland is more effective than the degenerated, 2) the extract of the normal gland has a longer-lasting effect than the extract of the degenerated gland.

The Toronto researchers believed that SCOTT was the first to have treated the intact pancreas with alcohol. They were not aware of the older works of ZÜLZER (19, 20, 21), who attempted to extract the antidiabetic agent from the pancreas with alcohol. In two experiments on pancreatictomized dogs and in 8 cases of human diabetes, ZÜLZER showed that his preparation reduced sugar excretion and acidosis. However, the preparation also had toxic effects, which ZÜLZER described in detail. When his first article appeared in 1907, the editor remarked in a footnote that he had held back the publication for three years at the request of the author. Obviously, ZÜLZER had prolonged this delay in the hope that he would be in a position to write in his article that he had, in the meantime, produced a nontoxic preparation for the treatment of diabetes. He was doubtless on the right track. But although the outstanding help of his colleagues at the Berlin Physiological Institute and the support of the experienced chemists of SCHERING & Co. had been available to him for four years, he could not reduce the toxicity of his preparation sufficiently to make it suitable for clinical purposes. In 1909, FORSCHBACH (22), from MINKOWSKI's clinic in Breslau, demonstrated the striking antidiabetic effect of the preparation in a panreatectomized dog. In the 12 hours in which the urine was collected before the injection of the "hormone", total sugar excretion was 16.4 g and the quotient D/N was 3.6. In the 12 hours after injection the sugar excretion fell to 1.3 g and the D/N quotient to 0.31. However, the temperature rose to 39.2°C. The preparation made by SCHERING was then given to two diabetic patients. In the first case, in which a 16-day-old product was used, no effect at all was seen. In the second case the temperature rose to 40°C and the patient was unable to urinate for 12 hours. After this unpleasant episode the use of the preparation was completely abandoned in MINKOWSKI's clinic and I have found no further reports in the German literature or elsewhere. The marked toxicity of the preparation is probably to be ascribed to the lytic products of protein, peptones and albumoses produced by autolysis.

When BANTING (22) reported to the New Haven Convention of the American Physiological Society on the results of his work, carried out with BEST during the previous seven months, he was in a position to show that they had prepared pancreatic extracts which restored the blood-sugar of pancreatectomized dogs to normal levels, and eliminated sugar excretion and acidosis. At this time, BANTING and BEST had not yet given their preparation to patients. When this was tried some weeks later in a small number of diabetics, fever developed and aseptic abscesses formed at the injection sites, so that use of the extract had to be abandoned. BANTING and BEST were thus producing a pancreatic extract which was no more successful in the tratment of diabetes than that of ZÜLZER four years before them. In fact, in his Cameron Prize Lecture at Edinburgh in 1929, BANTING (24) gave generous praise by admitting that the first results of ZÜLZER with diabetics were better than those of BEST and himself. This was a misleading statement, since both ZÜLZER's and BANTING's extracts were so toxic as not to be admissible for the treatment of human diabetes.

In December 1921, Professor MACLEOD enlarged his group by adding the biochemist JAMES B. COLLIP. COLLIP (26, 27) had only been engaged in the work for a few weeks when he accidentally poured a clear weak alcoholic extract of fresh pancreas into 4–5 volumes of 95% and absolute alcohol. A precipitate formed and this precipitate was assayed. It emerged that it contained the internal secretion of the pancreas and was to the greatest part free from toxic products. The toxic substances had dissolved in the alcohol. This preparation was the first insulin to be used successfully in the treatment of diabetics and gave the Toronto workers well-earned great renown. When its success was reported to the Congress of American Physicians in May 1922, FREDERICK M. ALLEN (25), whose laboratory studies of diabetes and its treatment were probably more extensive than those of any other scientist, stated in the discussion of this epoch-making report: "Others have reduced glycosuria and hyperglycemia with pancreatic extracts. I have done so myself. But the obvious reason why these experiments proved nothing is the great toxicity of such extracts, so that the animals that received them were injured and not improved, and the blood-sugar reduction ascribed to the toxicity. If, as seems to be the case, the Toronto workers have obtained the internal secretion of the pancreas free from toxic material, they possess without doubt the priority for one of the greatest achievements of modern medicine."

What the group of Berlin chemists and physiologists could not achieve in 4 years, namely to rid the internal secretion of the pancreas from contaminating toxic products to such an extent that it could be used in the treatment of diabetes, was achieved by the Canadian chemists in a few weeks. The success overwhelmed COLLIP so completely that neither he nor his coworkers MACLEOD, BANTING and BEST recognized the great significance of his discovery. What COLLIP had discovered was that the precipitation of insulin from a weak alcoholic solution with absolute alcohol freed the extract from impurities, and thereby made possible for the first time the preparation of a product which could be successfully used in the treatment of diabetes. Credit for the discovery belongs to the Torontoans BANTING, BEST, COLLIP and MACLEOD, who worked together as a close-knit team. Each one of them made an important contribution. As one of his biographers says, BANTING was "the captain of the team".

It was BANTING's conviction that an internal secretion could be obtained from the pancreas that stimulated COLLIP to participate in the work. But it must be expressly emphasized that it was COLLIP who first produced an extract of the pancreas which contained the internal secretion and freed it sufficiently from toxic products that it could be used successfully in the management of the sugar disease.

References

1. BANTING, F. G., BEST, C. H., COLLIP, J. B., CAMPBELL, W. R., FLETCHER, A. A., MACLEOD, J. J. R., and NOBLE, E. C., The Effect Produced on Diabetes by Extractions of Pancreas. Transact. Ass. Amer. Physicians, 37:337, 1922.
2. HEIDENHAIN, R., Beiträge zur Kenntnis des Pankreas. Arch. Physiol., Bonn 10:557, 1875.
3. BAYLISS, W. and STARLING, E. H., The Proteolytic Activities of the Pancreatic Juice. J. Physiology, 30:61, 1903–04.
4. DÉLÉZENNE, C. and. FROUIN, A., La sécrétion physiologique du pancréas ne possède pas d'action digestive propre vis-á-vis de l'albumine. Compt. rend. Soc. Biol., Paris 691, 1902.
5. STEVENSON, L., Sir Frederick Banting. Toronto 1946. pp. 67n, 68n, 74.
6. MACLEOD, J. J. R., Insulin. Encyclopedia Britannica. 14. Edit. 12:451.

7. CECIL, R. L. and LOEB, R. F., A Textbook of Medicine. Philadelphia 1951. p. 615.
8. MILNE, L. S. and PETERS, H. L., Atrophy of the Pancreas after Occlusion of the Pancreatic Duct. J. Med. Res., Boston 26:405, 1912.
9. ALLEN, F. M., Studies Concerning Glycosuria and Diabetes. Boston 1913.
10. PRATT, J. H., The Relation of the Pancreas to Diabetes. J. Amer. Med. Ass. 55:2112, 1910.
11. BEST, C. H., Diabetes and Insulin and Lipotropic Factors. The Beaumont Lecture. Springfield, Ill. 1948.
12. SSOBOLEW, L. W., Zur normalen und pathologischen Morphologie der inneren Secretion der Bauchspeicheldrüse. Virchows Arch. path. Anat. 168:122, 1902.
13. DE WITT, L. M., Morphology and Physiology of Areas of Langerhans in some Vertebrates. J. Exper. Med. 8:193, 1906.
14. SCOTT, E. L., On the Influence of Intravenous Injections of an Extract of the Pancreas on Experimental Diabetes. Am J. Physiol. 29:306, 1912.
15. MURLIN, J. R., CLOUGH, H. D., GIBBS, C. B. F., and STOKES, A. M., Aquecous Extracts of Pancreas. I. Influence on the Carbohydrate Metabolism of Depancreatized Animals. J. Biol. Chem. Baltimore 56:253, 1923.
16. PRATT, J. H., LAMSON, P. D., and MARK, H. K., The Effect of Excluding Pancreatic Juice from the Intestines. Transact. Ass. Amor. Physicians 24:266, 1909.
17. BANTING, F. G. and BEST, C. H., The Internal Secretion of the Pancreas. J. Laborat. Clin. Med., S. Louis 7:251, 1922.
18. ROBERTS, F., Insulin. Brit. Med. J. 2:1193, Dec. 16, 1922.
19. ZUELZER, G., Experimentelle Untersuchungen über den Diabetes. Berliner klin. Wschr. 474, 1907.
20. ZUELZER, G., Über Versuche einer spezifischen Fermenttherapie des Diabetes. Zschr. exper. Path., Berlin 5:307, 1908.
21. ZUELZER, G., DOHRN, M. and MARXER, A., Neuere Untersuchungen über den experimentellen Diabetes. Dtsch. med. Wschr. 34, 1380, 1908.
22 FORSCHBACH, J., Versuche zur Behandlung des Diabetes Mellitus mit dem Zuelzerscher Pancreas Hormone. Dtsch. med. Wschr. 2053, 1909.
23. BANTING, F. G., BEST, C. H. and MACLEOD, J. J. R., The Internal Secretion of the Pancreas. Amer. J. Physiol. 59:479, 1922.
24. BANTING, F. G., The History of Insulin. Edingburg Med. J. 36:1, 1929.
25. ALLEN, F. M., Discussion of paper by Banting et al. Transact. Ass. Amer. Physicians 37:337, 1922.
26. COLLIP, J. B., The History of the Discovery of Insulin. Northw. Med. 22:267, 1923.
27. COLLIP, J. B., Frederick Grant Banting. The Scientific Monthly 55:472, 1941.

in: *Sudhoff's Archiv 38 (1954) 48–57.*

Problems of Priority in the Discovery of Insulin

by Eric Martin

Summary

The 50th anniversary of Banting's and Best's discovery of insulin will be celebrated this year. Although the Canadian physicians demonstrated the hypoglycemic effect of a pancreatic extract further purified by J. B. Collip, and introduced its use in the treatment of human diabetes, contemporary research elsewhere was approaching the same results. A Rumanian physiologist, Paulesco, had prepared a pancreatic extract which lowered blood sugar, urea and ketone bodies in the diabetic animal. Due to unfavorable circumstances this author was unable to employ a purified extract in diabetic humans. Since the discovery of insulin will be revived this year, it will be the occasion to redress the injustice done to the Rumanian physiologist.

It is exceptional in the 20th century for an important scientific discovery to have been the work of one man. Generally, it is the result of the work of a team inspired by very many preceding studies. Nevertheless, a basic idea is required and someone to bring it to life. The problem is posed, the idea is in the air; some individual or small team will go further than the precursors and will exploit a discovery to its consequences and applications before anyone else.

Such was the case with the discovery of insulin, attributed to Banting and Best, but which had been preceded by many approximative studies. A Scottish physician, Ian Murray, tells us this exciting story just as we are about to celebrate the fiftieth anniversary of the discovery of the Canadian doctors.

We have received from Professor I. Pavel of Bucharest a letter and documents which stress the merits of his compatriot Paulesco in this matter without possibility of denial. Let us blaze the trail that led to the discovery of insulin.

PAUL LANGERHANS, in 1869, revealed the existence within the pancreas of cellular islets to which LAGUESSE gave the name of islets of LANGERHANS in 1893, suspecting that these structures had a special function differing from that of the acinous glands.

Various observations in the 19th century drew attention to the possible relation between diabetes and a disorder of the pancreas, observations based particularly on cases where the diabetes was associated with lithiasis of the pancreatic duct and sclerosis of the gland. But long before, as far back as 1682, a Swiss, J. C. BRUNNER, had shown that massive extirpation of the pancreas in the dog was accompanied by polyuria and intense thirst.

But it was the experiments of MINKOWSKI and MERING in 1889 which advanced our knowledge: total extirpation of the pancreas in the dog led to diabetes with a fatal outcome after a few weeks, but MINKOWSKI showed that an isolated pancreatic graft protected the operated animal from diabetes.

In the following years, two lines of research emerged:

What was the origin of the islets? Could they originate by transformation of the acinous cells and what was the condition of the islets in human diabetes? Could diabetes be influenced by pancreatic extracts? Many attempts were made, with disappointing or confusing results. In fact, these extracts caused local reactions at the site of injection, general reactions, particularly fever, and ill-understood manifestations which could in some cases have been due to hypoglycemia. The difficulty in interpreting the "toxic" manifestation secondary to the injection of pancreatic extracts is easily understood in view of the inadequacy of the methods used to determine the blood-sugar; they were unreliable, and also they required considerable amounts of blood (50 ml) which limited the repetition of sampling in the experimental animal.

It is certain that in 1908 L. G. ZUELZER obtained very promising results by injection of a pancreatic extract, first in the pancreatectomized animal and then in some diabetic patients, but the treatment could not be pursued because of toxic reactions and a lack of available extract. After two years of research a purified extract was prepared but unfortunately an approach to the chemical industry did not secure commercialization of the product. However this may be, ZUELZER may be considered as one of the first to have obtained a positive result, insufficient as it was.

Other experimenters, including E. L. SCOTT (1912), rightly convinced that the digestive enzymes destroyed the antidiabetic factor, sought to destroy the exocrine part of the gland by ligature of WIRSUNG's duct so as to be able to extract the hormone causing hypoglycemia. If the atrophy was incomplete, the residual acini were destroyed with concentrated alcohol. Unfortunately, the alcoholic extract seemed to inhibit the hypoglycemic effect. It was at this time that a Rumanian physiologist, PAULESCO, became interested in the problem. He had previously made his name by developing a technique of hypophysectomy which was used by HARVEY CUSHING, the neurosurgical pioneer. PAULESCO's studies of the pancreas were interrupted by the occupation of Bucharest by enemy armies in 1916, and he was unable to publish his results until 1921.

In June 1921, at the Rumanian Biological Association, PAULESCO presented a communication published in the Reports of the French Society of Biology.[1] He described the consequences of pancreatectomy in the dog: hyperglycemia, hyperazotemia and increase of ketone bodies in the blood and urine, and showed that his pancreatic extract, injected into the jugular vein, reduced or suppressed the hyperglycemia and diminished the levels of urea and acetone in the blood and urine. The effect of the extract began immediately after the injection, was maximal after 2 hours and continued for about 12 hours. The hypoglycemic action of the pancreatic extract varies with the amount of gland used as primary material. In the normal dog, the extract produced a noticeable reduction of blood-sugar and of blood and urinary urea.

A second publication in the August 1921 number of the *Archives Internationales de Physiologie* (manuscript received 22 June) reported the same experiments more thoroughly and gave instructions on the preparation of the extract. Similar effects were not obtained by an intravenous injection of normal saline, nor by an intravenous injection of an extract derived from another organ than the pancreas, nor by an intraspinal injection of a solution of nuclein and soda, which caused a febrile attack. The anti-diabetic *hormone* was called by PAULESCO *pancreatin*. The pancreatic extract could not be given in man by injection as it produced a local reaction and fever; it was inactive by the oral or rectal route.

It is beyond denial that PAULESCO was the first to provide an exemplary demonstration of the antidiabetic and antiketogenic effect of a pancreatic extract. Because of the war, and for lack of

---

[1] C. R. Soc. Biol. (Paris) 85, 555–559 (1921)

the necessary support to pursue his study, his work was largely forgotten.

It was at this time that the Canadian authors began their studies. BANTING, a Canadian surgeon with few patients, had learned of a paper by MOSES BARRON of Minneapolis, entitled: "The relation of the islets of LANGERHANS to diabetes, with special reference to cases of pancreatic lithiasis". This idea haunted him and he was fortunate enough to be admitted as an assistant into the laboratory of Professor J. J. MACLEOD, an eminent biochemist specializing in diabetes. The original idea was as follows: it was the external secretion of the pancreas which destroyed that of the islets, so it was necessary to get rid of the exocrine part of the gland and preserve the islets. Thanks to an excellent operative technique, BANTING ligatured the pancreatic duct and obtained complete atrophy of the exocrine gland while preserving the integrity of the islets. To pursue the biochemical part of his study, he was able to rely on a young physiologist whom MACLEOD assigned to him, CHARLES BEST. In June 1959, BEST related the history of this fruitful collaboration to the Royal Society under the title: "A Canadian trail of medical research".

It was a happy combination of circumstances: an idea in the air – that the islets of LANGERHANS have some connexion with diabetes; a skilled operator, BANTING, concerned to prevent the inhibitory action of the digestive part of the gland on the islets; a somewhat sceptical but highly qualified chief, MACLEOD, who made his laboratory available and provided the young and enthusiastic biochemical collaborator whom BANTING needed.

BEST began his collaboration with BANTING on 17 May 1921, the day after finishing his examination in physiology and biochemistry; he was 22. For 8 months they developed the extraction of the pancreatic hormone from the gland of the dog, then of the adult or fetal ox. Ligature of the duct proved unnecessary.

The first results were produced at the Medical Faculty of Toronto on 14 November 1921: the protocol showed an unquestionable effect of 30 ml of pancreatic extract on the glycemia in the pancreatectomized dog. The hypoglycemia so produced was corrected by the injection of glucose. The product was called *isletin*, a term replaced by *insulin* at MACLEOD's instance.

These results were communicated in a preliminary note to the American Society of Physiology at Christmas 1921. To comply with the rules of the Society, MACLEOD added his name to those of BANTING and BEST, who, in their turn in 1922, related their discovery in an article that appeared in the *Journal of Laboratory* and Clinical Medicine in February 1922.[2] This was a very complete study, entitled "The internal secretion of the pancreas". The essential conclusions corresponded exactly to those noted by PAULESCO the year before.

The discovery of BANTING and BEST soon became known and patients flocked, but the experimenters hesitated because the most active extract seemed that derived from the pancreas of the fetal calf. The effects in man were sometimes dramatic, inconstant and accompanied by toxic manifestations. The first use of the pancreatic extract in a diabetic was in January 1922. The patient was a boy aged 12 whose diabetes had appeared a year before. The effect of the injection on the hyperglycemia was favorable, but the subcutaneous reaction was such that the treatment had to be discontinued.

With the help of an eminent biochemist, J. B. COLLIP, who worked with MACLEOD at Toronto, the extract was purified and its production developed. It was COLLIP's essential merit to have developed a purified extract that could be used in the treatment of human diabetes.

By 1922, several physicians were using the product around the world: DALE, MINKOWSKI, FRASER, etc. BEST obtained a miraculous result in a case of diabetic coma and employed the treatment for a young patient who was still alive 37 years later. Enthusiasm ran high in every medical center and a contact was made between BEST and the ELI LILLY Company. The manufacture of insulin, still difficult and expensive, was well on the way. The progress made since in developing the range of insulins required to balance the different types of diabetics is well-known.

It is time to ask the expected question: Were BANTING and BEST aware of PAULESCO's work, consistent with but preceding theirs?

Certainly, since they referred to it in their report of February 1922 in the following terms: "PAULESCO has recently demonstrated the effect of a total extract of pancreatic gland on the levels of sugar, urea and ketone bodies in the blood and urine of the animal made diabetic". Then they continued: "PAULESCO has established that injection of the extract produces *no effect if it is given into the peripheral vein*, and that a second injection has a lesser effect than the first".

This was an absolutely erroneous interpretation by the Canadian authors of the Rumanian experiments. As there was no question of doubting the good faith of BANTING and BEST, Profes-

---

[2] J. Lab. clin. Med. 7, 251–266 (1922)

sor PAVEL of Bucharest wrote to BEST to ask for an explanation of this misleading quotation of the work of his compatriot. We have a copy of the reply from BEST, a sympathetic and loyal personality beyond all others. He replied to Professor PAVEL: "I very much regret that there was an error in our translation of Professor PAULESCO's article. I cannot recollect after this length of time exactly what happened. As it was almost fifty years ago I do not remember whether we relied on our own poor French or whether we had a translation made."

Thus, probably due to an ignorance of French, the achievement of the Rumanian author was reduced to zero.

In 1923, not without difficulty, the Nobel Prize was awarded jointly to BANTING and MACLEOD for their discovery of insulin, a decision that was not accepted by the laureates, BANTING giving half the amount of his prize to BEST and MACLEOD doing the same for Collip.

BANTING had been the instigator of the research, MACLEOD the well-known personality, director of the laboratory where the research was carried out; he had attached his name to the first report of the preliminary results. COLLIP had engaged in the tentative measures necessary to the purification of a poorly tolerated extract and gone on to the first trials in man. BEST had been BANTING's collaborator from the start. They had all deserved well of science and humanity.

But in this list of discoverers the merits of PAULESCO were passed over silently. Now, if we accept, according to statements in the notebook of BEST and BANTING, that on 30 July 1921 they obtained a reduction in the blood-sugar of the dog by means of injection of a pancreatic extract, we must also note that in June of the same year PAULESCO had already presented a very well-documented communication to the Rumanian Biological Association and sent an important report to the *Archives Internationales de Physiologie*.

Thus, it is not correct to write, as did N. S. PAPASPYROS in *The History of Diabetes Mellitus*,[3] "With the precious liquid BANTING and BEST succeeded on the 30th July 1921, for the first time in the history of diabetes, in lowering the level of blood-sugar by giving the diabetic organism the hormone which controls carbohydrate metabolism." For PAULESCO had obtained the same result previously.

[3] Georg Thieme Verlag, Stuttgart 1964

If we compare the techniques employed by the Canadian authors, on the one hand, and Paulesco on the other, we can make the following remarks: The pancreatectomy was made by Paulesco without any previous maneuver, but at Toronto after ligature of the pancreatic duct to produce atrophy of the exocrine gland. This technique was not subsequently adhered to. Preparation of the extract was made by mincing the gland and adding normal saline in the ice-box. The solution was neutral and active in intravenous injections, but provoked toxic manifestations; it reduced the glycemia and the glycosuria diminished as well as the levels of blood and urinary urea and the acetonuria. Note that Paulesco used Pflüger's method to estimate the blood-sugar, which required 25 ml of blood, while Best had at his disposal the Lewis-Benedict technique which required only 0.2 ml of blood, which facilitated repeated sampling and allowed monitoring in man.

To sum up: If we adhere to the chronology of events, it is certain that Paulesco obtained an insulinic effect in the pancreatectomized dog before the Toronto team, and that his experiments were conducted and interpreted in an irreproachable manner. It is probable that positive results had been obtained before him, but were difficult of interpretation.

The success of the Toronto team lies in having led to the elaboration of an insulin usable in man, which has allowed the survival of millions of diabetics.

At a time when we are preparing to celebrate the 50th anniversary of the discovery of insulin, it is right and proper, without detracting from the merits of Banting and Best, that we should stress the cardinal importance of the discovery of Paulesco, a discovery known to the Canadian physicians but poorly interpreted by them, with the result that the determinative studies of the Rumanian physiologist have been left in the shade.

References

1. Scot. med. J. 14, 286 (1969)
2. C. R. Soc, Biol. (Paris) 85, 555–559 (1921)
3. Arch. int. Physiol. 17, 85–109 (1921)
4. J. Endocr. 19, I–XVII (1959)
5. J. Lab. clin. Med. 7, 251–266 (1922)

in: *Schweizerische Medizinische Wochenschrift 101 (1971) 164–167*

Right and Wrong Avenues of Exploration in German Insulin Research

by PAULA DRÜGEMÖLLER and LEO NORPOTH

The history of German insulin research is permeated by something of the fatefulness of ancient tragedy. Promising high points are often followed by peripeteia and finally not only is there no happy ending but, if you like, the battle of the gods still goes on even then. The various stages in insulin research have been described elsewhere (23, 36, 39, 49, 52, 68), but neither the reasons for the German failure nor the tragic elements in this have been appreciated.

In their search for insulin Banting and Best found four preconditions:

1. that diabetes is a disease of the pancreas (as had been recognized since the classic pancreas extirpation experiments of v. Mering and Minkowski (41));

2. that the special function of the pancreas is the production of an internal secretion (as had been demonstrated by the transplantation experiments of Minkowski (44,45), the parabiotic experiments of Forschbach (16, 17) and the vessel anastomosis experiments of Hédon (24));

3. that the site at which the secretion is formed is related to the islets of Langerhans (which few still doubted following the anatomic studies after ligation of the pancreatic duct carried out by Schulze (66) and Ssobolew (67)), and

4. that the active product of the islets is inactivated by the external secretion of the pancreas (since experience had shown that the enteral administration of pancreatic- or islet-extracts was always ineffective).

Banting was stimulated to take up this field of research through a study by Barron (7) who was able to show, on the basis of pancreatic duct lithiasis corresponding to the ligation experiments of Schulze (66) and Ssobolew (67), that the glandular parenchyma atrophied whereas the islets remained intact, and that as long as the islets were intact no diabetes developed. Although basically this study did not conribute anything new, yet it pointed the way to the design of the first experiment. In collaboration with Best (3, 4, 5, 6), Banting ligated the excretory ducts of the pancreas in dogs; after atrophy of the glands he made up extracts with Ringer's solution which, after intravenous injection into dogs with pancreatic diabetes brought about a fall in the blood-sugar and regression of the glycosuria and ketonuria. Later, in 1921, he used the pancreas of calf embryos to make up the extracts, since Ibrahim (27) had shown that up to the 4th month the acini are not yet sufficiently developed to secrete trypsin. Extraction with alcohol and slight acidification also proved particularly useful; as a result of further refinements in the extraction process and, following a suggestion of Macleod (40), the use of extracts made up from the islet apparatus of selachian fishes, where this is localized separately from the pancreas, things had progressed so far by 1922 that insulin, as the extract was called following de Meyer (42), was given to patients for the first time with convincing results.

The preconditions used as a working hypothesis by Banting and Best were meagre. This forces one to ask the question therefore of why, following the pancreas extirpation experiments of v. Mering and Minkowski in 1889 which clearly demonstrated the significance of the pancreas in the pathogenesis of diabetes, it still took 30 years before insulin was isolated? We shall be examining the German contribution to this research in particular here, especially since the initial foundations for this area of research were laid by German investigators.

The first attempts made to try and influence diabetes through oral pancreas administration, following the discoveries of v. Mering and Minkowski, were a failure. This avenue was explored in happy anticipation of being successful, since it had just become known that hypofunctioning of the thyroid gland could be treated through oral thyroid administration.

– Thesen and Lauritzen (69) reported very good results, but these were mainly due to an effective diet. Lüthje (38), Sandmeyer (64), and Pflüger (55) did not achieve any therapeutic success, and nor did Goldscheider (22) with keratinized pancreatic tablets. With oral medication the pancreas itself destroys its active principle.

Looking back today one would think that this mode of administration would very soon have been given up because of its lack of efficacy. And yet one finds reports on oral organ therapy of diabetes up to 1922 and even after this date. In 1909 Vahlen

(72) had produced the zymogenic enzyme "Metabolin" from the pancreas and had allegedly used this with good results. Later Vahlen (73) was able to obtain the same effective enzyme from yeast and in 1921 Loening (37, 74) was still reporting good results. It could be confirmed that this enzyme led to improved digestive activity, but other authors did not observe any antidiabetic action. The hypothetical basis for their work was the theory postulated in 1890 by Lepine (33), which assumed that in diabetes glycolysis was disordered due to the absence of pancreatic activity. As Macleod (39) and his pupils were able to show, however, the site of action of insulin is not the glycolysis in the blood.

The initially hopeful experiments of Cohnheim (12, 13, 14, 15) from 1903 to 1906 therefore also had to come to nothing. In his search for a glycolytic enzyme in the expressed muscle juice he observed a considerable amount of sugar disappear through the addition of pancreatic extract so that it could no longer be demonstrated through reduction. Since the glucose could also be demonstrated after heating and alcohol-treatment of the pancreatic juice, Cohnheim considered that the active product was not an enzyme but rather an internal secretion. Since the experiments did not always succeed he expressed the possibility that the external secretion might upset the internal secretion. With a view to the therapeutic possibilities which he expected in the treatment of diabetes he took out a patent for his extraction process. – Claus and Embden (28, 29) were unable to completely confirm these experiments of Cohnheim however. In 1903 de Meyer (43) and also Hirsch (26) similarly found a more than 100% increase in glucose after the addition of pancreatic extract. Later, from 1909 to 1912, Levene and Meyer (35) were able to establish that this in no way consisted of a glycolysis, but rather of a polymerization of the glucose through lactic acid and that the reducing property was lost through this. – The problem of glycolysis and the search for the glycolytic enzyme took up a grat deal of research effort for almost 10 years, from 1902 to 1912, before it was realized that this was the wrong approach.

Minkowski (45) was the first to carry out experiments with the injection of pancreatic extracts in animals with pancreatic diabetes. He observed severe necroses at the injection sites due to his extract with physiological saline solution however, so that the excretion of sugar was secondarily reduced. The glycerin extracts, expressed juices and sodium chloride extracts of

Goldschneider (22) and Fürbringer (19) proved to be ineffective, and the foreign authors Gley and Thiroloix (21), Hale and White (75), and Hédon (25) reported the same. The results of the Italians Caparolli (11), Vanni (71) and Battistini (8) were somewhat more encouraging, but they did not stand up to Pflüger's verification and criticism (57, 58).

Blumenthal (10) was the first to come close to the active principle in 1898. He produced pancreatic expressed juices which he treated with alcohol to remove the proteins, whereby he unintentionally inactivated the trypsin as well. When injected into diabetic animals and people this extract distinctly increased assimilation, but could not be generally used because of the development of necroses at the injection sites. – Although Blumenthal assessed his experiments very optimistically, no further investigations were carried out either by him or stimulated by his work. He finally gave up.

Leschke's (34) attempts at the treatment of diabetes with a pancreatic extract in 1910 were very discouraging. Although he clearly recognized that only the continuous administration of pancreatic extract promised to be successful, and also thought of the possibility that the external secretion might disturb the internal secretion, he did not observe a decrease but rather an increase in the excretion of sugar through his heated pancreatic extract. He was then completely sceptical about the internal secretion of the pancreas – and in this he was a true pupil of Pflüger – and considered that organ therapy was hopeless. Zuelzer (76) had commenced his experiments two years before the work done by Leschke. After adrenaline-diabetes had become known in 1906 through Blum (9) he based his work on the assumption of an antagonism between the function of the adrenals and of the pancreas. He worked with calves' pancreas which was removed at the height of digestion after ligature of the veins for one hour, in order to achieve maximally optimal accumulation of the active substance. From this he prepared an extract which he treated with alcohol, thereby removing the protein and inactivating the trypsin. This extract led to a considerable improvement in an adrenaline-glycosuria and a dog with pancreatic diabetes for some time. Zuelzer now allowed this preparation to be tested clinically by Forschbach at the recognized centre, at the Minkowski clinic. Forschbach (18) was able to confirm the decrease in the excretion of sugar and in the ketonuria. The patients exhibited very severe symptoms of intoxication however with attacks of shivering, fever, a racing pulse, vomiting and sweating attacks. The toxic symptoms were alarming in some patients so that Forschbach understandably rejected the idea of its clinical use for fear of even worse effects, but without doubting the antidiabetic active substance itself. Following the publication of the work of Abderhalden (1) on protein chemistry, his chemical colleague Camille Reuter (62) was able to produce a protein-free insulin in 1914. After the laboratory experiments had been completed Reuter undertook the first processing of the material at the Hoffmann–La Roche company, but he altered the extraction process a little here. The preparation obtained induced convulsions in dogs so that it was thought that a convulsant had also been extracted. Retrospectively, Zuelzer (77) believed that this reaction was hypoglycemic in nature. No checks on the blood-sugar were reported. With the start of the first world war no further studies were carried out.

Zuelzer experienced a second misfortune however. He knew about the islet apparatus being in a separate localization in selachian fishes and, with the intention of producing extracts from these islets which would not be under the influence of the trypsin and steapsin and then investigating these, he applied to the Berlin faculty to grant him the Countess Bose endowment for the necessary work in Naples. He did not receive it.

Zuelzer had certainly had insulin in his hands, and a preparation which could have been used therapeutically would undoubtedly have been developed soon after the first reports if more attention had been paid to the intensive study of laboratory experiments than to the trials in patients. Zuelzer did not recognize the hypoglycemic complex of symptoms, even though sufficiently reliable blood-sugar determinations were available by this time (2). He also carried out blood-sugar determinations, but with no systematic approach. The toxicity of his preparations was caused first of all by the content of protein substances, and later by their efficacy itself – which became all too good. In addition there was the fact that the recognized authority in Germany, Minkowski, had a very cautious attitude to Zuelzer's experiments. No lucky star watched over Zuelzer's work; he did not have any fortunate Toronto coalition. It is understandable therefore that he was bitter when Banting and Best, Macleod and Collip received the Nobel prize in 1923.

As early as 1905 the Frenchman Gley (20) and in 1910/11 E. Scott (65) had already come close to discovering insulin. Like Banting and Best they prepared extracts from atrophic pancreatic glands. Gley observed very favorable results with such an extract. No further investigations were carried out because of other research work however. He deposited his observation in a sealed letter with the Societé de Biologie and allowed it to be opened when the first reports came from Toronto. Scott had already observed very favorable results with pancreas soaked in alcohol which he concentrated by evaporation in a vacuum and then produced an aqueous solution from this. He was satisfied with this but he himself doubted whether this extract contained the hormone.

Rennie and Fraser (61) obtained extracts from the isolated islet apparatus of selachian fishes for the first time in 1907, but unfortunately they administered these orally. In the single experiment with injection of the extract they observed no effect. – The experiments set up by Murlin and Kramer (50, 51) from 1913 to 1916 also came close to grasping insulin. Murlin was kept from further study of this by his military service. Kleiner and Meltzer (30, 31, 32) in 1915 and Paulesco (54) in 1921 also observed good antidiabetic results, but these preparations showed marked toxicity.

Not all of those who were involved in the search for insulin can be mentioned in this report. Nevertheless one is struck by their small number, with the exception of those who were involved in this during the first years after the discovery of pancreatic diabetes. As Macleod (39) once reported, since 1910 and the reports of Zuelzer and Forschbach and following the very critical investigation of Leschke, who belonged to the school of Pflüger, things had come to such a pass that it was no longer generally believed that diabetes could be treated through organ therapy. The question forces itself upon us here of whether it might not have been the influence of Pflüger, who in the first decade of this century was one of the bitterest opponents of pancreatic diabetes and who disputed with Minkowski using violent polemics against him (55, 56, 57, 58, 59, 60 and 46, 47, 48, 49). Pflüger supported the theory of nervous diabetes, postulated by Thiroloix in 1892 (70), and thought that there was an antidiabetic centre situated in the duodenum, injury of which during pancreatic extirpation led to the development of diabetes. He was all the more energetic in support of his theory since up until then no successful results had been seen with pancreatic therapy in diabetes, and he constantly emphasized that he could only be convinced through the isolation of the hypothetical hormone. Minkowski was able to prove to Pflüger (46) that his theory was wrong by removing the entire duodenum after creating a gastroenterostomy. The animals did not become diabetic however until the pancreas had been completely removed as well. Despite his authority Pflüger stood on his own to some extent in so strongly denying pancreatic diabetes, and yet even so it must be admitted that he had an inhibiting influence in this area of research. A great deal of time and energy was wasted on unfruitful criticism and counter-criticism. It would appear however that the indirect influence of Pflüger was even greater. He was an excellent experimenter and through his authority he would have deterred many, whose theory did not conform to his, from becoming involved in the study of the pancreas.

Conclusion

To sum up, we have seen that even before Banting and Best insulin came close to being isolated. Apart from the unfavorable external circumstances at the time, the fact that this did not happen is due to the lack of any large-scale systematic organization of the research work. In 1923, following the discovery of insulin, Hermann Sahli (63) said that here once again we had a typical, instructive example from the history of medicine which showed how an important invention or discovery can sink into complete oblivion again if it is not adequately worked through, so that with the loss of intellectual energy it does not reemerge until after a period of years when it is then brought to fruition through more consistent work. Ostwald (53) drew attention to the fact that it is often young researchers who have the great stroke of luck, precisely because they tackle the job without being inhibited by the difficulties to be expected and often in ignorance of previous discouraging failures.

And yet the German contribution to research into pancreatic diabetes after v. Mering and Minkowski for the development of insulin is by no means slight. Even though the goal was not finally reached, through their detailed work they were able to contribute towards the ripening of the fruits.

Literature

(1) Abderhalden, E.: Lehrbuch der physiologischen Chemie. (Berlin–Wien 1906). – (2) Bang, J. Chr.: Der Blutzucker. (Wiesbaden 1913.) – (3) Banting, F. G., Best, C. H.: The internal secretion of the pankreas. (J. Laborat. Clin. Med., St. Louis, 7 [1922], S. 251.) – (4) Banting, F. G., Best, C. H.: Pankreatic extracts. (J. Laborat. Clin. Med., St. Louis, 7 [1922], S. 464.) – (5) Banting, F. G., Best, C. H.: Pancreatic extracts in the treatment of diabetes mellitus. (Canad. Med. Ass. J. 12 [1922], S. 141.) – (6) Banting, F. G., Best, C. H., Macleod, J. J. R.: The internal secretion of the pancreas. (Amer. J. Physiol. 69 [1922], S. 479). – (7) Barron, O. M.: The relation of the islets of Langerhans to diabetes with special reference to cases of pancreatic lithiasis. (Surg. Gyn. Obstetr., Chicago 11 [1920], S. 437). – (8) Battistini, F.: Über zwei Fälle von Diabetes mellitus mit Pankreassaft behandelt. (Therap. Mhefte, Okt. 1893, S. 494.) – (9) Blum, F.: Über Nebennierendiabetes. (Dtsch. Arch. klin. Med. 71 [1901], S. 146.) – (10) Blumenthal, F.: Über Organsafttherapie bei Diabetes mellitus. (Zschr. diät. phys. Therap. 1 [1898], S. 250.) – (11) Caparelli, A.: Über die Funktion des Pankreas. (Biol. Zbl. 12 [1892], S. 606.) – (12) Cohnheim, O.: Die Kohlehydratverbrennung in den Muskeln und ihre Beeinflussung durch das Pankreas. (Zschr. physiol. Chemie 39 [1903], S. 336.) – (13) Cohnheim, O.: Über die Kohlehydratverbrennung. (Zschr. physiol. Chem. 42 [1904], S. 401.) – (14) Cohnheim, O.: Über Kohlehydratverbrennung. (Zschr. physiol. Chem. 43 [1905], S. 547.) – (15) Cohnheim, O.: Über Glykolyse. (Zschr. physiol. Chem. 47 [1906], S. 253.) – (16) Forschbach, J.: Parabiose und Diabetes mellitus. (Dtsch. med. Wschr. 34 [1908], S. 910.) – (17) Forschbach, J.: Zur Pathogenese des Pankreasdiabetes. (Arch. exper. Path. Pharmak., Leipzig 60 [1909], S. 131.) – (18) Forschbach, J.: Versuche zur Behandlung des Diabetes mellitus mit dem Zuelzerschen Pankreashormon. (Dtsch. med. Wschr. 35 [1909], S. 2053.) – (19) Fürbringer, M.: Über die moderne Behandlung von Krankheiten mit Gewebsflüssigkeiten. (Dtsch. med. Wschr. 20 [1894], S. 293.) – (20) Gley, E.: Action des extraits de pancréas sclérosé sur des chiens diabétiques (par exstirpation du pancréas). (Compt. rend. Soc. biol., Paris 87 [1922], S. 1322.) – (21) Gley, E., Thiroloix, J.: Contribution à l'étude du diabète pancréatique; des effects de la greffe extra-abdominal du pancréas. (Compt. rend. Soc. biol., Paris 4 [1892], S. 686.) – (22) Goldscheider, A.: Zur Gewebssafttherapie. (Dtsch.med. Wschr. 20 [1894], S. 376.) – (23) Grafe, E.: Über die praktische und theoretische Bedeutung des Insulins. (Dtsch. med. Wschr. 49 [1923], S. 1141.) – (24) Hédon, E.: Transfusion carotienne croisée entre chiens diabétiques chiens normaux. (Compt. rend. Soc. biol., Paris 67 [1910], S. 792). – (25) Hédon, E.: Greffe sous-cutanée du pancréas et ses résultats au point de vue la théorie du diabète pancréatique. (Compt. rend Soc., biol., Paris 44 [1892], S. 678.) – (26) Hirsch, R.: Über die glykolytische Wirkung der Leber. (Hofm. Beitr. 4 [1903], 535.) – (27) Ibrahim, J.: Trypsinogen und Enterokinase beim menschlichen Neugeborenen und Embryo. (Biochem. Zschr. 22 [1909], S. 24.) – (28) Klaus, R., Embden, G.: Pankreas und Glykolyse. (Hofm. Beitr. 6 [1905], S. 214.) – (29) Klaus, R., Embden, G.: Über Beziehungen zwischen Kohlehydraten und stickstoffhaltigen Produkten des Stoffwechsels. (Hofm. Beitr. 6 [1905], S. 303.) – (30) Kleiner, J. S., Meltzer, S. J.: On the rapid disappearance from the blood of large quantities of dextrose injected. Intravenously. (Amer. J. Physiol. 33 [1914], S. 17.) – (31) Kleiner, J. S., Meltzer,

S. J.: The influence of depancreatization upon the state of glycemia following the intravenous injection of dextrose in dogs. (Amer. Physiol. 36 [1951], S. 361.) – (32) Kleiner, J. S.: The action of intravenous injections of pancreas-emulsions in experimental diabetes. (J. Biol. Chem., Baltimore 40 [1919], S. 153.) – (33) Lépine, R., Barral: Sur le variations du pouvoir glycolytique et sacharifiant du sang dans lo diabète phlorhizique et dans le diabète de l'homme. (Compt. rend Soc. biol., Paris 113 [1891], S. 1044.) – (34) Loschke, E.: Über die Wirkung des Pankreasextrakts auf pankreasdiabetische und auf normale Tiere. (Arch. Anat., [Physiol. Abtlg.] [1910], S. 401.) – (35) Loveno, P. A., Meyer, G. M.: On the action of leucocytes on glycose. (J. Biol. Chem., Baltimore 12 [1912], S. 265.) – (36) Lieben, F.: Geschichte der physiologischen Chemie. (Leipzig und Wien 1935.) – (37) Loening, K.: Organotherapie des Diabetes mellitus. (Vorh. Dtsch. Ges. inn. Med. 33 [1921], S. 297.) – (38) Lüthje, H.: Die Zuckerbildung des Eiweiß. (Dtsch. Arch. klin. Med. 79 [1904], S. 498.) – (39) Macloed, J. J. R.: Kohlehydratstoffwechsel und Insulin. (Berlin 1927.) – (40) Macloed, J. J. R.: The source of insulin: a study of the effect produced on blood suggar by extracts of the pancreas and principal islets of fishes. (J. Metabol. Res., Morristown 2 [1922], S. 149.) – (41) Mering, I., Minkowski, O.: Diabetes und Pankreasexstirpation. (Arch. exper. Path. Pharmak., Leipzig 26 [1890], S. 371.) – (42) De Meyer, J.: Action de la sécrétion interne du pancréas sur différentos organos et on particulior sur la sécrétion renale. (Arch. fisiol. 7 [1909], S. 96.) – (43) De Meyer, J.: Sur la signification physiologique de la sécretion interne du pancréas. (Zbl. Physiol. 18 [1904], S. 826.) – (44) Minkowski, O.: Weitere Mitteilungen über den Diabetes mellitus und Exstirpation des Pankreas. (Berliner klin. Wschr. 1892, Nr. 5.) – (45) Minkowski, O.: Untersuchungen über den Diabetes mellitus nach Exstirpation des Pankreas. (Arch. exper. Path. Pharmak., Leipzig 31 [1893], S. 85.) – (46) Minkowski, O.: Bemerkungen über den Pankreasdiabetes. (Arch. exper. Path. Pharmak., Leipzig 53 [1905], S. 331.) – (47) Minkowski, O.: Über die Zuckerbildung im Organismus bei Pankreasdiabetes. (Arch. Physiol., Bonn 111 [1906], S. 13. – (48) Minkowski, O.: Zur Kenntnis der Funktion des Pankreas beim Zuckerverbrauch. (Arch. exper. Path. Pharmak., Leipzig, Suppl.-Bd. [1900], S. 395.) – (49) Minkowski, O.: Die Lehre vom Pankreasdiabetes in ihrer geschichtlichen Entwicklung. (Münch. med. Wschr. 76 [1929].) – (50) Murlin, J. R., Kramer, B.: The influence of pancreatic and duodenal extracts on the glycosurie and the respiratory metabilism of depancreatized dog. (J. Biol. Chem., Baltimore 15 [1913/14], S. 365.) – (51) Murlin, J. R., Kramer, B.: Pancreatic diabetes in the dog. (J. Biol. Chem., Baltimore 27 [1916], S. 534.) – (52) Murlin, J. R.: Progress in the preparation of pancreas extract for the treatment of diabetes. (Endocrinology 7 [1923], S. 519.) – (53) Ostwald, W.: Zit. n. Sahli, H.: – (54) Paulesco, N. C.: Action de l'extrait pancréatique infecté – dans le sang chez un animal diabétique. (Compt. rend. Soc. biol., Paris 85 [1921], S. 555.) – (55) Pflüger, E.: Ein Beitrag zur Frage nach dem Ursprung des im Pankreasdiabetes ausgeschiedenen Zuckers. (Arch. Physiol. 108 [1905], S. 123.) – (56) Pflüger, E.: Prof. O. Minkowskis Abwehr gegen meine ihn treffende Kritik. (Arch. Physiol., Bonn 110 [1905], S. 1.) – (57) Pflüger, E.: Untersuchungen über den Diabetes mellitus. (Arch. Physiol., Bonn 118 [1907], S. 265.) – (58) Pflüger, E.: Untersuchungen über den Pankreasdiabetes. (Arch. Physiol., Bonn 118 [1907], S. 267.) – (59) Pflüger, E.: Untersuchungen aüber den Pankreasdiabetes. (Arch. Physiol., Bonn 118 [1907], S. 406.) – (60) Pflüger, E.: Über die

Natur der Kräfte, durch welche das Duodenum den Kohlehydratstoffwechsel beeinflußt. (Arch. Physiol., Bonn 119 [1907], S. 227.) – (61) Rennie, J., Fraser, T.: Tho islets of Langerhans in relation to diabetes. (Biochem. J., London 2 [1907], S. 7.) – (62) Reuter, C.: Zit. nach Zuelzer, G.: Über Acomatol, das deutsche Insulin. (Med. Klin. 19 [1923], S. 1551.) – (63) Sahli, H.: Prolegomena zur Einführung der Insulintherapie des Diabetes mellitus. (Schweiz. med. Wschr. 53 [1923], S. 813.) – (64) Sandmeyer, W.: Über die Folgen der partiellen Pankreasexstirpation beim Hund. (Zschr. Biol. 31 [1895], S. 12.) – (65) Scott, E. L.: On the influence of intravenous injections of an extract of the pancreas on experimental pancreatic diabetes. (Amer. J. Physiol. 29 [1911/12], S. 306.) – (66) Schulze, W.: Die Bedeutung der Langerhansschen Inseln im Pankreas. (Arch. mikrosk. Anat. 56 [1900], S. 491.) – (67) Ssobolew, L. W.: Zur normalen und pathologischen Morphologie der inneren Sekretion der Bauchspeicheldrüse. (Arch. path. Anat., Berlin 168 [1902], S. 91.) – (68) Staub, H.: Insulin. (Berlin 1925.) – (69) Thesen, J. E., Lauritzen, M.: Pankreas und Diabetes. (Ref. in Dtsch. Med.-Ztg. 18 [1897], S. 62.) – (70) Thiroloix, J.: Le diabite pancréatique. (Thèse, Paris 1892.) – (71) Vanni, L.: Sugli effetti dell'estirpazione del pancreas. (Arch. ital. clin. med. 33 [1894], S. 157.) – (72) Vahlen, E.: Über das Einwirken bisher unbekannter Bestandteile des Pankreas. (Zschr. physiol. Chem. 50 [1900], S. 194.) – (73) Vahlen, E.: Über Metabolin und Antinelabolin aus Hefe. (Zschr. physiol. Chem. 106 [1919], S. 133.) – (74) Vahlen, E., Loening, K.: Über Organtherapie des Diabetes mellitus. (Dtsch. med. Wschr. 48 [1922], S. 217.) – (75) White, W. Hale: On the treatment of Diabetes mellitus by feeding on raw pancreas and by the subcutaneous injection of liquor pancreaticus. (Brit. Med. J. [1893/1], S. 452. – (76) Zuelzer, G., Dorn, M., Marxer, A.: Neuere Untersuchungen über den experimentellen Diabetes. (Dtsch. med. Wschr. 34 [1908], S. 1880.) – (77) Zuelzer, G.: Über Acomatol, das deutsche Insulin. (Med Klin. 19 [1923], S. 1551.)

Aus: *Deutsche Medizinische Wochenschrift 78 (1953) 919–922.*

50 Years of Insulin Treatment at the Vienna Hospital for Children – the Fate of Diabetic Children from the First Insulin Era*

by W. KORP and ERNST ZWEYMÜLLER

Summary

A follow-up report is presented of the 91 juvenile-onset diabetics who had been treated by Priesel and Wagner at the Paediatric Clinic of the University of Vienna during the early insulin era (1922 to 1932) and the course taken by the diabetes described. During the first two decades coma, tuberculosis and infections were the main causes of death, superseded later on by diabetic nephropathy and arteriosclerosis. The incidence of diabetic micro-angiopathy in the suviving cases is comparatively low. It is concluded that the careful control and education of the patients during the first years of their disease were the main causes for the excellent long-term prognosis of this group.

Key words: Juvenile-onset diabetes, long-term prognosis, causes of death, microangiopathy, arteriosclerosis.

Historical Aspects

The beginnings of insulin therapy in Vienna [32, 53] go back to the first month of the year 1923. Since commercial insulin preparations were not yet available at that time, the physician Leo Pollak [34] together with Susi Glaubach at the Pharmacology Institute had started to produce insulin in accordance with the instructions of the Toronto research group [20]. In June 1923 the girl B. A., born 5th July 1909 (Tabelle 1), was the first child at the Vienna Hospital for Children to receive the insulin produced by Pollak, after she had lapsed into a precoma

* Extracts read at the meeting of the Vienna Medical Association on January 21st 1972.

Table 1. Mortality and causes of death in the patients

Year of obs.	No. of cases	No. of deaths	a) Age b) Duration of diabetes of pats. who died a)	b)	Causes of death Coma and hypo-glycemia	Infectious diseases inc. TBC	Uremia	Arterio-sclerosis	Other causes
1923–1925	27	1	14	1	1	–	–	–	–
1926–1935	90	8	8,6 ± 6	2,7 ± 3	4	3	–	–	1
1936–1950	82	37	23,3 ± 5	15,0 ± 4	10	17	4	–	6
1951–1971	45	21	39,1 ± 8	31,2 ± 7	1	2	10	4	4
Total	91	67			16	22	14	4	11

following an almost 9-month stay in hospital and despairing attempts at dietetic treatment [19]. The rescue of this child, who incidentally is still alive today after suffering from her diabetes for over 50 years and who is in a relatively good state of health, initiated a fruitful period of diabetic research at the Pirquet clinic, which was soon to make the diabetes unit founded by Priesel and Wagner in 1924 into one of the leading centres in Europe for the treatment of diabetic children. In the autumn of 1925 an out-patient department was set up [35], followed a few years later by the creation of places in a childrens' home for cases with social difficulties. The scientific knowledge gained from their observations was recorded by Priesel and Wagner between 1924 and 1932 in numerous papers and publications [38–42, 51] and summarized in a monograph in 1932 [43]. In 1933 Wagner [52] reported on the first ten years of insulin therapy to the Vienna Medical Association, as did Priesel [35] in 1935 on the occasion of his inaugural lecture at Innsbruck. The subsequent fate of these children was reported on in a monograph by Trude Rohracher [45] in 1951, 30 years after the discovery of insulin. We have to thank this interimassessment, produced under extremely adverse circumstances, for important clues which led to the discovery and identification of the earliest cases in the hospital who, since 1930, had been under the further care of the metabolic department founded by Carl von Noorden in the Lainz hospital. The 50th anniversary of the start of insulin therapy at the Vienna Hospital for Children has stimulated this report on the fate of the patients treated during the first ten years (1923 to 1932), who have already formed the subject of some previous publications [21–26].

Case
Case 1: the first child in the hospital treated with insulin, the patient B. A. who is still alive today.

Patients and Method

Out of ca. 120 patients of Priesel and Wagner [45] who were treated in the first ten years of the insulin era, we were able to obtain adequate information about the subseqent fate of 91 cases (51 boys and 40 girls). The diabetes of all 91 patients had become manifest before the 15th year of life, in 21 cases before the 5th year of life (5 of these between the 1st and 3rd year of life), 29 between the 6th and 10th year of life and in 37 between the 11th and 15th year of life. The age at which the disease became manifest was not known for 4 patients. The mean *age of manifestation* was 8.7 ± 3.9 years and was one year lower for the boys at 8.2 ± 3.8 years than for the girls (9.2 ± 4.1 years). The mean *duration of the disease* for all patients up until death or up until the time of the follow-up examination (1st January 1972) was 25.8 ± 15.1 years (range 0 to 50 years); that for the male patients was 26.7 ± 14.1, and for the female patients 24.9 ± 16.3 years. The patients' *age* was 34.4 ± 15.9 years (range 2 to 63 years), that of the men 34.9 ± 14.9 and that of the women 33.6 ± 17 years.

67 patients (38 men and 29 women) had died, 24 patients (13 men and 11 women) were still alive.

The cause of death could be ascertained by autopsy for 45 of the 49 patients who died in hospitals. Reports on the cause of death by the general practitioner last in attendance were available for 10 patients, 4 patients were killed in the war or died in a concentration camp. Only for 4 patients was the cause of death not known.

Table 1 shows the age and duration of the diabetes of the patients who died at various intervals of time.

The age of the 24 surviving patients at the cut-off date of January 1st 1972 was 54.5 ± 5.3 (range 42 to 63) years, the duration of the diabetes was 44.8 ± 3.1 (40 to 50) years.

21 of the surviving patients could be followed up in the year 1971. In addition, angiologic findings were available for 32 of those who had died. Prior to 1938 examination of the fundus of the eye was only carried out in exceptional cases, but after the war it was routinely performed in almost all patients. Only in

recent years have neurologic investigations been routinely carried out on the patients.

The following definitions were used:

Retinopathy was divided into

a) minimal retinopathy (discrete disorders often with spots of bleeding only demonstrable in a transitory way),
b) simple retinopathy (corresponding to Retinopathia simplex or so-called background-retinopathy in Anglo-American terminology) and
c) proliferative retinopathy [7].

Neuropathies were divided into

0a) slight stationary forms with discrete disorders of sensibility and abnormal reflexes without motor activity being affected and
b) severe progressive neuropathies [23] possibly developing further up to diabetic pseudotabes.

The diagnosis of a diabetic *nephropathy* was only made if a nephrotic syndrome was present with constant proteinuria or if the histologic findings showed a diabetic glomerulosclerosis (Kimmelstiel–Wilson-lesion).

Results

Table 1 show the behaviour of the mortality and causes of death of the patients in the various periods of observation between 1923 and 1971.

In the years between 1925 and 1946 14 patients died in a diabetic coma, half of these in the war years because of a lack of insulin or the lack of medical care. The age at death was 18.4 ± 8.4 (2 to 31) years, the duration of the diabetes was 10.3 ± 6.7 (0 to 18) years.

Two patients succumbed to hypoglycemic shock in 1939 and 1951. In both cases previous excessive physical effort (mountain climbing) seemed to have been a precipitating factor.

Nine patients died between 1930 and 1947 from infectious diseases (2 patients from diphtheria) or from sepsis (otogenic sepsis in 2 cases, sepsis after buccal phlegmon once and after gluteal phlegmon once). One patient died following acute enterocolitis in 1945, 1 patient died from chronic gangrenous pneumonia. The age at death of these patients was 19.6 ± 7.5 (5 to 29) years, the duration of the diabetes was 12.0 ± 8.2 (0 to 21) years.

In 13 patients who died between 1931 and 1956 at an age of 24.0 ± 4.9 (16 to 33) years and after a mean duration of their diabetes of 15.0 ± 6.0 (7 to 27) years, the cause of death was a cavernous pulmonary tuberculosis which in three cases was complicated by tuberculosis of the larynx and in three patients by an intestinal tuberculosis.

The cause of death "Renal failure" first appeared in the patient collective in 1941, in a 19 year old male patient who, after his diabetes had lasted for 10 years, died following nephrectomy of one kidney from a pyonephrosis of the second kidney. Two other patients succumbed to severe urinary tract infections with terminal renal failure.

Since 1951 eleven patients have died from a diabetic nephropathy, and here a Kimmelstiel-Wilson lesion could be demonstrated on histology in 6 cases. The duration of the diabetes in the patients with Kimmelstiel-Wilson syndrome was 20 to 41 years, that for the entire group was 26.7 ± 9.8 (10 to 41) years, the mean age was 34.3 ± 3.7 (19 to 47) years.

Four patients died from arteriosclerotic vascular complications, two from myocardial infarction, one patient from a decompensated, coronarysclerotic myocardiopathy and one patient from a cerebral stroke. The age of the group was 43.5 ± 9.6 (33 to 56) years, the duration of the diabetes was 34.3 ± 6.6 (27 to 43) years.

One patient died from a cervical carcinoma at the age of 49, after the diabetes had lasted for 39 years, four patients died in the second world war or in a concentration camp. One patient died at the age of 9 years in a hepatic coma, after suffering from diabetes for 6 years, one patient died at the age of 38 years following a gastric operation after suffering from the diabetes for 26 years. Table 2 shows the frequency of occurrence of angiopathy in the patients who died, divided according to year of death, with the cut-off date of January 1st 1972 for the surviving patients.

Fifty-three out of 91 patients in our collective (58%) were investigated for vascular complications. Angiopathy was found in 42 patients (79% of those investigated).

Table 2. Frequency of angiopathy in the patient collective

Year of observ.	No. of causes	No. of those invest. by angiology	Patients with angiopathy
		Patients who died	
1925	1	–	–
1926–1935	8	2	–
1936–1950	37	11	2
1951–1970	21	19	19
		Surviving patients	
1971	24	21	21
Total	91	53	42

The breakdown by duration of the disease shows a frequency of microangiopathy of 14% for diabetes which had existed for up to 15 years, of 82% with diabetes for 16 to 30 years and of 93% for diabetes of 31 to 50 years in duration (Tabelle 3). Table 4 shows the severity of the vessel lesions.

28% of all those investigated by angiology and 36% of the cases of angiopathy showed a minimal retinopathy, 32% resp. 40% a simple retinopathy and 19 resp. 24% a proliferative retinopathy.

The 26 cases of neuropathy consisted of 20 slight and 6 severe progressive forms.

Table 3. Frequency of microangiopathy and duration of diabetes

		Duration of diabetes (years)		
		–15	16–30	31–50
Pats. who died				
with angiopathy	21	1	14	6
no angiopathy	11	6	3	2
Pats. who survived				
with angiopathy	21	–	–	21
no angiopathy	–	–	–	–
Total	53	7	17	29
with angiopathy	42	1 (14 %)	14 (82 %)	27 (93 %)

In 6 of the 11 patients with nephropathy a diabetic glomerulosclerosis was demonstrated on histology.

Table 5 gives information about the forms of arterial sclerotic occlusional disease affecting the cerebral, cardiac and extremity arteries in the patient collective.

Table 4. Forms of manifestation and degree of severity of the microangiopathy

	Patients who died			Patients who survived
Duration of diabetes	up to 15	16–30	31–43	41–50
Retinopathy				
minimal ret.	1	1	–	13
simple ret.	–	8	3	6
proliferative ret.	–	5	3	2
Neuropathy				
slight neur.	?	?	?	20
severe progressive neur.	?	1	4	1*
Nephropathy**	–	8 [5]	3 [1]	–

* Case with combined alcoholic polyneuritis
** Figures in brackets: histologically verified Kimmelstiel-Wilson lesion

Table 5. Form of manifestation of the arteriosclerosis

	Patients who died			Patients who survived
Duration of diabetes	up to 15	16–30	31–43	41–50
Cerebral insult	–	2	3	–
Myocardial infarction and severe coronary sclerosis	2	–	4	4
Obliterative arteriosclerosis of the leg arteries	–	2	2	4

In 5 cases (9% of those investigated by angiology) there was clinical or autopsy evidence of cerebrosclerosis, sometimes with an insult, 10 (19%) showed a severe coronary sclerosis with or without myocardial infarction, 8 (15%) an obliterating arteriosclerosis of the extremities with or without gangrene.

Discussion

Only one single patient, B. A. who is still alive (Tabelle 6, No.1), out of the diabetic children treated at the Vienna Hospital for children in the pre-insulin era [4], experienced the insulin era. All of the other children had already died after their diabetes

Table 6. The earliest cases in the hospital*

Case No.**	Initials/Sex and date of birth			Admission to hospital	Fate of the child. Last findings 1971 or cause of death
1	B. A.,	w,	05 07 09	13. 10. 1922	slight microangiopathy
2	G. F.,	w,	03 08 19	14. 8. 1923	Died 1923, cavernous upper lobe-TBC
3	M. E.,	m,	03 09 17	24. 11. 1923	minimal microangiopathy
4	P. F.,	m,	18 07 10	4. 2. 1924	minimal microangiopathy
5	O. O.,	m,	18 02 10	4. 2. 1924	Died 1931, cavernous phthisis
6	S. L.,	m,	30 09 11	12. 2. 1924	Died 1967, cerebral insult
7	S. G.,	w,	09 05 11	18. 2. 1924	slight microangiopathy
8	H. S.,	w,	02 12 12	15. 3. 1924	minimal microangiopathy
9	M. E.,	w,	19 11 11	24. 4. 1924	severe microangiopathy
10	K. K.,	w,	12 11 12	20. 5. 1924	severe microangiopathy
11	R. F.,	m,	06 02 21	19. 7. 1924	Died 1959, myocardial infarction
12	Z. J.,	w,	12 08 11	5. 9. 1924	Died 1925, coma
13	Z. H.,	w,	07 06 12	15. 9. 1924	Died 1961, uterine carcinoma
14	H. K.,	m,	10 02 18	17. 10. 1924	Died 1965, uremia with pyelonephritis
15	L. L.,	w,	03 09 14	14. 11. 1924	lost
16	W. W.,	m,	01 04 13	20. 11. 1924	Died 1942, cavernous phthisis

w = woman m = man

* see also Fig. 1.

** The case numbers are identical to those used by Priesel and Wagner in their 1926 publication [39]

had lasted for a few weeks or month, in rare exceptions after 2 to 3 years. Other European authors had similar experiences [33]. Only the Joslin school [30] was able to keep one-third of their patients alive into the insulin era through the consistent use of Allen's hunger treatment in the period from 1914 to 1922.

Altough the supply of insulin was still patchy in the years from 1923 to 1924 and the crude extracts which could be obtained were not without their dangers because of the high degree of contamination, not a single child was lost during the first years of treatment. As early as 1924 Priesel and Wagner [38] were able to report on their experience with the first 5 children, and in 1926 [39] on 39 cases in a detailed publication. At that time the patient B. A. had survived for 4 years – "a record figure for diabetes" [51].

The careful management of the diabetic children in the first insulin era in hospital (during these years the mean stay in hospital lasted for 18 (!) months) and the marvellous care given outside of hospital in the diabetic out-patient clinics set up in 1924, were visibly reflected in the reduction in the mortality from diabetes which was exemplary for the European [44, 50] and the American [10, 14] standard (mortality rate up to 1935 10%, virtually no cases of coma death, no cases of death due to insulin reactions), and also in the complete absence of any gross growth retardation, which had affected almost 15 % of the patients in other representative groups of patients, such as those of Joslin [6], Fanconi [47] and Joos and Johnston [12]. The only case of delayed pubertal development observed [35] could be completely rectified after more accurate therapy [36].

Only a few patients had died up to the year 1935, the end of the "old insulin era"; half of these from coma and half from infections. Up to the start of the antibiotic era after the end of the second world war tuberculosis in particular was to become one of the main causes of death in our patient collective. A similar trend was also seen in American publication [10, 11, 13–15, 54, 55], although the mortality from tuberculosis was not as great there as in our patient material, no doubt because of their better nutritional situation during the war years.

Whereas in Joslin's patients [15] coma fell to 8.8% of all causes of death at the end of the second world war, in our patient collective there was a sudden jump in the mortality due to coma in the 5 years between 1941 and 1946 because of the difficulties in obtainig supplies of insulin due to the war. During these years the number of deaths due to coma was twice as high as in the first two decades of insulin therapy taken together.

In collected statistics for West Germany Krainick and Struwe [27] had an even higher figure for mortality due to coma in the wartime and post-war period. In Austria the basic supply of insulin could already be guaranteed again shortly after the end of the war. Since 1946 not a single child has again fallen a victim to the lack of insulin. Similarly there was a fall in the mortality due to sepsis and tuberculosis in the post-war period through the use of antibiotics and tuberculostatic drugs. The last case of death due to sepsis was reported in 1950 and the last from tuberculosis in 1956.

Late vascular complications in the form of diabetic retinopathy, neuropathy and nephropathy made their appearance relatively late in our patient collective and were seen to a lesser extent than in other patient collectives. The first reports of diabetic vascular damage in children with diabetes originated from the cases of Joslin in the 30's [55]. As early as 1942 Eisele [6], at the follow-up investigation of children from the pre-insulin era observed that over half of the patients were suffering from a diabetic retinopathy after suffering from the disease for 20 years and that some cases showed renal lesions and neuropathies. The life-shortening role of diabetic nephropathy first became distinctly apparent in the patient material of Fanconi [47]. The harmful role of nephropathy has since been confirmed in numerous investigations since 1945 [3, 9, 11, 12, 15, 16, 28, 45, 56, 59, 60].

Diabetic angiopathy does not actually occur in childhood [58]. It is still rare in adolescence [6, 8, 10, 58] and first develops as the duration of the disease progresses [6, 17, 21, 57, 58]. When the diabetes has been present for between 15 and 20 years in fact there is a distinct increase in the frequency of angiopathy [15, 17, 57, 58]. Nephropathy is the main cause of death of diabetic children in the middle period when the diabetes has been present for about 20 years [54, 56], and is not overtaken by arteriosclerosis (especially coronary sclerosis) as the cause of death until the disease has been present for over 30 years [57].

In our own patient collective severe diabetic angiopathies were found in 15 patients, i.e. in 12 patients who died and in 3 surviving patients (Tabelle 4). Out of the 11 patients who died from nephropathy, 8 died already before the diabetes had been present for 30 years. Five cases were suffering from a proliferative retinopathy at the same time, in some cases with blindness. The total frequency of the severe forms of microangiopathy in

2the 32 patients who died (34% nephropathy, 25% proliferative retinopathy, 16% severe progressive neuropathy) and in the 21 surviving patients (nephropathy 0, proliferative retinopathy 10%, severe progressive neuropathy 5%) is slight compared with other collectives of long-term juvenile-onset diabetecs. White and Graham [58] in their figures for the incidence of nephropathy in the Boston collective quote 1.5% with diabetes for 10 years, 18% with diabetes for 20 years, 39% with diabetes for 30 qears and 63% for diabetes which has lasted for over 35 years.

They quote a frequency of 60% for proliferative retinopathy with a duration of the disease of over 30 years. Knowles [17] gives an incidence of blindness of ca. 30% when the diabetes has been present for 30 years. Whereas slight stationary forms of neuropathy [23, 30] can already be observed with a relatively short duration of the disease, so-called progressive forms [16, 23, 47], possibly in combination with autonomic neuropathies, are only ever seen in long-term diabetics. On the basis of our personal experience [21] the degree of severity of the concomitant neuropathy is of prognostic information value here.

As in other collectives [15–17] an increase in arteriosclerosis has been observed in our patient material over the past two decades. The mortality rate from myocardial infarction or coronary sclerotic myocardiopathies is relatively low however, White for example [56, 57] quoting a frequence of 31% for these after diabetes for 20 years and of 52% after the disease has been present for more than 30 years.

An astonishingly large number of patients (Tabelle 4), including some from the very first treatment period (Tabelle 6) have now survived diabetes for a period of 40 to 50 years with no major damage. Only recently Shepherd [49] has pointed out how rare such observations are [1,5].

Long-term diabetic survivors with only slight vascular complications have recently been reported from the Joslin clinic [2, 46, 48]. These consist of cases who have remained completely free of complications after suffering from the disease for up to 25 years. These and similar cases [1, 4, 24, 31] raise the question of what the causes of this relative freedom from complications are.

Whereas in the 50's discussion was only kindled by the question of a controlled diet [59, 60] or a free diet [28, 29], later on, besides the diet, the types of insulin used (long duration of treatment with old insulin [2, 31, 48]) and also genetic factors (long-lived parents [2, 48]) were said to be of decisive importance in preventing or postponing the devolpment of latc complications.

Like so many other authors [2, 4, 9, 12, 16, 18, 31, 48, 59, 60], we believe that the strictest possible control of the diabetes is of essential importance for their prevention. Until insulins become available with which metabolic control is automatically achieved, despite all the advances made in therapy the diabetic child will have to observe great discipline. We have to admit that ultimately, even 50 years after the discovery of insulin, we still do not know the causes of the development of late diabetic complications. The words written 20 years ago by Richard Priesel [37], are therefore still completely valid today:

"These patients who developed diabetes 30 years ago were kept under in-patient surveillance for years at a time in the Pirquet clinic at that time; this made continuous education and instruction possible with the result that later on most of these patients were able to maintain a well-compensated metabolic state successfully by themselves. This is undoubtedly what is needed."

References

1. Blöch, J. Korp, W.: Wien, klin. Wschr. *75*, 378–380 (1963).
2. Chazan, B. I., Balodimos, M. C., Ryan, J. R., Marble, A.: Diabetologia *6*, 565–569 (1970).
3. Chute, A. L.: Amer. J. Dis. Childr. *75*, 1–10 (1948).
4. Constam, G. R.: Méd. et Hyg. *26*, 1036–1037 (1968).
5. Csapó, G. Hódi, M.: Med. Klin. *62*, 871–873 (1967).
5. Eisele, H. E.: J. Amer. med. Ass. *120*, 188–190 (1942).
7. Fischer, F.: Bericht d. Ophthalm. Ges. *69*, 81–86 (1968).
8. Imerslund, O.: Acta Pediatrica *49*, 243–248 (1959).
9. Jackson, R. L., Hardin, R., Walker, G. L., Hendricks, A. D., Kelly, H. G.: Pediatrics *5*, 959–970 (1950).
10. John, H. E.: J. Pediatr. *6*, 211–225 (1935).
11. John, H. E.: J. Pediatr. *35*, 723–744 (1949).
12. Joos, T. H., Johnston, J. A.: J. Pediatr. *50*, 133–137 (1957).
13. Joslin, E. P.: J. Amer. med. Ass. *88*, 28–31 (1927).
14. Joslin, E. P.: Ann. int. Med. *11*, 1348–1353 (1938).
15. Joslin, E. P., Wilson, J. L.: Brit. Med. J. *11*, 1293–1296 (1950).
16. Kerr, R. B., Brown, G. D., Kalant, N.: Canad. M. A. J. *66*, 97–104 (1952).
17. Knowles, H. C., jr.: Long-term juvenile diabetes mellitus and unmeasured diet. In: Diabetes, Proceedings of the Seventh Congress of the International Diabetes Federation. Buenos Aires 1970 (Rodriquez, R. R., Vallance-owen, J., Hrsg.). Excerpta medica *1971*, 209–215.

18. Knowles, H. C., jr., Guest, G. M., Lampe, J., Kessler, M. Skillman, T. G.: Diabetes *14*, 239–273 (1965).
19. Korp, W.: Der Diabetesverlauf des ersten insulinbehandelten Kindes an der Wr. Kinderklinik. Mitteilung in der Österr. Gesellschaft für Kinderheilkunde am 11. Juni 1963.
20. 20. Korp, W.: 40 Jahre Insulintherapie in Österreich. Mitteilung in der Gesellschaft der Ärzte, Wien am 21. Juni 1963.
21. Korp, W.: Klinik und Verlauf der diabetischen Mikroangiopathie am Beispiel des jugendlichen Diabetes. Referat in der gemeinsamen Sitzung der österreichischen Arbeitsgemeinschaft für Angiologie und der österreichischen Diabetesgesellschaft am 4. Dezember 1971.
22. Korp, W., Lenhardt, A., Levetti, R. E., Neubert, J.: Wien. klin. Wschr. *83*, 814–817 (1971).
23. 23. Korp, W., Levett, R. E., Summer, K.: Verhandl. Deutsch. Ges. inn. Med. *72*, 1165–1167 (1966).
24. Korp, W., Nobis, H.: Jugendliche Diabetiker aus der ersten Insulinära. 5. Kongreß der Deutschen Diabetesgesellschaft, Bad Godesberg, 1970.
25. Korp, W., Statz, H.: Mortalität und Todesursachen diabetischer Kinder. 4. Kongreß der Deutschen Diabetesgesellschaft, Ulm, 1969.
26. Korp, W., Weikmann, E.: Sozialmedizinische Probleme des jugendlichen Diabetikers im Erwachsenenalter. In: Die Betreuung des diabetischen Kindes. Arbeitstagung der Deutschen Diabetesgesellschaft. Ausschuß Pädiatrie (Hungerland, H., Hrsg.). Beihefte zum Arch. Kinderheilk. *58*, 53–58 (1968).
27. Krainick, H. G., Struwe, F. E.: Deutsch. med. Wschr. *85*, 1632–1640 (1960).
28. Larson, Y., Lichtenstein, A., Ploman, K. G.: Diabetes *1*. 449–458 (1952).
29. Larsson, Y., Sterky, G., Christiansson, G.: Acta Pädiatr. *51*, (Suppl. 130), 1–76 (1962).
30. Lawrence, D. G., Locke, S.: Brit. Med. J. *I*, 784–785. (1963).
31. Lawrence, R. D.: Brit. Med. J. *II*, 1624–1625 (1963).
32. Lesky, E.: Österr. Ärztezeitung *27*, 242–244 (1972).
33. Noorden, C.: Diabetes mellitus. In: Handbuch der Kinderheilkunde (Pfaundler, M., Schlossmann, A., Hrsg.), 2. Aufl., S. 117–123. Leipzig: F. C. W. Vogel. 1910.
34. Pollak, L.: Wien. klin. Wschr. *37*, 55–60 (1924).
35. Priesel, R.: Wien. klin. Wschr. *48*, 1503–1506 (1935).
36. Priesel, R.: Zschr. Altersforschg. *1*, 310–324 (1939).
37. Priesel, R.: Wien. klin. Wschr. *67*, 665–666 (1955).
38. Priesel, R., Wagner, R.: Zschr. Kinderheilk. *38*, 103–117 (1924).
39. 39. Priesel, R., Wagner, R.: Ergebnisse inn. Med. und Kinderheilk. *30*, 537–730 (1926).
40. Priesel, R., Wagner, R.: Zschr. Kinderheilk. *46*, 62–104 (1928).
41. Priesel, R., Wagner, R.: Zschr. Kinderheilk. *48*, 516–551 (1929).
42. Priesel, R., Wagner, R.: Therapie d. Gegenw. 1930, 1–9.
43. Priesel, R., Wagner, R.: Die Zuckerkrankheit und ihre Behandlung im Kindesalter. Leipzig: G. Thieme. 1932.
44. Püschel, E.: Med. Welt 1940, 1090–1092.
45. Rohracher, T.: Spätschicksale zuckerkranker Kinder. Wien: Maudrich. 1951.
46. Root, H. F., Barclay, P. B.: J. Amer. med. Ass. *161*, 801–806 (1956).

47. Rosenbusch, H.: Prognose und Spätkomplikationen des Diabetes im Kindesalter. Basel–New York: Karger, 1945.
48. Ryan, J. R., Balodimos, M. C., Chazan, B. I., Root, H. F., Marble, A., White P., Joslin, A. P.: Metabolism *19*, 493–501 (1970).
49. Shepherd, G. R.: Arch. Int. Med. *128*, 284–290 (1971).
50. Trusen, M., Walenta, E.: Mschr. Kinderheilk. *51*, 15–21 (1931).
51. Wagner, R.: Wien. klin. Wschr. *39*, 581 (1926).
52. Wagner, R.: Wien. klin. Wschr. *46*, 602 (1933).
53. Wagner, R.: Österr. Ärztezeitg. *26*, 1501–1507 (1971).
54. Warren, S., Le Compte, P. M., Legg, M. A.: The pathology of diabetes mellitus, 4. Aufl. Philadelphia: Lea & Febiger. 1966.
55. White, P.: J. Amer. med. Ass. *95*, 1160–1162 (1930).
56. White, P.: Diabetes *5*, 445–450 (1956).
57. White, P.: Diabetes *9*, 345–355 (1960).
58. White, P., Graham, Ch. A.: The child with diabetes. In: Joslin's Diabetes mellitus, 11. Aufl. (Marble, A., White, P., Bradley, R. F., Krall, L. P., Hrsg.), S. 339. Philadelphia: Lea & Febiger. 1971.
59. 59. Wilson, J. L., Root, H. F., Marble, A.: Amer. J. med. Sci. *221*, 479–489 (1951). – 60. Wilson, J. L., Root, H. F., Marble, A.: Diabetes *1*, 33–36 (1952).

in: *Wiener Klinische Wochenschrift 85 (1973) 385–390.*

The Beginning of the Diabetic Association in England

by Robert Daniel Lawrence

"The love of money is the root of all evil" saith the prophet. But the need for money in a good cause can be a powerful stimulus; indeed it led to the beginning of *The* Diabetic Association in 1933. I make no apology for this title as it was the first and only Association then, although such organizations have now spread everywhere. Indeed it was the first time that a body of sufferers from any disease banded themselves toghether for mutual help.

I hope I may be forgiven for being personal in this story. In London, as elsewhere, insulin had produced by 1931 a vital snowballing of living diabetics. At King's College Hospital, I myself had been given charge of them in our small biochemical laboratory. They occupied all odd seats so extensively as to threaten the extinction of Bunsen burners and all other routine work. Our voluntary hospital had no money to spare for equipping a new department, so I started to raise money from some of my rich and grateful diabetic patients for a new diabetic department. Amongst these I approached the great writer, H. G. Wells, who, not feeling so affluent in his contribution as I expected, offered to write a letter of appeal to *The Times*. This is interesting in being the first public intimation of the profound debt diabetics felt for the progress of treatment and the discovery of insulin. I shall quote parts of Wells' letter of appeal.

The Select Company of Diabetics

"Sir, – May I make an appeal through your columns, not to all your readers, but to that select percentage of them who are diabetic and who 12 years ago would have been "suffering from diabetes"?

"Some hundreds of thousands of people to-day who have this physiological idiosyncrasy are living active and happy lives thanks either to a scientifically regulated dietary or to the use of insulin. Many of them – many of us, to be more personal – would either be dying slowly and uncomfortably or be already dead if it were not for the work of a small group of experimentalists and practitioners who have brought this particular maladjustment under control, and none of us can feel anything but the liveliest gratitude for that work.

"An opportunity occurs for expressing this gratitude in a very direct and effective fashion. We can contribute to the research that is still perfecting the very precise and beautiful treatment by which we have been restored to normality, and we can help to extend its benefits to many fellow diabetics not so well off as ourselves who would otherwise be obliged to cease work and so cease to be self-supporting.

"I suggest that it would be a becoming thing of the elect class of grateful diabetics to whom I appeal to tax themselves for the benefit of our cult. If 40 of us would put up £20 each the thing would be done. When I think of the relief our treatment has given us and the real invigoration, the bracing effect, of its clear and rational discipline, £20 seems to me a small sum. Indeed, as I think the matter over I am a little surprised we have not already formed a Diabetic Association, to watch over and extend this most benign branch of medical science to which we owe our lives. I will not, however, let my imagination run on to an Annual Dinner for Old Diabetics, or to the organized propaganda of our simple requirements among cooks and hotel and restaurant proprietors. The immediate business in hand is to raise that £800, and I shall be very glad to hear from all my fellow diabetics who are willing to assist in any measure in raising this not very considerable sum. The participation of friendly nondiabetics will rouse no resentment. Advice and suggestions may be freely tendered. The figure of £20 is given merely by way of illustration. Cheques should be made out to "H. G. Wells Diabetic a/c," King's College Hospital, S.E.5."

Sincerely yours,
H. G. Wells.

This letter raised enough money from some 30 subcribers for my immediate hospital purposes and put into mind the idea of an Association of diabetics for self-help in social matters and to raise money for research, really my main interest. This was the start of our Diabetic Association and the movement was soon inaugurated at our annual hospital dinner where we diabetic subscribers ate our special privileged food and talked over the idea.

Next the sympathy of various doctors specially interested was sought and, with them and the patients they brought, the movement was started, almost entirely in London. I soft-pedaled my interest in starting the movement, an interest which (as a diabetic myself), was really altruistic but might have been, and in some quarters was, considered a Lawrence "stunt".

I shall never forget the first meeting in Wells' apartment of some 50 earnest people, diabetics from all ranges of life. We knew we wanted to do something good and important for the lives of diabetics and the progress of knowledge. But how and where and what, was vaguely tentative in our minds. However, we formed a Diabetic Association on the spot with Wells as President, an advertising expert as Secretary, an accountant as Treasurer, a small Council of lay diabetics with a few doctors, and determined to publish a Journal to unify and spread our efforts, at first in such diabetic clinics as were in being throughout the country.

So it started and spread slowly but surely and our quarterly journal consisted of useful simple advice to patients on diet and insulin. Soon it became incorporated legally in law as a philanthropic non-earning association by which means income tax is avoided and other privileges gained. Fundamentally the organization and directive power has always been in the hands of lay diabetics and our constitution insists on a preponderance of lay diabetics on the governing council in excess of the interested dators who also cooperate – only one-third of the total council can be practising physicians earning money from the treatment of diabetics. This has proved a good rule which we have never seen reason to change. The conjoined work of doctors and laymen has always remained happily co-ordinated with no divergent strains and stresses – perhaps a unique situation, though common enough in the practical compromise ingrained in this country when occasional divergent interests meet.

Perhaps an unusual feature in our Association was the different grades of membership we created for the relatively rich and poor. The former became full members with voting rights for an annual subscription of one pound (5 dollars then) and the others paid two shillings (half a dollar) for membership which included their receipt of the same quarterly journal established in 1934.

Such was the beginning – an association essentially for lay diabetics: to help them in their social and personal problems –

but not to advise them on their personal treatment which was their own doctors' concern: to educate and encourage them to lead a normal life without handicap from their disease and to dispel invalidism: to fight old-standing prejudices concerning their employment and insurance.

Since the early days, with an ever-growing membership, we have done more and more. Before the war we had holiday homes for children on a small scale and these are now happily recreated for some 300 children. Other fields of activity have been set up with two convalescent homes for men and women. Five educational homes have been established for children from 3 to 16 whose lack of care at home in poor families make their lives and education impossible. We have strained our finances lately – almost to bankruptcy – by setting up a home for elderly poor and uncared-for diabetics. And we endow at present five young and keen research workers on diabetes in different hospital laboratories.

But enough of our present efforts. It was the beginning 20 years ago that I set out to describe. But it is good to feel that the little fire we lit has led to Diabetic Associations all over the civilised world and, indeed, recently to an International Diabetes Federation of all national associations which met this year in Holland.

in: *Diabetes 1 (1952) 420–421.*

The Early History of the American Diabetes Association

by Cecil Striker

I have had the honor and privilege to have been intimately associated with the formation and early period of the American Diabetes Association. In view of the fact that I was its first President, and then its Secretary for seven consecutive years, I have had the opportunity of seeing the flourishing development of this unique organization.

Let us go back to the spring of 1939, when a small group of physicians gathered around a lunch table in New Orleans, where they had been attending the annual meeting of the American College of Physicians. A few of them had been exchanging letters as to why there was not a common meeting place for discussion by men who were interested in diabetes. A great deal of correspondence had taken place so the stage was set to create some sort of machinery to develop such an organization. It is important to record the names of Dr. Herman O. Mosenthal of New York City, Dr. Joseph H. Barach of Pittsburgh, Dr. Joseph T. Beardwood, Jr., and Dr. E. S. Dillon of Philadelphia and a few others, whose names should not be slighted but whose record is not complete. Following this meeting I met with Dr. Mosenthal to delineate specific machinery for the establishment of the American Diabetes Association. This machinery consisted of obtaining representatives from the five known existing local diabetes associations in the United States and, on April 2, 1940, the first meeting of a formal committee for the establishment of an American Diabetes Association was held. Various committees were appointed and as a result of the activities of this initial committee a second meeting was held on June 12, 1940, in New York City. There were twentysix physicians at this meeting. Following this, various committees were expanded and a national membership list was established. At this time it is fitting to pay great tribute to the activities of Dr. Herman O. Mosenthal, Dr. Joseph H. Barach, Dr. Joseph T. Beardwood, Jr., and Dr. William H. Muhlberg. The author is confident that, had it not been for the wise counseling of these men and their work and inexhaustible enthusiasm, the American Diabetes Association might not have been established.

The first Annual meeting of the American Diabetes Association was held on June 1, 1941, in Cleveland, Ohio. It was felt by those of us who were actively engaged in the formation of the Association that we would be most happy to have an attendance of about 250 as the program was very attractively arranged with Drs. Best, Joslin, Mosenthal and others presenting scientific papers. Much to our amazement instead of the hopeful 250, there was an attendance of over 300 physicians. This indicated to us that the progress and development of the American Diabetes Association would be assured.

In reviewing the files of the early history of the Association, one is confronted with the problem of having to omit interesting and important facts but among many important letters I wish to point out four that may be of particular interest. I quote:

UNIVERSITY OF TORONTO
Toronto 5, Canada
Department of Physiology

November 20, 1940.

Dr. Cecil Striker, President,
American Diabetes Association,
Cincinnati, Ohio.

Dear Dr. Striker:

I am very pleased to receive your letter of November 16, and I accept with a great deal of pleasure your invitation to become an Honorary Member of The American Diabetes Association.

I am keenly interested in increasing in every way possible our knowledge of the diabetic state and look forward to investigating a great many points when peace is restored. In the meantime we are able to keep a small group of workers busy in this field.

With all good wishes for the success of The Association,

Yours most sincerely,
C. H. Best
Professor of Physiology.

I would now like to quote a second letter:

UNIVERSITY OF TORONTO
Toronto 5, Canda

Department of Medical Research
Banting Institute

November 20, 1940.

Dr. Cecil Striker,
1019 Provident Bank Bldg.,
Cincinnati, Ohio.

Dear Dr. Striker:

Please accept my sincere thanks for your recent letter, for the honour that you have conferred on me in asking me to be an Honorary Member of your proposed Diabetic Association.

May I say, however, that I belong to so many organizations at the present time that I cannot contribute my share to their welfare. In addition, may I say that I have not engaged either in practice or experimental work on diabetes since 1924. For these reasons, you can readily understand that hesitate to accept your kind offer, as I desire to get out of responsibilities rather than into added responsibilities.

Yours very truly,
F. G. Banting.

UNIVERSITY OF TORONTO
Toronto 5, Canada

Department of Medical Research
Banting Institute

December 2nd,1940.

Dr. Cecil Striker,
1019 Provident Bank Bldg.,
Cincinnati, Ohio.

Dear Dr. Striker:

I have received your letter of November 28th, and whereas I would again remind you that I have no right to be honoured in the manner suggested in your letter, if it would be of any assistance to you, I would lend my name, provided always that it does not involve any responsibility or work.

Yours very truly,
F. G. Banting.

I would now like to quote another letter:

The
DIABETIC ASSOCIATION
9, Manchester Square, London W. 1.

January 13, 1942.

149 Harley St.,
London, W. 1.
England.

Dear Dr. Striker:

I am delighted to hear from you and the friendly contact your letter inaugurates is most welcome to our Association. They have asked me as their Chairman to convey their deep appreciation of the feelings you express and hope that our future co-operation may be close and helpful. Diabetes is universal, its progressive treatment and conquest international and calls for optimism and not sterilisation –. This sounds rather too like a Chairman, doesn't it?
My last visit (1936) to the United States was so enjoyable that the idea of another visit to your meeting in June 1942, raises fond dreams of better times. As you can imagine, a visit by myself or any of us seems impossible under present conditions but we hope your congress will still go on and be a success. Here we diabetics have had some anxious times over food and even insulin supplies, but provision and special arrangements in which our Association has been most useful, have prevented serious hardships. On the whole, diabetics have been as healthy and fit as usual and we trust the war will bring no serious difficulties to your side of the Atlantic.
I am glad to tell you that I personally am very well and busy and that life in London seems almost humdrum in its recent quiet. Our Association offices have been bombed, but our work and membership are expanding every year.
We are greatly cheered by your letter and hope our contacts may grow and expand as years go on. We are glad to be allied in every way.

With best wishes,
Very sincerely yours,
R. D. Lawrence.

One could record many human interest events in the early development of the Association. Among these, one is of sufficient interest and importance to merit special mention. Through the kind efforts of the late Dr. John R. Williams of Rochester, New York, I received this communication, which speaks for itself.

UNITED STATES MARITIME COMMISSION
WASHINGTON

Dezember 24, 1946

Office of the Chairman

The Honorable
James W. Wadsworth
House of Representatives

Dear Congressman Wadsworth:

Subject: SS FREDERICK BANTING

This will acknowledge receipt of your letter of December 16, 1946, in which you inquire regarding the SS FREDERICK BANTING.

The FREDERICK BANTING was delivered to the British Government, under Lend-Lease, on December 30, 1943. She has since been operated by them to ports in Japan, China, Australia, India, and the Mediterranean. The most recent information in our possession reflects the fact that she left Liverpool on December 5th, bound for Halifax, N. S., and is probably now at that port.

Sincerely yours,
(signed)
W. W. Smith
Chairman

This needs no comment.

Soon after the early scientific meetings, various committees were developed. Always the interest and activities of these committees were aimed toward the benefit of the diabetic patient. The committees have studied various problems such as quack remedies, improvements of insulin, establishment of summer camps for diabetic children, statistical investigations to ascertain more information concerning the prevalence and complications of diabetes and, in the early period of World War II, the creation of identification tags for diabetics to be used in the event of a catastrophe, and the question of establishing lay diabetes associations in which the problems of the patiens could be discussed at their own meetings.

In the early days when the war was at its peak the American Diabetes Association took a leaf from the activities of The British Diabetic Association. Their experience was of great benefit to us in reference to methods of allocation of insulin, provision for emergency treatment for diabetics and the issuance of proper rations. We pay tribute and thanks to them for the lessons we learned from them.

Probably one of the greatest events in the history of the American Diabetes Association was the commemorative meeting under the joint auspices of the University of Toronto and the American Diabetes Association on September 16, 17, and 18, 1946, at Toronto, Canada, on the Twenty-fifth Anniversary of the discovery of insulin. This meeting brought together many of the leading men interested in diabetes. It was unparalleled in that the only missing members of the earlier workers in the field were Sir Frederick Banting and Professor J. J. R. Macleod. Among those in attendance were Professor C. H. Best, Professor J. B. Collip, Drs. Walter R. Campbell, A. A.Fletcher, Russell M. Wilder, Seale Harris, Elliott P. Joslin, Rollin T. Woodyatt, as well as Dr. R. D. Lawrence of London, Dr. H. C. Hagedorn of Gentofte, Denmark, and Dr. B. A. Houssay of Buenos Aires and a host of others long interested in the field of carbohydrate metabolism. This meeting attracted over 500 physicians from all parts of the world. I think it can be said that never again will it be possible to bring together a group of men so fully representative of a single field of medicine and science. It was a memorable event.

In the early history of the Association two separate publications were issued. They were *Diabetes Abstracts* and the *Proceedings*. More recently they have been combined in the Association's scientific journal *Diabetes*.

It should be publicly recorded that in the early development of this Association the activities of Mr. J. K. Lilly, Mr. Eli Lilly and Dr. F. Bruce Peck of Indianapolis, were of invaluable assistance. Their efforts, foresight and enthusiasm make the American Diabetes Association forever indebted to them.

So that one may have a perspective on its phenomenal growth and development it should be noted that the initial budget was $35.00 a month and I am reliably informed that in 1955–56 it totals approximately $250.000.00 annually.

The continued success and enthusiasm of the American Diabetes Association has been due to the religious devotion to service for the diabetic by its officers, Council and committees. Its present Executive Director, Mr. J. Richard Connelly, and his staff have the same devotion to service. Living testimony proves this, as there are now over, 2,100 members of the American Diabetes Association from all over the world and thousands of individuals belonging to lay associations.

Any effort that was extended in the early development of this Association has been amply repaid by the service that it is giving and the distinguished position that it holds in the scientific world.

in: *Diabetes 5 (1956) 317–320.*

Bibliography of Primary Sources

The following reference works, arranged alphabetically by author, comprise the most important primary sources in the scientific literature on diabetes and its therapy from classical antiquity until 1922, the year insulin was discovered. In the eighteenth and nineteenth centuries there was a dramatic increase in the number of publications. For a survey of this material, see J. Schumacher's *Index zum Diabetes mellitus. Eine internationale Bibliographie*, Munich 1961.

ᶜAbd al-Laṭīf al-Baġdādī (1162–1231): l-Maraḍ al-musammā diyābīṭā, in: Ms. Bursa Hüseyin Çelebi 823, fol. 140v-149r; arab. u. dt., in: H.-J. Thies: Der Diabetestraktat ᶜAbd al-Laṭīf al-Baġdādī's, Untersuchungen zur Geschichte des Krankheitsbildes in der arabischen Medizin, Bonn, 1971, S. 83–170.

Actuarius, Joannes (13. Jhdt.): De urinis libri septem, Basel 1529, S. 123, 170 u. 236.

Aëtius von Amida (6. Jhdt.): De diabeta, in: De cognoscendis et curandis morbis sermones, lib. XI, cap. I, Basel 1535.

Alexander Trallianus (525–605): De arte medica, lib. 9, cap. 8, Lausanne 1772, S. 34, dt.: Ein Beitrag zur Geschichte der Medizin, Bd. 2, Wien 1879, S. 493.

Amatus Lusitanus (1511–1568): De diabetes curatione, in: Curationes medicinales, tom. I, cent. II, cap. 4, Venezia 1566, S. 208f; port., Lisboa 1944.

Apollonius von Memphis (3. Jhdt. v. Chr.), in: Caelius Aurelianus: De morbis acutis et chronicis libri VIII, Amsterdam 1709, S. 469; engl., Chicago 1950.

Aretaios von Kappadozien (81–138 n. Chr.): De diabete, in: De causis et signis diuturnorum morborum liber secundus, cap. II, in: Opera quae extant, Leipzig 1828 (= Medicorum graecorum opera, Bd. 24), S. 131–134; Curatio diabetis, in: De curatione morborum diuturnorum liber secundus, cap. 2, a.a.O., S. 329–331, dt.: Von den Ursachen und Kennzeichen chronischer Krankheiten, 2. Buch, 2. Kapitel, Wiesbaden 1858, Nachdruck 1969, S. 85–87; Therapie der chronischen Krankheiten, 2. Buch, 2. Kapitel; a.a.O., S. 214–215; engl., in: The extant works, London 1856, S. 338–340.

Avicenna (Ibn Sina) (980–1037): De diabete, in: Liber canonis, lib. 3, fen. 19, tract. 2, cap. 17f, Basel 1556, Nachdruck, Teheran 1976, S. 684 f; engl., Chicago 1950.

Baglivi, Giorgio (1668–1705): Epistola IV. De rara diabetis curatione, in: Opera omnia medico-practica et anatomica, Antwerpen 1710, S. 717–720; ital., Firenze 1841.

Banting, Frederick Grant (1891–1941), u. Charles Herbert Best (1899–1978): Pancreatic extracts in the treatment of diabetes mellitus, in: Canadian Medical Association Journal 12 (1922) 141–146.

Bernard, Claude (1813–1878): Du suc pancréatique et de son rôle dans les phénomènes de la digestion, in: Comptes Rendus des Séances et Mémoires de la Société de Biologie, (1849) 1850, 99–119.

Bernard, Claude (1813–1878): in: Leçons sur le diabète et la glycogenèse animale, Paris 1877; dt., Vorlesungen über den Diabetes und die tierische Zuckerbildung, Berlin 1878.

Bouchardat, Apollinaire (1806–1886): Du diabète sucré ou glycosurie, son traitment hygiénique, Paris 1851.

Brunner, Johann Conrad (1653–1727): Experimenta nova circa pancreas, Amsterdam 1683; engl. z. T. in: Annals of Medical History 3 (1941) 91–100.

Cantani, Arnaldo (1837–1893): Diabete mellito, Milano 1875 (= Patologia e terapia del recambio materiale); dt., Der Diabetes mellitus, Berlin 1877, [2]1880; franz., Le diabète sucré, Paris 1876.

Cardano, Geronimo (1501–1576): Cura morborum superstitiosa, in: De rerum veritate, lib. 8, cap. 44, Basel 1557, S. 577–579.

Cardano, Geronimo (1501–1576): De vita propria, Paris 1643; dt., München 1969, S. 27; engl., London 1934; franz., Paris 1935; ital., Torino 1945.

Cawley, Thomas (18. Jhdt.): A singular case of diabetes, consisting entirely in the quality of the wine, with an inquiry into the different theories of that disease, in: London Medical Journal 9 (1788) 286–308, dt.: Von einer Harnruhr, bey der bloß die Eigenschaft des Urins verändert wurde, nebst einigen Bemerkungen über die verschiedenen Theorien von dieser Krankheit, in: Neue Sammlung auserlesener Abhandlungen zum Gebrauche praktischer Aerzte 13 (1789) (1) 112–133; franz.: Observation singulière sur un diabètes, consistant entièrement dans la qualité de l'urine; avec des recherches sur les différentes théories de cette maladie, in: Journal de Médecine, Chirurgie, Pharmacie 79 (1789) 211–238.

Celsus, Aulus Cornelius (1. Jhdt. v. Chr.): De urinae nimia profusione, in: De Medicina, lib. IV, cap. 20, Leipzig 1915 (= Corpus Medicorum Latinorum, Bd. 1); dt.: Von der übermäßigen Absonderung des Urins, in: Über die Arzneiwissenschaft in acht Büchern, Braunschweig [2]1906, Nachdruck Hildesheim 1967, S. 204 f. engl.; London 1819; franz., Paris 1855.

Chevreul, Michel Eugène (1786–1889): Note sur le sucre de diabète, in: Annales de Chimie 95 (1815) 319–320.

Cullen, William (1710–1790): Synopsis nosologiae methodicae, genus 62, Edinburgh 1769, [2]1790, S. 188–191; dt.: Kurzer Inbegriff der methodischen Nosologie oder systematische Einteilung aller Krankheiten, Leipzig 1786, S. 326; engl., London 1800.

De le Boë-Sylvius, Franciscus (1614–1672): Diabetis causa et curatio, in: Praxeos medicae appendix, in: Opera medica, cap. 5, Amsterdam [2]1680, S. 725.

Demetrios von Apameia (2. Jhdt. v. Chr.), in : Caelius Aurelianus: De morbis acutis et chronicis, libri VIII, Amsterdam 1709, S. 469 f; engl., Chicago 1950.

Dobson, Matthew (1731–1784): Experiments and observations on the urine in a diabetes, in: Medical Observations and Inquiries by a Society of Physicians in London, Bd. 5, London 1776, S. 298–316, dt.: Versuche und Erfahrungen, die mit dem Urin bey einer Harnruhr sind angestellt worden, in: Medicinische Bemerkungen und Untersuchungen einer Gesellschaft von Aerzten in London, Bd. 6, Altenburg 1778, S. 248–263.

Dodonaeus, Rembert (1517–1585): Praxis medica, cap. XLII, Amsterdam 1616, S. 424–429.

Dolaeus, Johann (1651–1707): Diabetem observavi, in: Decas epistolarum de rebus medicis et philosophicis, Frankfurt a. M. 1689, S. 220 f.

Ettmüller, Michael (1644–1683): Diabetes, in: Opera omnia theoretica et practica, pars 2, Lyon 1685, S. 188–192; engl., London 1703.

Frank, Johann Peter (1745–1821): Diabetes, in: De curandis hominum morbis epitome, Bd. 5, § 476, Mannheim 1794, S. 38–67; dt.: Harnruhr (Diabetes), in: Behandlung der Krankheiten des Menschen, Bd. 5, Berlin 1830, S. 22–42; ital., Milano 1832.
Galen, Claudius (129–199): Opera omnia, Bd. 1, Leipzig 1821 (= Medicorum Graecorum Opera), S. 781; Bd. 3, Leipzig 1822, S. 344; Bd. 8, Leipzig 1824, S. 394.
Helmont, Jan Baptista van (1574–1644): Retenta, in: Opera omnia, Frankfurt a. M. 1682, S. 589; engl., London 1664; franz., Lyon 1675.
Home, Francis (1719–1813): Diabetes, in: Clinical experiments, histories and dissections, sect. 16, Edinburgh 1780, [3]1787; dt.: Von der Harnruhr (Diabetis), in: Clinische Versuche, Krankengeschichten und Leichenöffnungen, Leipzig 1781, S. 338–372.
Jaksch, Rudolf von (1855–1947): Ueber Acetonurie und Diaceturie, Berlin 1885.
Kratzenstein, Christian Gottlieb (1732–1795): Theoria fluxus diabetici ejusque sanandi methodus more geometrico explicata, Halle 1746.
Kußmaul, Adolf (1822–1902): Zur Lehre vom Diabetes mellitus. Ueber eine eigenthümliche Todesart bei Diabetischen, über Acetonämie, Glycerin-Behandlung des Diabetes und Einspritzungen von Diastase in's Blut bei dieser Krankheit, in: Deutsches Archiv für Klinische Medizin 14 (1874) 1–46.
Laguesse, Gustave Edouard (1861–1927): Sur la formation des îlots de Langerhans dans le pancréas, in: Comptes Rendus des Séances et Mémoires de la Société de Biologie 45 (1893) 819–820.
Lancereaux, Etienne (1829–1910): Le diabète maigre, ses symptomes, son évolution, son pronostic et son traitement, in: Union Médicale, 3. sér., 29 (1880) 161–167, 205–211.
Langerhans, Paul (1847–1888): Beiträge zur mikroskopischen Anatomie der Bauchspeicheldrüse, Diss. med., Berlin 1869; engl. Baltimore 1937.
Latham, John (1761–1843): Facts and opinions concerning diabetes, London 1811.
Lister, Martin (1638–1712): De diabete, in: Sex exercitationes medicinales, London 1694, S. 71–103, auch in: Octo extercitationes medicinales, Amsterdam 1698, S. 63–89.
Medicus, Friedrich Casimir (1736–1808): Die periodische Harnruhr, in: Geschichte periodischer Krankheiten, Bd. 1, Karlsruhe 1764, [2]1792, S. 161–165; franz., Paris 1790.
Mering, Joseph von (1849–1908): Über experimentellen Diabetes, in: Verhandlungen des Congresses für Innere Medicin 5 (1886) 185–189.
Mering, Joseph von (1849–1908), u. Oscar Minkowski (1858–1931): Diabetes mellitus nach Pankreasexstirpation, in: Archiv für experimentelle Pathologie und Pharmakologie 26 (1890) 371–387.
Morton, Richard (1637–1698): De tabe a diabete, seu nimio fluxu urinae, in: Phthisiologia, lib. I, cap. VIII, Genf 1696, S. 17–19; dt., Helmstedt 1780; engl., London 1694, [2]1720.
Naunyn, Bernard (1839–1925): Der Diabetes mellitus, Wien 1898, [2]1906.
Noorden, Carl Harko von (1858–1944): Die Zuckerkrankheit und ihre Behandlung, Berlin 1895, [8]1927; engl., New York 1905.
Oribasios (325 – Anf. 5. Jhdt.): Peri diabetou, in: Synopsis ad Eustathium, lib. 9, Leipzig 1926 (= Corpus Medicorum Graecorum, Bd. 6, 3), S. 297 f; franz., Paris 1876.
Papyrus Ebers (1500 v. Chr.), engl., Berlin 1890, London 1937.
Paracelsus (1493–1541): De diabetica, in: De morbis ex tartaro oriundis, lib. II, tract. III, cap. II, Sämtliche Werke, 1. Abt., 5. Bd., München 1931, S. 103–105.

Paulos von Aegina (7. Jhdt.): De arte medendi, lib. 2, cap. 13, lib. 3, cap. 45, Leipzig 1921 (= Corpus Medicorum Graecorum, Bd. 9, 1), S. 94 f. u. S. 247; dt.: Des besten Arztes sieben Bücher, Leiden 1914, S. 282; engl., London 1844.

Rhazes (850–992): De his qui inuiti urinam reddunt, in: Opera, lib. IX, cap. 78, Basel 1544, S. 263 f.

Rollo, John (gest. 1809): An account of two cases of the diabetes mellitus, London 1797, ^{2}1798, auch London 1806; dt.: Abhandlung des Diabetes oder zuckerartigen Harnruhr, Wien 1801; franz., Paris 1798.

Rufus von Ephesus (1. Jhdt. n. Chr.): De la diarrhée d'urine, in: Oeuvres, Paris 1879, Nachdruck Amsterdam 1963, S. 35–37.

Sauvages, François Boissier de (1706–1767): Diabetes, in: Nosologia methodica sistens morborum classes, genera et species, tom. 3, pars 2, Amsterdam 1763, S. 184–188; engl., Philadelphia 1793; franz., Paris 1771.

Susruta Samhita (500 n. Chr.): Bd. 1–3, Calcutta 1907–16.

Sydenham, Thomas (1624–1689): De diabete, in: Processus integri in morbis fere omnibus curandis, in: Opera universa medica, Leipzig 1837 (= Scriptorum classicorum de praxi medica nonnullorum opera collecta, Bd. 1), S. 503; dt.: Medizinische Werke, Bd. 2, Wien 1787, S. 650, engl., London 1696.

Trincavelli, Vittore (1496–1563): De causis diabetae, epistolae medicae XV–XVI, in: Consilia medica, Basel 1587, Sp. 824–827.

Trnka z. Křovic Václav (1739–1791): De diabete commentarius, Wien 1778.

Wedel, Georg Wolfgang (1645–1721): Diabetes a potu succi betulae lethalis, in: Miscellanea curiosa medico-physica academiae naturae curiosorum sive ephemerides (1671), observatio 198, S. 300–301.

Willis, Thomas (1621–1675): De Diuresi nimia, ejusque remedio, et speciatim de Diabete, in cujus theoriam, et therapiam inquiritur, in: Pharmaceutice rationalis sive diatriba de medicamentorum operationibus in humano corpore, sect. 4, cap. 3, London 1674, S. 163–182; engl.: Pharmaceutice rationalis or an exercitation of the operations of medicine in human bodies, chap. 3, London 1679, S. 79ff.

Zacutus Lusitanus (1576–1642): De diabete, in: Opera Omnia, Bd. 1, Lyon 1649, S. 420–423; De diabete, in: Opera Omnia, Bd. 2, Lyon 1649, S. 443–446.

Zuelzer, Georg Ludwig (1870–1949): Ueber Versuche einer specifischen Fermenttherapie des Diabetes, in: Zeitschrift für experimentelle Pathologie und Therapie 5 (1908) 307–318.

Bibliography of Secondary Literature

This bibliography lists publications that have appeared since the beginning of the nineteenth century about the history of research on diabetes from classical antiquity until the discovery of insulin in 1922. Historical studies on the lives of diabetics have also been included. The original titles of publications in German, English, French, and Italian are listed; the titles of publications in other languages are given in English. Dissertation Abstracts offfer information on dissertations in the United States.

anonym: (Rezension): R. T. Williamson: The geographical distribution of Diabetes Mellitus. The Medical Chronicle. July 1909, in: Janus 17 (1912) 335–336.

anonym: Diets in use in the Edinburgh Royal Infirmary in 1843, in: Edinburgh Medical Journal 22 (1919) 234–236.

anonym: Note on the history of diabetic gangrene, in: New York Medical Journal 111 (1920) 72.

anonym: Historical diagnosis (Herod the Great), in: St. Bart's Hospital Journal 63 (1959) 260.

anonym: R. D. Lawrence (a diabetic patient, a research worker in diabetes and one of the founders of the British Diabetic Association), in: British Medical Journal (1962) 1310.

anonym: Forty years of insulin therapy, in: Chemist and Druggist 179 (1963) 487–505.

anonym: Poterii spinosi cortex radicis, in: Quarterly Journal of Crude Drug Research 4 (1964) 582–588 (dt., engl., franz.).

anonym: Oscar Minkowski (1858–1931), designer of experimental diabetes, in: Journal of the American Medical Association 199 (1967) 754–755.

anonym: Matthew Dobson (1735–1784), clinical investigator of diabetes mellitus, in: Journal of the American Medical Association 205 (1968) 698.

anonym: Robert Daniel Lawrence, in: Lancet (1968) (2) 579.

anonym: Robert Daniel Lawrence, in: British Medical Journal (1968) 621–622.

anonym: Josef von Mering (1849–1908). Clinical chemist, in: Journal of the American Medical Association 204 (1968) 1188–1189.

anonym: Is diabetes mellitus neglected by philatelic agencies?, in: Scalpel & Tongs (Journal of Medical Philately) 15 (1971) 72–75.

anonym: Hommage au premier découvreur de l'insuline: Paulesco, in: La Semaine des Hôpitaux de Paris (1971) (2.6) 11.

anonym: Insulin: fifty years ago, in: Annals of Internal Medicine 75 (1971) 797–800.

anonym: Diabetes: Discovery of insulin 1921–1971. 1. Early descriptions of diabetes, in: Update Plus 1 (1971) 413–420.

anonym: Diabetes: Discovery of insulin 1921–1971. 3. Adolf Kussmaul, in: Update Plus 1 (1971) 603–604.

Ackerknecht, Erwin H.: Histoire du diabète, in: Médecine et Hygiène 19 (1961) 545–546.

Ackerknecht, Erwin H.: Geschichte und Geographie der wichtigsten Krankheiten, Stuttgart 1963 (S. 144).

Adlersberg, David: Adolf Kussmaul, in: Diabetes 4 (1955) 76–78.

Adlersberg, David: Frederick William Pavy, in: Diabetes 5 (1956) 491–492.

Ahmad, Suhail: Diltiazem and hyperglycemia – coma (letter), in: Journal of the American College of Cardiology 6 (1985) 494.

Ajgaonkar, Shreedhar Shantaram: Diabetes mellitus as seen in the ancient Ayurvedic medicine, in: Jasbir S. Bajaj, Hg.: Insulin and metabolism, Bombay 1972, S. 1–19.

Ajgaonkar, Shreedhar Shantaram: Diabetes mellitus as seen in the ancient Ayurvedic medicine, in: Madhumeh 12 (1972) suppl., 1–19.

Allan, Frank N.: The history of the treatment of diabetes by diet, in: Journal of the American Dietetic Association 6 (1930) 1–9.

Allan, Frank N.: The history of diabetes, in: Diabetes 1 (1932) 7–9.

Allan, Frank N.: J. J. R. Macleod, in: Diabetes 4 (1955) 491–492.

Allan, Frank N.: Diabetes before and after insulin, in: Medical History 16 (1972) 266–273.

Allan, Frank N.: The writings of Thomas Willis, M. D.; diabetes three hundred years ago, in: Diabetes 2 (1953) 74–78.

Allen, Frederick M.: The history of diabetes, in: Diabetes 1 (1932) 7–9.

Allen, Frederick M.: Arnaldo Cantani; pioneer of modern diabetes treatment, in: Diabetes 1 (1952) 63–65.

Allen, Frederick M.: Edgar Stillman u. Reginald Fitz: Total dietary regulation in the treatment of diabetes, New York 1919 (= Rockefeller Institute for Medical Research, Monograph 11), S. 30–33.

Ammon, Robert: E. J. Lesser's Beitrag zur Insulin-Forschung, in: Medizinische (1954) 397–398.

Ammon, Robert: Ernst Josef Lesser und sein Beitrag zur Entdeckung des Insulins, in: Mannheimer Hefte (Boehringer) (1968) 29–37.

Anderson, Fanny J.: John Rollo's patient, in: Journal of the History of Medicine 20 (1965) 163–164.

Andersson, Bo: (Diabetes mellitus – a historical retrospect, swed.), in: Opuscula Medica 13 (1968) 379–390.

Andral, Léon (?): Documents pour servir à l'histoire de la glycosurie, in: France Médicale 22 (1875) 233–236; auch in: Courrier Médical 25 (1875) 124–130; auch in: Tribune Médicale 8 (1875) 363–367.

Angeli, István: (50th anniversary of the death of Oskar Minkowski, discoverer of pancreatic diabetes, hung.), in: Orvosi Hetilap 122 (1981) 1726–1729.

Angrisani, Vincenzo: Evoluzione storica della malattia diabetica alla luce delle recenti acquisizioni degli ultimi cento anni, in: 21st International Congress of the History of Medicine, Siena 1968, Atti, Bd. 1, Roma 1970, S. 648–658.

Annes, Dias Heitor: (Diabetes; the evolution of its concept, port.), in: Dia Médico 15 (1943) 905–908.

Antiseri, Dario, u. Giovanni Federspil: Verisimiglianza, verità e approssimazione alla verità. Criteri epistemologici di preferibilità tra teorie; verità come ideale regolativo; ed esemplificazione storica del progresso nella conoscenza sul diabete, in: Medicina nei Secoli 13 (1976) 505–545.

Appermann, Isaac, u. George Alonzo Abbott: Some modern aspects of diabetes mellitus, in: Hospital News 5 (1938) (6) 1–22.

Aszódi, Zoltán: Twenty-five years of insulin, in: Orvosi Lapja 3 (1947) 1601–1610.

Ault, K., M. Sheta u. F. Vinicor: Diabetic Ketoacidosis: changing views of treatment, in: Indian Medical Journal 80 (1987) 719–725.

Baacke, Ulrich: Die Geschichte der wissenschaftlich begründeten oralen Antidiabetika, Diss. med. dent., Berlin 1977.

Banse, Hans-Joachim: Über die Behandlung der Zuckerkrankheit. Die Geschichte des Insulins, in: Der Diabetiker 6 (1956) 65–67.

Banting, Frederick Grant: The history of insulin, in: Edinburgh Medical Journal 36 (1929) (1) 1–18.

Banting, Frederick Grant: Early work on insulin, in: Science 85 (1937) 594–596.

Baquet, R.: Les conseils aux diabétiques d'Apollinaire Bourchardat, in: Maroc Médical 51 (1971) 517–520.

Barach, Joseph H.: Historical facts in diabetes, in: Annals of Medical History 10 (1928) 387–401.

Barach, Joseph H.: President's address (including excerpts from first paper on insulin treatment of diabetes mellitus published in USA, 1923), in: Proceedings of the American Diabetes Association 5 (1946) 65–78.

Barach, Joseph H.: Diabetes and its treatment, New York 1949 (History of the disease, S. 1 ff.)

Barach, Joseph H.: Diabetes in industry, diabetes in history, in: Industrial Medicine and Surgery 19 (1950) 257–262.

Barach, Joseph H.: Paul Langerhans 1847–1888, in: Diabetes 1 (1952) 411–413.

Baranov, Vasilij Gavrilovič: (History of the discovery of insulin, russ.), in: Kliničeskaja Medicina 27 (1949) 21–23.

Bartsocas, Christos: Goiters, dwarfs, giants and hermaphrodites, in: Progress in Clinical and Biological Research 200 (1985) 1–18.

Battle, Constance Urciolo: The beginning of the insulin era in historical context, in: Journal of the American Medical Women Association 22 (1967) 327–332.

Baumann, Evert Dirk: De diabete antiquo, in: Janus 37 (1933) 257–270.

Baumann, Evert Dirk: Der Spasmos Kunikos der Antiken, in: Janus 40 (1936) 34–42.

Baumel, Léopold: Un mot d'historique sur le diabète sucré. – Sa théorie pancréatique, in: Mémoires de l'Academie des Sciences et Lettres de Montpellier, Section Médecine 6 (1885–92) 451–465; auch in: Gazette Hebdomadaire de Médecine et de Chirurgie 28 (1891) 341–345; auch Montpellier 1891.

Becker, Henricus: Scriptorum et sententiarum de diabete mellito conspectus historicus, med. Diss., Rostock 1844.

Becker Volker: Paul Langerhans – 100 Jahre nach seiner Doktorarbeit, in: Deutsche Medizinische Wochenschrift 95 (1970) 358–362.

Beek, Cornelia van: Leonid V. Sobolev 1876-1919, in: Diabetes 7 (1958) 245–248.

Beek, Cornelia van: S. G. Chassovnikov, in: Diabetes 7 (1958) 413–414.

Belicza, Biserka: (Beginnings of the socio-medical approach to the problem of diabetes mellitus in Croatia, serbocroat. u. engl.), in: Diabetologica Croatia 6 (1977) 211–220.

Berg, Alexander: Die Entwicklung der Lehre vom Diabetes bis zur Gewinnung des Insulins, in: Münchener Medizinische Wochenschrift 104 (1962) 807–815.

Besson, Suzanne: La priorité de la découverte de l'insuline, in: Moniteur des Pharmacies et des Laboratoires 25 (1971) 2607.

Best, Charles Herbert: The discovery of insulin, in: Proceedings of the American Diabetic Association 6 (1947) 85–93).

Best, Charles Herbert: Reminiscences of the discovery of insulin. The first clinical use of insulin, in: Diabetes 5 (1956) 65–67.

Best, Charles Herbert: Elliott Proctor Joslin. June 6, 1869 – January 28, 1962. First Honorary President of the American Diabetes Association, in: Diabetes 11 (1962) 242–244.

Best, Charles Herbert: Selected papers, London 1964.

Best, Charles Herbert: Nineteen hundred twenty-one in Toronto, in: Diabetes 21 (1972) (suppl. 2) 385–395.

Best, Charles Herbert: Philosophy and outlook, in: Advances in Metabolic Disorders 7 (1974) 141–154.

Bett, Walter Reginald: A short history of some common diseases, London 1934, Norman ²1954.

Béttica-Giovannini, Renato: Il diabete e il pancreas prima del diabete, in: Annali dell'Ospedale Maria Vittoria di Torino 20 (1977) 93–129.

Biechteler, Walter: Krankheiten und Todesursachen berühmter Männer, Diss. med., München 1938.

Binder, Gerhard: Darf ich vorstellen. Kleine Motivphilatelie am Beispiel „Diabetes und Insulin", in: Briefmarkenwelt (1979) (4) 200–201.

Bliss, Michael: The discovery of insulin, Edinburgh 1983.

Bliss, Michael: The aetiology of the discovery of insulin, in: Health, disease and medicine. Essays in Canadian history, Hannah Conference on the history of medicine, 1982, Toronto 1984, S. 333–346.

Braun, Adolf: Krankheit und Tod im Schicksal bedeutender Menschen, in: Münchener Medizinische Wochenschrift 80 (1933) 1981–1985.

Brillante, Carlo, u. Giancarlo Laffi: Profilo storico-sintetico della malattia diabetica (dal papiro di Ebers a Banting e Best), in: Minerva Medica 73 (1982) 1087–1106.

Buhač, Ivo: Über die Erkrankung und den Tod des Herodes, in: Deutsche Medizinische Wochenschrift 88 (1963) 287–288.

Buxton, Roger St. John: Diabetes mellitus through the ages, in: Black Bag (Bristol Univ.) 17 (1961) 50–56.

Cabanés, Augustin: Quelle était la maladie de M...?, in: Cabanés: Cabinet secret, Bd. 1, Paris 1897, S. 133–138.

Cammidge, Percy John, u. Hubert A. Harry Howard: New views on diabetes mellitus, London 1923.

Canadell i Vidal, José Maria: La historia de la diabetes, in: Canadell i Vidal: Libro de la diabetes, Barcelona 1973, S. 21–40.

Campbell, Walter R.: Paul Langerhans 1847–1888, in: Canadian Medical Association Journal 79 (1958) 855–856.

Campbell, Walter R.: Anabasis, in: Canadian Medical Association Journal 87 (1962) 1055–1061.

Carlström, Sven: (Documents of diabetes in the history of medicine, swed.), in: Sydsvenska Medicinhistoriska Sallskapets Arsskrift (1979) 54–61.

Carrasco-Formiguera, Rosendo: From the preinsulin age to the Banting and Best era. Reminiscences of a witness and participant, in: Israel Journal of Medical Sciences 8 (1972) 484–487.

Cawley, Thomas: A singular case of diabetes, consisting entirely in the quality of urine; with an inquiry into the different theories of that disease, in: London Medical Journal 9 (1788) 286–308, dt.: Von einer Harnruhr, bey der bloß die Eigenschaft des Urins verändert wurde, nebst einigen Bemerkungen über die verschiedenen Theorien von dieser Krankheit in: Neue Sammlung auserlesener Abhandlungen zum Gebrauche praktischer Aerzte 13 (1789) (1) 112–133; franz.: Observation singulière sur un diabète, consistant entièrement dans la qualité de l'urine; avec des recherches sur les différentes théories de cette maladie, in: Journal de Médicine, de Chirurgie, Pharmacie etc. 79 (1789) 211–238.

Celso, Alfonso: O Imperador no Exilio, Rio de Janeiro ca. 1915.

Charcot, Jean Martin: Quelques documents concernant l'historique des gangrènes diabétiques, in: Gazette Hebdomadaire de Médecine et de Chirurgie 8 (1861) 539–545.

Chesley, Leon Carey: History and epidemiology of praeclampsia – eclampsia, in: Clinical Obstetrics and Gynecology 27 (1984) 801–820.

Chevers, Norman: The mild treatment of diabetes in the seventeenth century, in: Indian Medical Gazette 9 (1874) 121.

Chevrel, Bernard: A propos du cinquantenaire de la découverte de l'insuline. Hommage tardif à N. Paulesco, in: La Presse Médicale 79 (1971) 1512.

Chevrillon, André: Portrait de Taine. Souvenirs, Paris 1958.

Cheymol, Jean: A propos de „la découverte de l'insuline“ par Banting et Best il y a cinquante ans, in: Bulletin de l'Académie de Médecine de Paris 155 (1971) 836–852.

Cheymol, Jean: Il y a cinquante ans Banting et Best découvraient l'insuline, in: Histoire des Sciences Médicales 6 (1972) 133–151.

Cheymol, Jean: Il y a un siècle. Apollinaire Bouchardat montrait le rôle primordial du régime alimentaire dans le traitement du diabète sucré, in: Bulletin de l'Académie Nationale de Médecine 159 (1975) 760–769.

Chirife, Alejandro V., u. Fernando S. Chirife: (The discoverers of insulin, span.), in: Prensa Medica Argentina 59 (1972) 363–368.

Clapp, Sylvanus: Diabetes mellitus, 1854, in: The Rhode Island Medical Journal 51 (1968) 493–499.

Clemow, Frank.: Zur Geschichte des Pankreasdiabetes, in: Schering-Kahlbaum A. G. Berlin, Medizinische Mitteilungen 1 (1929) (2) 31–33.

Cockle, John: On some points connected with the past and present history of diabetes, and on a less common form of death in this disease, in: Transactions of the Medical Society of London 2 (1862) 17–19; auch in: The Lancet (1862) (1) 37–38.

Cohen, J., H. Lipman u. E. Lipman: Doctor Marat and his skin, in: Medical History 2 (1958) 281–286.

Cohn, Max: Jean Paul Marat: Ein Beitrag zur Lösung des von ihm gebotenen Problems seines Charakters und seiner Krankheit, in: Zeitschrift für Psychotherapie 8 (1920) 35–56.

Coignard, Augustin: Un point de l'histoire du diabéte sucré, in: Journal de Thérapeutique 9 (1882) 41–47.

Coleman, Vernon: The history of diabetes, in: Nursing Mirror and Midwives Journal 140 (1975) 70.

Collip, James Bertram: The history of the discovery of insulin, in: Northwest Medicine 22 (1923) 267–273.

Collip, James Bertram: Reminiscences on the discovery of insulin, in: Canadian Medical Association Journal 87 (1962) 1045.

Colwell, Arthur R.: Rollin Turner Woodyatt, in: Diabetes 3 (1954) 164–165.

Colwell, Arthur R.: Fifty years of diabetes in perspective, in: Diabetes 17 (1968) 599–610.

C(one), Thomas E., jr.: Dr. John Lovett Morse of Boston on a child with diabetes mellitus (1916), in: Pediatrics 54 (1974) 135.

C(one), Thomas E., jr.: Abraham Jacobi on juvenile diabetes mellitus – 1896, in: Pediatrics 60 (1977) 830.

Conklin, Groff: Diabetics unknown, New York 1961 (=Public Affairs Pamphlets, Nr. 312).

Conn, Jerome W.: Expanding concepts of diabetes mellitus, in: Modern Medicine of Canada (1964) (ang.) 49–58.

Coturri, Enrico: Il diabete insipido dalla conoscenza della melattia ad oggi, in: Castalia 20 (1964) 38–41.

Crawford, E. M.: Death rates from diabetes mellitus in Ireland 1833–1983: a historical commentary, in: Ulster Medical Journal 56 (1987) 109–115.

Cumston, Charles Greene: Notes on the life and writings of Geronimo Cardano, in: The Boston Medical and Surgical Journal 146 (1902) 77–81; auch Boston 1902.

Cumston, Charles Greene: The history of diabetes, in: Medical Journal and Record 120 (1924) 336–338.

Debeyre, Albert: Comment fût déclenchée la découverte de l'insuline? Corollaire des savantes recherches du Dijonnais G. A. Laguesse, alors professeur éminent de la Faculté de Médecine de l'Université de Lille, in: Le Progrès Médical 84 (1956) 442–445.

Decourt, Philippe: La véritable histoire de la découverte de l'insuline, in: Archives Internationales Claude Bernard (1976) (9) 17–29.

De Kruif, Paul Henry: Men against death, New York 1932, dt.: Kämpfer für das Leben, Berlin 1946, 1951.

De Kruif, Paul Henry: Banting, der das Insulin fand, in: Der Diabetiker 3 (1953) 57–60, 75–76.

Dérot, Maurice: La découverte de l'insuline, in: La Vie Médicale (1971) (nr. spéc. 52) 13–22.

Dérot, Maurice: Perspectives en diabétologie (d'hier à demain), in: Bulletin et Mémoires de l'Académie Royale de Médecine de Belgique 136 (1981) 435–442.

Diabetes: A medical Odyssey, New York 1971.

Diamare, Vincenzo: Documenti per la storia della teoria insulare del diabete e sui precedenti dell' „insulina", in: Archivio di Fisiologia 22 (1924) 141–157.

Dinguizli, ?: Robin, Albert: Rapport sur un travail de M. le Dr. Dinguizli (de Tunis), intitulé: Diabète sucré et son traitment sans régime, d'après les auteurs arabes anciens, par Albert Robin, in: Bulletin de l'Académie de Médecine de Paris 70 (1913) 629–635.

Dittrich, Hans-Michael: Zur Geschichte der Pankreasforschung von Bichat bis zur Entdeckung des Insulins – unter besonderer Berücksichtigung des Greifswalder Anteils. Ein Beitrag zur Geschichte der Anatomie, med. Diss., Greifswald 1975.

Dittrich, Hans-Michael: Alfred Lublin (1895–1956) und sein Beitrag zur Diabetologie, in: Zeitschrift für Ärztliche Fortbildung, Jena 79 (1985) 361–363.

Dittrich, Hans-Michael, u. Herwig Hahn von Dorsche: Ein Jahrhundert Erforschung der Langerhansschen Inseln. Ein Beitrag zur Periodisierung der Diabetes-mellitus-Forschung, in: Anatomischer Anzeiger, Jena 137 (1975) 470–478.

Dittrich, Hans-Michael, u. Herwig Hahn von Dorsche: Zur Entwicklung der anatomischen Erforschung des Pankreas von Vesal bis Bichat. I. Mitteilung: Von Vesal bis Kerkring, in: Anatomischer Anzeiger, Jena 137 (1975) 11–25.

Dittrich, Hans-Michael, u. Herwig Hahn von Dorsche: Zur Entwicklung der anatomischen Erforschung des Pankreas von Vesal bis Bichat. II. Mitteilung: Von Borelli bis Bichat, in: Anatomischer Anzeiger, Jena 143 (1978) 21–36.

Dittrich, Hans-Michael, u. Herwig Hahn von Dorsche: Die anatomisch-histologische Erforschung des Pankreas vom Beginn des 19. Jahrhunderts bis zur Entdeckung des Insulins durch Banting und Best (1921) unter Berücksichtigung physiologischer Aspekte. 1. Die anatomische Pankreasforschung vom Beginn des 19. Jahrhunderts bis zur Entdeckung des Inselorgans (1869), in: Anatomischer Anzeiger, Jena 143 (1978) 221–230.

Dittrich, Hans-Michael, u. Herwig Hahn von Dorsche: Die anatomisch-histologische Erforschung des Pankreas vom Beginn des 19. Jahrhunderts bis zur Entdeckung des Insulins durch Banting und Best (1921) unter Berücksichtigung physiologischer Aspekte. 2. Die Pankreasforschung von der Entdeckung des Inselorgans (1869) bis zur Entdeckung des Pankreasdiabetes (1889), in: Anatomischer Anzeiger, Jena 143 (1978) 231–241.

Dittrich Hans-Michael, u. Herwig Hahn von Dorsche: Die anatomisch-histologische Erforschung des Pankreas vom Beginn des 19. Jahrhunderts bis zur Entdeckung des Insulins durch Banting und Best (1921) unter Berücksichtigung physiologischer Aspekte. 3. Die Entdeckung des Pankreasdiabetes durch v. Mering und Minkowski (1889), in: Anatomischer Anzeiger, Jena 143 (1978) 509–517.

Dittrich, Hans-Michael, u. Herwig Hahn von Dorsche: Die anatomisch-histologische Erforschung des Pankreas vom Beginn des 19. Jahrhunderts bis zur Entdeckung des Insulins durch Banting und Best (1921) unter Berücksichtigung physiologischer Aspekte. 4. Die Pankreasforschung nach der Entdeckung des Pankreasdiabetes (1889) bis zur Entdeckung des Insulins, in: Anatomischer Anzeiger, Jena 144 (1978) 260–272.

Dittrich, Hans-Michael, u. Herwig Hahn von Dorsche: Untersuchung über die Kenntnis des Pankreas in der Zeit vor Vesal mit besonderer Berücksichtigung der anatomischen Technik im 16. und 17. Jahrhundert, in: Anatomischer Anzeiger, Jena 142 (1977) 145–150.

Dörzbach, Eugen: Geschichte des Insulins, in: Medizinische Klinik 61 (1966) 1122–1123.

Dotz, Warren: Jean Paul Marat. His life, cutaneous disease, death, and depiction by Jacques Louis David, in: American Journal of Dermatopathology 1 (1979) 247–250.

Dougherty, Alexander N.: Observations on glycosuria, historical and clinical, in: Transactions of the Medical Society of New Jersey (1878) 52–119.

Drügemöller, Paula, u. Leo Norpoth: Wege und Irrwege der deutschen Insulin-Forschung, in: Deutsche Medizinische Wochenschrift 78 (1953) 919–922.

Drury, M. I.: The golden jubilee of insulin, in: Journal of the Irish Medical Association 65 (1972) 355–363.

Drury, M. I.: Diabetes in pregnancy. Matthews Duncan revisited, in: Irish Journal of Medical Science 153 (1984) 144–151.

Drury, M. I.: Corrigan Memorial Lecture. The pissing evile, in: Irish Journal of Medical Science 154 (1985) 1–13.

Dudziński, Wacław: (Illness and death of King Michal Korybut Wiśniowiecki, pol.), in: Wiadomosci Lekarskie 32 (1979) 55–58.

Dudziński, Wacław: (Illness and death of the King of Poland and Prince Elect of Saxony August II, called the Strong, pol.), in: Wiadomosci Lekarskie 32 (1979) 129–131.

Duncan, Leslie James Park, u. B. F. Clarke: Changing concepts of the cause of diabetes mellitus, in: Res Medica 5 (1967) 21–25.

Dziob, J. S.: Diabetes among the moderns, in: Rhode Island Medical Journal 20 (1937) 87–91.

Ebstein, Erich: Die Toxintheorie des Diabetes mellitus. Historische Notiz, in: Deutsche Medizinische Wochenschrift 26 (1900) 170–171.

Ebstein, Erich: Sollen wir Diabetes mellitus oder melitus schreiben?, in: Mitteilungen zur Geschichte der Medizin, der Naturwissenschaften und Technik 6 (1907) 194–195.

Ebstein, Erich: Zur Vorgeschichte des Coma diabeticum, in: Wiener Klinische Wochenschrift 25 (1912) 885–886.

Ebstein, Erich: Zur Entwicklung der klinischen Harndiagnostik in chemischer und mikroskopischer Hinsicht, Leipzig 1915.

Ebstein, Erich: Geschichte des Diabetes mellitus mit besonderer Berücksichtigung des Pankreas, in: Janus 28 (1924) 368.

Ebstein, Erich: Aus der Geschichte der Zuckerkrankheit mit besonderer Berücksichtigung der Bauchspeicheldrüse, in: Archiv für Verdauungskrankheiten 33 (1924) 215–226.

Ebstein, Erich: Zuckerkrankheit, Zuckerverbrauch und Luxus im Wandel der Jahrhunderte. Eine Fragestellung aus der Geschichte, in: Medizinische Welt (1928) (49) 1840–1842; auch in: Zentralblatt für die Zuckerindustrie 37 (1929) 13.

Ebstein, Wilhelm: Die Krankheit des Magus im Norden, in: Süddeutsche Monatshefte 9 (1912) (2) 162–178.

Endtz, Lambertus Jacobus: Note pour servir à l'histoire de la neuropathie diabétique. A la mémoire de Charles-Jacob Marchal, in: Journées Annuelles Diabétologie de l'Hôtel Dieu 9 (1968) 51–53.

Evans, Colin: Taine. Essay de Biographie intérieure, Paris 1975.

Fabre, Augustin. Les étapes de la question du diabète, in: Union Médicale de la Provence, Marseille 1 (1864) 117–128.

Fajans, Stefan S.: Diabetes mellitus, Bethesda 1976.

Falta, Wilhelm: Praktisches und Historisches zur Mehlfrüchtekur bei Diabetes mellitus, in: Deutsche Medizinische Wochenschrift 47 (1921) 889–891.

Farmer, Laurence: Notes on the history of diabetes mellitus. Views concerning its nature and etiology up to the discovery of the role of the pancreas, in: Bulletin of the New York Academy of Medicine 28 (1952) 408–416.

Farmer, Laurence: Notes on the history of diabetes mellitus. II: search for the antidiabetic principle, in: Bulletin of the New York Academy of Medicine 29 (1953) 636–641.

Feasby, William Richard: The discovery of insulin, in: Journal of the History of Medicine 13 (1958) 68–84.

Federspil, Giovanni: Lo sviluppo delle teorie sulla glicogenesi e il diabete in Claude Bernard e oggi, in: Medicina nei Secoli 16 (1979) 31–50.

Felig, Philip: Landmark perspective: Protamine insulin. Hagedorn's pioneering contribution to drug delivery in the management of diabetes, in: Journal of the American Medical Association 251 (1984) 393–396.

Fischer, Franz: Einst und jetzt: Die historische Entwicklung der Retinopathia diabetica, in: Münchener Medizinische Wochenschrift 96 (1954) 1287–1289.

Fischer, Franz: Der erste Fall von Retinopathia diabetica (Eduard von Jaeger, Wien 1855), in: Wiener Medizinische Wochenschrift 107 (1957) 969–972.

Fitzgerald, Patrick J.: Medical anecdotes concerning some diseases of the pancreas, in: Monographs in Pathology 21 (1980) 1–29.

Fleckenstein, Albrecht: Die Lebenslage der Diabetiker im Krieg, med. Diss., Würzburg 1942.

Fleckles, Leopold: Die Geschichte der gangbaren Theorien vom Diabetes mellitus, von Willis 1674 bis auf Pavy 1864, in: Deutsche Klinik 17 (1865) 89–93.

Foit, Richard, u. Jiři Syllaba, Hg.: Diabetes mellitus, Historické poznamky, Prag 1970, S. 13–32.

Forrest, D.: Diabetes, ancient and modern, in: Newcastle Medical Journal 2 (1921/22) 118–124.
Forssman, Hans: The recognition of nephrogenic diabetes insipidus. A very small page from the history of medicine, in: Acta Medica Scandinavia 197 (1975 (1–2) 1–6.
Frank, Erich: Die Entdeckung des Pankreasdiabetes (Zugleich Bemerkungen zu dem Aufsatz von H. Winternitz in Nr. 41 dieser Wochenschrift), in: Medizinische Klinik 46 (1931) 1692–1693.
Frank, Erich: Zur Entdeckung des Pankreasdiabetes. Schlußbemerkung zu der Stellungnahme von H. Winternitz in Nr. 4, 1932 dieser Wschr. zu meiner Erwiderung (M. Kl. 1931, Nr. 44) auf seinen Aufsatz (M. Kl. 1931, Nr. 35), in: Medizinische Klinik 28 (1932) 603–604.
Frank, Ludwig L.: Diabetes mellitus in the texts of old Hindu medicine (Charaka, Susruta, Vagobata), in: American Journal of Gastroenterology 27 (1957) 76–95.
Frank, Mortimer: The history of the discovery of the secretory glands and their function, in: Bulletin of the Johns Hopkins Hospital 27 (1916) 302–09.
Frankl, W.: Die wichtigsten Momente aus der Geschichte des Diabetes, in: Wiener Medizinische Presse 41 (1900) 1105–1112, 1155–1160.
Freshwater, Michael Felix: La pharmacie rustique. Sketched by Gottfried Locher in 1774; engraved by Barthelemy Huebner in 1775, in: Journal of the History of Medicine 25 (1970) 477.
Freyler, Heinrich: Ophtalmochirurgische Behandlungsmöglichkeiten der diabetischen Retinopathie, in: Wiener Klinische Wochenschrift 95 (1983) 257–261.
Fritz, Reginald H., u. Elliot Proctor Joslins: Diabetes mellitus at the Massachusetts General Hospital from 1824 to 1898. A study of the medical records, in: Journal of the American Medical Association 31 (1898) 165–171.
Fröhlich, Jürgen: Kußmaulsche Atmung und diabetische Ketoazidose, in: Friedrich Kluge, Hg.: Adolf Kußmaul. Seine aktuelle Bedeutung für Innere Medizin und Neurologie, Stuttgart 1985, S. 39–46.
Fulton, John F.: Reminiscences of the discovery of Insulin. Sir Frederick Banting 1891–1941, in: Diabetes 5 (1956) 64–65.
Furfaro, Domenico: La terapia del diabete prima e dopo la scoperta dell'insulina, in: Atti del I. Congresso Nazionale di Storia della Terapia, Roma 15–16 ottobre 1961, Roma 1963, S. 779–785.
Garreton-Silva, Alejandro: (The significance of the discovery of insulin by Banting and Best in 1921, span.), in: Revista Medica de Chile 100 (1972) 458–459.
Garrison, Fielding H.: Historical aspects of diabetes and insulin, in: Bulletin of the New York Academy of Medicine 1 (1925) 127–133.
Gaspar de Freitag, Divaldo: Les voyages de l'empereur Pierre Second (D. Pedro II) en France, in: Histoire des Sciences Médicales 13 (1979) (1) 91–99.
Gemmill, Chalmers L.: The Greek concept of diabetes, in: Bulletin of the New York Academy of Medicine 48 (1972) 1033–1036.
Genes, Semen Grigorevič: (Evolution of the concepts of the pathogenesis of diabetes, russ.), in: Arkiv Patologii 31 (1969).
Genes Semen Grigorevič: (Evolution of diet therapy in patients with diabetes mellitus, russ.), in: Terapičeskij Arkiv 46 (1974) 120–127.
Gerlach, Erich: Historische und kritische Beiträge zum experimentellen Pankreas-Diabetes, med. Diss., Berlin 1929.
Giacometti, Luigi, u. Margaret Barss: Paul Langerhans: A tribute, in: Archives of Dermatology 100 (1969) 770–772.

Gilbert, Judson Bennett: Bibliography of medical references to the famous, London 1962.

Giordano, Carmelo, N. G. De Santo, M. G. Lamendola u. G. Capodicasa: The genesis of the Armanni-Ebstein lesion in diabetic nephropathy, in: Journal of Diabetic Complications 1 (1987) (1) 2–3.

Goḍbole, Arvinda Sādasiva, u. Neelkanth G. Talwalkar: The history of diabetes mellitus, in: Goḍbole u. Talwalkar: Diabetes mellitus for practitioners, Bombay 1974, S. 1–9.

Goldman, Jean: Introduction à l'histoire du diabète, in: Revue d'Histoire de la Médecine Hébraique 21 (1968) 5–11, 71–75, 125–133, 715–719.

Goldner, Martin G.: Adolf Magnus-Levy, 1865-1955, in: Diabetes 4 (1955) 422–424.

Goldner, Martin G.: Historical review of oral substitutes for insulin, in: Diabetes 6 (1957) 259–262.

Goldner, Martin G.: Theorien und Fakten im Wandel der Diabetes-Forschung, in: Der Diabetiker 19 (1969) 166–168.

Goldner, Martin G.: History of insulin, in: Annals of Internal Medicine 76 (1972) 329.

Goldstein, Asher: (The history of diabetes mellitus – heredity and prophylaxis, hebr.), in: Koroth 5 (1971) 713–715.

Gori, Mario: Alla scoperta dell'insulina: Zuelzer, Paulesco, Banting, in: Il Policlinico, Sez. Med. 86 (1979).

Gori, Mario: Zuelzer: Primi tentativi di terapia ormonale del diabete mellito, in: Medicina nei Secoli 15 (1978) 423–426.

Graef, Irving: John Brisbane, M. D., in: Diabetes 6 (1957) 196–202.

Graham, George: Diabetes mellitus; a survey of changes in treatment during the last 45 years, in: Lancet (1938) (2) 1–7, 62–68, 121–125.

Grant, D. M.: Banting and Best – the men who tamed diabetes, in: Canadian Nurse 67 (1971) 27–30.

Gregory, John: Diabetes a century ago, in: Canadian Medical Association Journal 14 (1924) 432.

Grenfell, A.: Diabetic nephropathy: historical aspects, in: Clinical Endocrinology and Metabolism 15 (1986) 727–731.

Greydanus, Donald E., u. Adele D. Hofmann: Psychological factors in diabetes mellitus. A review of the literature with emphasis on adolescence, in: American Journal of Diseases of Children 133 (1979) 1061–1066.

Grmek, Mirko Dražen: Examen critique de la genèse d'une grande découverte: La piqûre diabétique de Claude Bernard, in: Clio Medica 1 (1965/66) 341–350.

Grmek, Mirko Dražen: La glycogenèse et le diabète dans l'oeuvre de Claude Bernard (jusqu'a la découverte du glycogène), in: Claude Bernard: Leçons sur le diabète, Paris 1968 (Nachdruck der Ausgabe Paris 1877), S. 187–234.

Grmek, Mirko Dražen: First steps in Claude Bernard's discovery of the glycogenic function of the liver, in: Journal of the History of Biology 1 (1968) 141–154.

Groen, Joannes Juda: Discovery of insulin told as a human story, in: Israel Journal of Medical Sciences 8 (1972) 476–483.

Grote, Louis Ruyter Radcliffe: Neuzeitliche Diabetisbehandlung, in: Ergebnisse der Gesamten Medizin 18 (1933) 301–458.

Grott, Józef Wacław, u. Ewa Swiezawska: (Frederick Madison Allen (1879–1964) and his contributions to the knowledge of diabetes mellitus, pol.), in: Polski Tygodnik Lekarskie 20 (1965) 1872.

Gutman, Jacob: Modern views on the causation and treatment of diabetes mellitus, in: Medical Record 148 (1938) 151–154.

Hahn von Dorsche, Herwig, u. Hans-Michael Dittrich: Die Diabetesforschung in Greifswald im 19. Jahrhundert und am Beginn des 20. Jahrhunderts in ihrer Bedeutung für die Diabetologie, in: Anatomischer Anzeiger, Jena 152 (1982) 435–448.

Haring, Wilhelm: Die Entwicklung der Diabetestherapie seit Naunyn und Minkowski, in: Zeitschrift für Innere Medizin 7 (1952) 148–154.

Harmsen, Ernst: Zur Entdeckung des Glykogens vor 75 Jahren, in: Münchener Medizinische Wochenschrift 27 (1932) 1075.

Harmsen, Ernst: Victor Hensen, der deutsche Entdecker des Glykogens, in: Medizinische Welt 8 (1934) 1783–1784.

Harris, Seale: Reminiscences of Banting, discoverer of insulin, in: Mississippi Doctor 20 (1943) 430–440.

Harris, Seale: Banting's miracle. The story of the discoverer of insulin, Philadelphia 1946; holl. Hoorn 1947.

Hauk, Joachim: Carl Harko Hermann Johannes von Noorden (1858–1944). Sein Leben und Werk unter besonderer Berücksichtigung seiner Theorien über die Ursachen des Diabetes mellitus, med. Diss., München 1980.

Harrower, Kate: Mouse pie, in: British Medical Journal (1962) (2) 994.

Hazard, René: Un précurseur oublié dans la découverte de l'insuline, in: Le Moniteur des Pharmacies et des laboratoires 25 (1971) 2607.

Hejda, Bedřich: (Beginnings of the insulin therapy of diabetes at the 2nd Internal Clinic of Prof. Pelnar, czech.), in: Casopis Lékařů Českých 112 (1973) 936.

Heinzemann, Gisela: Geschichte der Erforschung des Diabetes insipidus, med. Diss., Göttingen 1948.

Henderson, Alfred R.: Frederik M. Allen, M. D., and the Physiatric Institute at Morristown, H. J. (1920–1938), in: Academy of Medicine of New Jersey Bulletin 16 (1970) 40–49.

Henschen, Folke: The term „diabetes“ according to Aretaios and Galenos, in: Opuscula Medica 12 (1967) 167–169.

Henschen, Folke: On the term „diabetes“ in the works of Aretaeus and Galen, in: Medical History 13 (1969) 190–192.

Herold, Arthur Anselm: History of conceptions of etiology and therapy of diabetes mellitus, past and present, in: Journal Louisiana State Medical Society 109 (1957) 355–357.

Heuel, Josef: Über die Geschichte der Diabetestherapie, med. Diss., Bonn 1929.

Hoef, Joseph Pierre: Gustave Edouard Laguesse. His demonstration of the significance of the island of Langerhans, in: Diabetes 2 (1953) 322–324.

Hoff, Ferdinand: Diabetesforschung. In fünf Jahrzehnten Blütezeit deutscher Medizin, Festschrift 50. Kongreß für Innere Medizin, hg. v. Hans Spatz, Berlin 1938, S. 85–105.

Hoffmann, Joachim Peter Heinz: Die Geschichte des Diabetes mellitus, med. Diss., Düsseldorf 1960.

Hoffmann, Karl Franz: Erinnerungen an den Diabetologen Elliot Proctor Joslin (1869–1962), in: Der Diabetiker 19 (1969) 372.

Hofmeier, Heinrich: Zur Geschichte von Leber und Pankreas, in: Materia Medica Nordmark 12 (1960) 537–544.

Hogarth, Jean: An historical account of Toronto's contribution to the study and control of diabetes, in: Royal Free Hospital Journal 24 (1961) 17–19.

Holscher, Helmut D., u. René Kende: Diabetes. Aus der Geschichte seiner Erforschung und Behandlung, in: Grünenthal-Waage 10 (1971).

Holt, Anna C.: Elliott Proctor Joslin: a memoir, 1869–1962, Worcester 1969.

Hornor, Albert A.: Diabetes mellitus, 1880–1940, in: Frank Howard Lahey birthday volume, Springfield, Ill., 1940, S. 231–236.
Hornor, Albert A.: History of insulin, in: Annals of Internal Medicine 76 (1972) 330.
Horowitz, Philip: The history of diabetes mellitus, in: New York Medical Journal 111 (1920) 807–812.
Houssay, Bernardo Alberto: History of hypophysical diabetes, in: Essays in biology in honor of Herbert M. Evans, Berkeley 1943, S. 245–256.
Houssay, Bernardo Alberto: The discovery of pancreatic diabetes. The role of Oscar Minkowski, in: Diabetes 1 (1952) 112–116.
Hughes, Joseph: Eugene L. Opie, in: Diabetes 7 (1958) 496–499.
Jackson, James Godfrey Lambert: The British Diabetic Association, in: Guy's Hospital Gazette 85 (1971) 322–323.
James, Theodore: History of diabetes, in: South African Medical Journal 44 (1970) 1394–1395.
Johnsson, John William Schibbye: (History of diabetes, dan.), in: Ugeskrift for Laeger 87 (1925) 352–353.
Joslin, Elliot P.: Story of evolution of treatment of diabetes at New England Deaconess Hospital Boston, in: Nordisk Medicin (1939) (2) 1261–1267.
Joslin, Elliot P.: Banting memorial adress; diabetes yesterday, today and tomorrow, in: Proceedings of the American Diabetes Association 1 (1942) 117–137.
Joslin, Elliot P.: Diabetes, past, present and future, in: Proceedings of the American Diabetes Association 6 (1947) 159–169.
Joslin, Elliot P.: Apollinaire Bouchardat, 1806-1886, in: Diabetes 1 (1952) 490–491.
Joslin, Elliot P.: Reminiscences of the discovery of insulin. A personal impression, in: Diabetes 5 (1956) 67–68.
Jung, Georg Friedrich: Die Geschichte der Zuckerkrankheit. Nach Übersetzungen von Dr. Seidenberger, Frankfurt-Höchst, aus dem Buch von N. S. Papaspyros ‚The History of Diabetes mellitus', in: Der Diabetiker 17 (1967) 4–10, 83–88.
Kaiser, Wolfram, u. Arina Völker: Oskar Minkowski (1858–1931), in: Zeitschrift für die Gesamte Innere Medizin 36 (1981) 973–979.
Kalbfleisch, Karl: Diabetes, in: Sudhoffs Archiv 42 (1958) 142–144.
Kenéz, Janos: Zur Frühgeschichte der Insulin-Forschung, in: Münchener Medizinische Wochenschrift 114 (1972) 2003–2006.
Kho Peng Kiat: Historical aspects of diabetes mellitus, in: Berita Jururawat 13 (1973) 42–44.
King, Lester S.: Empiricism, rationalism, and diabetes, in: Journal of the American Association 187 (1964) 521–526.
Kleinsorge, Hellmut: Die Entdeckung der oralen Antidiabetika, in: Deutsche Medizinische Wochenschrift 101 (1976) 467–468.
Kloppe, Wolfgang: Paul Langerhans (1847-1888) und seine Berliner Dissertation (1869), in: Deutsches Medizinisches Journal 20 (1969) 581–583.
Kloppe, Wolfgang: Die Zuckerkrankheit – historisch betrachtet, in: Diabetiker 20 (1970) 252–254.
Knick, Bernhard: Zur Geschichte der diätetischen Behandlung der Zuckerkrankheit, in: Therapiewoche 23 (1973) 905–911.
Knoche, Bernhard: Die Geschichte der Zuckerkrankheit, in: Der Diabetiker 17 (1967) 434–435, 480–481, 18 (1968) 23–24, 61–63, 101–103, 146–149.
Knowles, Harvey C.: Max Rubner 1854-1932, in: Diabetes 6 (1957) 369–371.
Kolditz, W.: Historische Betrachtungen zum Diabetes mellitus – 50 Jahre nach der Entdeckung des Insulins, in: Literatur-Eildienst Roche 39 (1971) (8) 49–53.

Koopman, J.: (Of what disease died King Herodes the Great?, dutch), in: Bijdragen tot de Geschiedenis der Geneeskunde (1930) 330–332, auch in: Nederlands Tijdschrift voor Geneeskunde 74 (1930) 5951–5953.

Koopman, J.: (From the history of diabetes, dutch), in: Bijdragen tot de Geschiedenis der Geneeskunde 14 (1934) 81–91, auch in: Nederlands Tijdschrift voor Geneeskunde 78 (1934) 1973–1983.

Korczowski, M. M.: Dietary control of diabetes: reality or myth?, in: Southern Medical Journal 78 (1985) 979–986.

Korec, Rudolf: (50th anniversary of discovery and isolation of insulin, Banting, Best and Collip 1922, czech.), in: Časopis Českého Lékárnic 110 (1971) 416–418.

Korec, Rudolf: More comments on „Who discovered insulin?“, in: News in Physiological Sciences 1 (1986) 211–212.

Korp, W., u. Ernst Zweymüller: 50 Jahre Insulinbehandlung an der Wiener Kinderklinik – das Schicksal zuckerkranker Kinder aus der ersten Insulinära, in: Wiener Klinische Wochenschrift 85 (1973) 385–390.

Korseck, Carl: Historica de diabete mellito, med. Diss., Berlin 1840.

Kraus, W.: Kurze Geschichte des Diabetes Mellitus, in: Krankenpflege Journal 24 (1986) (11) 7–8.

Kudva, B. T.: On diabetes mellitus, in: Journal of the Association of Physicians of India 32 (1984) 320 u. 375.

Kühne, Willie: Notiz zur Geschichte des künstlichen Diabetes, in: Archiv für Anatomie und Physiologie 27 (1860) 261–262.

Květenský, Josef: (Historical evolution of knowledge of diabetes mellitus before the discovery of insulin, pol.), in: Vnitrni Lékarstvi 18 (1972) 67–72.

Labhart, Alexis: Intuition, luck and misfortune in diabetes research, in: Diabetologia 14 (1978) 353–358.

Labhart, Alexis: Diskursives Denken und Intuition in der medizinischen Forschung, in: Helvetica Chirurgica Acta 47 (1981) 859–872.

Laguesse, Édouard: Endocrine Inselchen und Diabetes; einige Worte über den ersten Ursprung der Inseltheorie, in: Zentralblatt für Allgemeine Pathologie 15 (1904) 865–869.

Latham, John: Facts and opinions concerning Diabetes, London 1811.

Lausch, Erwin: Diabetes: Siege, Hoffnungen und immer neue Rätsel, Weinheim 1971.

Lawrence, Robert Daniel: The beginning of the Diabetic Association in England, in: Diabetes 1 (1952) 420–421.

Lazarow, Arnold: Robert Russell Bensley, 1867–1956, in: Diabetes 5 (1956) 492–495.

Lebensohn, James E.: The semicentenary of insulin, in: American Journal of Ophtalmology 72 (1971) 1155–1157.

Leibowitz, Joshua O.: Maimonides on the incidence of diabetes, in: Israel Journal Medical Sciences 2 (1966) 714.

Leibowitz, Joshua O.: The concept of diabetes in historical perspective, in: Israel Journal Medical Science 8 (1972) 469–475.

Leickert, Karl Heinz: Insulin-Vorläufer – ein historischer Abriss. Erste Diabetes-Behandlungs-Versuche mit Pankreasextrakten, in: Arzneimittel-Forschung 25 (1975) 439–442.

Lenné, Albert Antony August: Der Diabetes Mellitus im Rück- und kurzen Ausblick, in: Veröffentlichungen aus dem Gebiete der Medizinalverwaltung, Berlin 15 (1922) (3) 217–222.

Leopold, Eugene J.: Aretaeus the Cappadocian. His contribution to diabetes mellitus, in: Annals of Medical History, n. ser., 2 (1930) 424–435.

Lépine, Raphael: Du coma diabétique, in: Rapport Congrès Français de Médecine, Lyon 12 (1911) 1–11, auch in: Gazette des Hôpitaux Civils et Militairs 84 (1911) 1784–1788.

Lesky, Erna: Etappen in der Erforschung des Diabetes mellitus, in: Österreichische Ärztezeitung 24 (1969) 2373–2376.

Lestradet, Henri: A propos du cinquantenaire de la découverte de l'insuline, in: Bulletin d'Information de l'Aide aux Jeunes Diabétiques 16 (1971) (2).

Lévêque, Theodore F.: The endocrine hypothalamus: an historical review, in: Canadian Journal of Neurological Sciences 1 (1974) 24–28.

Levine, Rachmiel: History of etiology of diabetes mellitus, in: Archives of Pathology 78 (1964) 405–408.

Levine, Rachmiel: Insulin – The biography of a small protein, in: New England Journal of Medicine 277 (1967) 1059–1064.

Levine, Rachmiel: Editorial: the fascinations and frustrations of diabetes mellitus, in: Western Journal of Medicine 121 (1974) 426–427.

Levine, Rachmiel: Charles Herbert Best (1899–1978), in: Physiologist 21 (1978) 43–44.

Levine, Rachmiel: Diabetes, the pancreas and insulin, a retrospective view, in: Canadian Journal of Biochemistry 57 (1979) 447–454.

Levine, Rachmiel: The endocrine pancreas, past and present, in: Advances in Experimental Medicine and Biology 124 (1979) 1–13.

Levine, Rachmiel: Historical view of the classifications of diabetes, in: Clinical Chemistry 32 (1986) 84–86.

Lietzmann, Alfred: Zur Geschichte des Diabetes mellitus, nebst Obductionsberichten des Berliner Pathologischen Institutes, med. Diss., Berlin 1877.

Liljestrand, Göran: Paul Sjöquist and the discovery of insulin, in: Svenska Läkaresällskapets Handlingar 69 (1947) 5–11.

Lippmann, Edmund O. v.: Geschichte des Zuckers, Leipzig 1890, vgl. a. ders.: Abhandlungen und Vorträge, Leipzig 1906, S. 261–274, 326–334.

Lippmann, Edmund O. v.: Zur Geschichte des diabetischen Zuckers, in: Chemiker Zeitung 29 (1905) 1197–1198; 30 (1906) 55; auch in: v. Lippmann: Beiträge zur Geschichte der Naturwissenschaften und der Technik, Berlin 1923, S. 211–213.

Lockwood, B. C.: Milestones in our knowledge of diabetes mellitus, in: Journal of the Michigan State Medical Society 51 (1952) 1295–1297.

Loubatières, August-Louis: Zur Geschichte der Entdeckung der oralen Antidiabetica, in: Ernst Friedrich Pfeiffer, Hg.: Handbuch des Diabetes mellitus, Bd. 2, München 1969, S. 1179–1197.

Loubatières, August-Louis: Evolution de la pathogénie et du traitement du diabète sucré, in: Bulletin de l'Académie Nationale de Médecine 135 (1971) 302–305.

Lowenstein, Bertrand E.: u. Paul D. Preger: Diabetes: new look at an old problem, New York 1976.

Lozoya, Mariana: (Historical antecedents of diabetes mellitus, span.), in: Medicina Tradicionale 3 (1980) (10) 5–9.

Lukens, Francis D. W.: William C. Stadie 1886–1959, in: Diabetes 8 (1959) 476–478.

Lund, Fred Bates: Galen on malingering, centaurs, diabetes and other subjects more or less related, in: Proceedings of the Charaka Club 10 (1941) 52–70.

Lundboek, Knud: Current trends in diabetes mellitus. Introduction, in: Acta Medica Scandivica 476 (1967) (suppl.) 15–16.

Macdonald, Eleanor (?) J.: The historical trend of diabetes, in: Common-health, Boston 21 (1934) 57, 24 (1937) 87.
McCradie, Andrew R.: The discoveries in the field of diabetes mellitus and their investigators, in: Medical Life 31 (1924) 215–250.
McGee, Lemuel Clide, u. J. E. Martin: Hagedorn era in diabetes mellitus, in: West Virginia Medical Journal 35 (1939) 361–368.
MacLaren, Noel Keith, u. Marvin Cornblath: Insulin, in: American Journal of Diseases of Children 128 (1974) 610–612.
MacNalty, Arthur Salusbury: Distinguished diabetics, in: Nursing Mirror and Midwives Journal 121 (1965).
Magnus-Levy, Adolf: Diabetikerdiäten der Vorinsulinära, in: Bulletin of the History of Medicine 3 (1944) (suppl.) 161–169.
Maiello, M., Ennio Guarnieri u. Maria Assunta Mannelli: Evoluzione storica delle conoscenze sulla sindrome poliuro-polidipsica insipida (Dall'antica civiltá egiziana al secolo XVIII. Da C. Bernard alle conoscenze della prima metà del secolo XX. La neurosecrezione), in: Rassegna di Neurologia Vegetatica 21 (1967) 311–326.
Maiwald, Karl-Heinz: Johann Peter Frank 1745–1821. Sein Beitrag zur Kenntnis des Diabetes mellitus, in: Therapie des Monats (Boehringer Mannheim) 10 (1960) 14–20.
Maiwald, Karl-Heinz: (Johann Peter Frank 1745–1821 and diabetes mellitus, hung.), in: Orvosi Hetilap 102 (1961) 1812–1814.
Major, Ralph Hermon: Johann Conrad Brunner and his experiments on the pancreas, in: Annals of Medical History, 3. s., 3 (1941) 91–100.
Major, Ralph Hermon: Classic descriptions of disease, Springfield 1932, ²1939, ³1945, ⁴1959.
Mani, Nikolaus: Die Entdeckung des Glykogens durch Claude Bernard, in: Zeitschrift für Klinische Chemie 2 (1964) 97–104.
Mann, Ruth J.: Historical vignette. ‚Honey urine' to pancreatic diabetes – 600 B. C. – 1922, in: Mayo Clinic Proceedings 46 (1971) 56–58.
Maragliano, Edoardo: Arnaldo Cantani, in: Le Scuole Italiane di Clinica Medica 1 (1894) 3–29.
Marble, Alexander: Otto Folin. Benefactor of diabetics through biochemistry, in: Diabetes 2 (1953) 503–505.
Marble, Alexander: John Rollo, in: Diabetes 5 (1956) 325–327.
Marble, Alexander: Late complications of diabetes. A continuing challenge. The Elliot P. Joslin Memorial Lecture of the German Diabetes Federation, in: Diabetologia 12 (1976) 193–199.
Marchal de Calvi, Charles-Jacob: Remarques historiques sur la gangrène diabétique, in: Union Médicale 2. sér., 11 (1861) 164, 193, 226, 258, 294.
Marinelli, Luigi: Vecchio e nuovo in tema di diabetologia, in: Riforma Medica 60 (1946) 545–547.
Martin, Eric: Problèmes de priorité dans la découverte de l'insuline, in: Schweizerische Medizinische Wochenschrift 101 (1971) 164–167.
Marwood, S. Francis: Notes on the history of diabetes mellitus, in: History of Medicine 6 (1975) 18–24.
Marwood, S. Francis: Personalities and progress in the story of diabetes mellitus, in: St. Bart's Hospital Journal 54 (1950) 108–111, 128–131, 158–163.
Marwood, S. Francis: Diabetes mellitus – some reflections, in: Journal of the Royal College of General Practitioners 23 (1973) 38–45.
Mastbaum, L.: Diabetes mellitus. Past, present and future, in: Minnesota Medicine 62 (1979) 9–11.

McQuillan, John, u. Marcia S. McQuillan: The discovery of insulin and control of Diabetes mellitus, in: Janus 69 (1982) 97–118.

Meindl, Rudolf: Zur Geschichte der Zuckerharnruhr, (Quellensammlung und textkritische Betrachtungen zur gesamten Geschichte der Zuckerharnruhr unter besonderer Berücksichtigung der frühen und mittleren Geschichte der Diabeteskenntnisse), med. Diss., Göttingen 1948; auch Berlin 1950.

Mellinghoff, Klaus Helmut: Georg Ludwig Zuelzers Beitrag zur Insulinforschung, med. Diss., Düsseldorf 1971 (= Düsseldorfer Beiträge zur Geschichte der Medizin, H. 36).

Mellinghoff, Klaus Helmut: Georg Ludwig Zuelzers Beitrag zur Pankreasextraktforschung, in: Medizinische Welt 23 (1972) 622–626.

Merchant, C. C.: Short historical review of the development of present knowledge of diabetes mellitus, in: Antiseptic 37 (1940) 441–454.

Mering, Joseph von, u. Oscar Minkowski: Diabetes mellitus nach Pankreasexstirpation, in: Archiv für experimentelle Pathologie und Pharmakologie 26 (1890) 371–387.

Messini, Mariano: Fegato e diabete. Il centennario della morte di Claude Bernard, in: Clinica Terapeutica 85 (1978) 335–360.

Meyshan, Yosef: (The disease of Herod the Great, King of Judea, hebrew., engl. and french summ.), in: Harefuah 53 (1957) 155.

Minkowski, Oscar: Die Lehre vom Pankreas-Diabetes in ihrer geschichtlichen Entwicklung, in: Arbeiten zur Kenntnis der Geschichte der Medizin im Rheinland und in Westfalen 1 (1929) ?; auch in: Münchener Medizinische Wochenschrift 76 (1929) 311–315.

Mirouze, Jacques: Histoire du coma diabétique et des son traitement, in: La Vie Médicale (1971) (nr. spéc. 52) 25–35.

Mirus, G.: Diabetes ‚einst und jetzt‘, in: Diabetiker 4 (1954) 8–9.

Miyasita, Saburo: An historical analysis of Chinese drugs in the treatment of hormonal diseases, goitre and diabetes mellitus, in: American Journal of Chinese Medicine 8 (1980) 17–25.

Molnár, Gábor: Historischer Überblick: Erste Versuche zur kontinuierlichen Blutzuckermessung, in: Verhandlungen der Deutschen Gesellschaft für Innere Medizin 93 (1987) 299–308.

Morgenstern, Leon: The „secret“ of the islets: a footnote to history, in: Mount Sinai Journal of Medicine 54 (1987) 197.

Mosenthal, Hermann O.: Charles F. Bolduan: His role in the attack on diabetes as a public health problem, in: Diabetes 3 (1954) 495–497.

Müller, Reinhold F. G.: Die Harnruhr der Alt-Inder, Prameha (unter besonderer Berücksichtigung der Carakasamhitá), in: Sudhoffs Archiv 25 (1932) 1–42.

Müller, Reinhold F. G.: Grundlagen altindischer Medizin, Halle 1942. (Nova Acta Leopoldina, N. F., Nr. 74).

Muir-Smith, L.: The advent of insulin (The experience of a diabetic before and after insulin), in: Guy's Hospital Gazette 76 (1962) 620–622.

Muntner, Süssmann: (Herod's disease, hebrew), in: Koroth 1 (1953) (3–4) 134–136.

Murlin, John R., u. Benjamin Kramer: A quest for the anti-diabetic hormone, 1913–1916, in: Journal of the History of Medicine 11 (1956) 288–298.

Murlin, Winifred R.: History of insulin, in: Annals of Internal Medicine 76 (1972) 330.

Murphy, H. B.: Historic changes in the sex ratios for different disorders, in: Social Science and Medicine 12 (1978) 143–149.

Murray, Ian: The search for insulin, in: Scottish Medical Journal 14 (1969) 286–288.

Murray, Ian: Paulesco and the isolation of insulin, in: Journal of the History of Medicine 26 (1971) 150–157.
Nelken, Ludwig: Insulin in retrospect. Chairman's remarks, in: Israel Journal of Medical Sciences 8 (1972) 467–468.
Nelken, Ludwig: The history of research, treatment and organization of diabetes in Isreael, in: Koroth 7 (1977) 497-503; LXVI–LXXXIV.
Nelles, Hans: Die Geschichte der Behandlung des diabetischen Coma, Diss. med., München 1982.
Ney, Denise, u. Dorothy Reycroft Hollingsworth: Nutritional management of pregnancy complicated by diabetes: historical perspective, in: Diabetes Care 4 (1981) 647–655.
Noble, Robert Laing: Memories of James Bertram Collip, in: Canadian Medical Association Journal 93 (1965) 1356–1364.
Noorden, Carl von: Die Zuckerkrankheit und ihre Behandlung, Berlin 1895.
Noorden, Carl von: Altes und Neues über Kostformen bei Diabetes, in: Therapie der Gegenwart 70 (1929) 241–244.
Notelovitz, Morris: Milestones in the history of diabetes – a brief survey, in: South African Medical Journal 44 (1970) 1158–1161.
Nothman, Martin M.: The history of the discovery of pancreatic diabetes. (By Minkowski in 1889), in: Bulletin of the History of Medicine 28 (1954) 272–274.
Oakley, Wilfried G.: The evolution of the management of diabetic pregnancy, in: Postgraduate Medical Journal 45 (1969) 802–805.
Oakley, Wilfried G.: R. D. Lawrence, M. D., F. R. C. P., 1892–1968, in: Diabetes 18 (1969) 54–55.
Oefele, Felix von: Zwanzig Jahre Diabeteserfahrung, in: New Yorker Medizinische Monatsschrift 23 (1912/13) 335–34, 24 (1913/14) 19–25, 35–43; auch in: Monatsschrift für Kolonialpolitik 24 (1913) 335–345.
Office of Health Economics: The pattern of diabetes, London 1964.
Oliaro, Tomaso: Le diabete e la sua storia, in: Minerva Medica 57 (1962) (varia).
Olmsted, James Montrose Duncan: Claude Bernard, 1813–1878. A pioneer in the study of carbohydrate metabolism, in: Diabetes 2 (1953) 162–164.
Orth, Hermann: Die antiken Diabetes Synonyme und ihre Wortgeschichte, in: Janus 51 (1964) 193–201.
Otten, Johannes-Hermann: Die Geschichte der oralen Diabetestherapie, med. Diss., Freiburg i. Br. 1966.
Otten, Johannes-Hermann: Zur Geschichte der oralen Diabetestherapie, in: Medizinische Klinik 63 (1968) 22–25.
Oyen, Detlef, Ernst A. Chantelau u. Michael Berger: Zur Geschichte der Diabetesdiät, Berlin 1985.
Padfield, Christopher J.: A review of the history of the treatment of diabetes mellitus and the search for oral hypoglycaemic agents, in: Guy's Hospital Reports 113 (1964) 45–54.
Palmer, F. S.: A sketch of the history and pathogenesis of sugar excretion, in: Westminster Hospital Reports 12 (1901) 33–40.
Papaspyros, Nikos S.: The history of diabetes mellitus, London 1952, Suttgart ^{2}1964.
Paton, Alexander: The English diabetes (1674–1877), in: St. Thomas Hospital Gazette 52 (1954) 189–191.
Paton, Alexander: Notes for a history of diabetes mellitus, in: British Journal of Clinical Practice 15 (1961) 37–39.
Patrick, Adam: The symptomatology of diabetic coma: a retrospect, in: Scottish Medical Journal 7 (1962) 153–158.

Páv, Jaroslav: (History of a world-wide priority orginating in Prague, czech.), in: Časopis Lekaru Českych 125 (1986) 784–785.

Pavel, Ion: Insuline: Priorité de Paulesco, in: Médecine et Hygiène 966 (1971) 954.

Pavel, Ion: Zur Frühgeschichte der Insulin-Forschung, in: Münchener Medizinische Wochenschrift 115 (1973) 729–730.

Pavel, Ion, H. Bonaparte u. Dan Sdrobici: The role of Paulesco in the discovery of insulin, in: Israel Journal of Medical Sciences 8 (1972) 488–490.

Pavel, Ion, u. Dan Sdrobici: Le cinquantenaire de la découverte de l'insuline. N. Paulesco, L'étape sociale dans l'assistance du diabète, in: Journées Annuelles de Diabétologie de l'Hôtel Dieu Paris 6. - 8.5.1971, Paris 1971, S. 7–11.

Pavy, Frederick William: Researches on the nature and treatment of diabetes, London 1862, ^{2}1869.

Pazzini, Adalberto: (Historical evolution of diabetes, span.), in: Prensa Médica Mexicana 39 (1974) 481–486.

Pazzini, Adalberto, u. Aroldo Baffoni: Storia delle malattie, Roma 1950 (S. 317–338).

Pedfield, C. J. A.: Review of the history of the treatment of diabetes mellitus and the search for oral hypoglycaemic agents, in: Guy's Hospital Reports 113 (1964) 45–54.

Peel, John: A historical review of diabetes and pregnancy, in: Journal of Obstetrics and Gynaecology of the British Commonwealth 79 (1972) 385–395.

Penchev, Ivan G.: Zakharna bolest, Sofia ^{2}1966 (S. 13-22 = history).

Perret, Louis: (Extracts of the history of diabetic research, swed.), in: Helsingfors Läkartidning (1962) (5) 1–10; auch in: Nordisk Medicinhistorisk Årsbok (1963).

Pestel, Maurice: Le cinquantenaire de la découverte de l'insuline. E. Gley, précurseur de F. J. Banting et C. H. Best, in: La Nouvelle Presse Médicale 1 (1972) 1527–1528.

Peton, A.: Notes for a history of diabetes mellitus, in: British Journal of Clinical Practice 15 (1961) 37–39.

Pinner, Max, u. Benjamin F. Miller: When doctors are patients, New York 1952; dt.: Was Ärzte als Patienten erlebten, Stuttgart 1953.

Pollack, Herbert: Stanley Rossiter Benedict: Creator of laboratory test for glycosuria, in: Diabetes 2 (1953) 420–421.

Pollack, Herbert: Antoine Laurent Lavoisier, in: Diabetes 5 (1956) 250–251.

Ponte, Euro: Passato e futuro per il diabete, in: Il Lanternino 8 (1985) (2) 4–6.

Porep, Rüdiger: Der Prioritätenstreit um die Entdeckung des Glykogens zwischen Claude Bernard und Victor Hensen, in: Medizinische Monatsschrift 25 (1971) 314–321.

Porges, Otto: Carl H. von Noorden 1858-1944, in: Diabetes 7 (1958) 326–328.

Porkert, Manfred: Epistemological fashions in interpreting disease. The deleterious effects of western terminology on the application of the scientific tradition of Chinese medicine (illustrated by the case of diabetes mellitus vs. sitis diffundens (hsiao-k'o)), in: Nihon Ishigaku Zasshi 23 (1977) 1–18.

Poulet, Jacques: Le diabète avant la découverte de l'insuline, in: La Vie Médicale (1971) (nr. spéc. 52) 5–10.

Pratt, Joseph H.: Zur Geschichte der Entdeckung des Insulins, in: Sudhoffs Archiv 38 (1954) 48–57; engl.: A reappraisal of researches leading to the discovery of insulin, in: Journal of the History of Medicine 9 (1954) 281–289.

Proosdij, Cornelis van, u. Andreas Julius Augustus de Looff: (From lethal to bearable: 300 years of diabetes history, dutch), in: Nederlands Tijdschrift voor Geneeskunde 121 (1977) 1974–1978.

Puschmann, Theodor: Nachträge zu Alexander Trallianus: Fragmente aus Philamenos und Philagruis, nebst einer bisher noch ungedruckten Abhandlung über Augenkrankheiten, Berlin 1886.
Pyke, David Alan: Claude Bernard et l'étiologie du diabète, in: Journées Annuelles de Diabétologie de l'Hôtel-Dieu (1981) 153–161.
Raghunathan, Komanduri: History of diabetes from remote to recent times, in: Bulletin of the Indian Institute of the History of Medicine 6 (1975) 18–24.
Raghunathan, Komanduri, u. Priya Urat Sharma: Oral hypoglycaemic agents – a brief survey, in: Nagarjun 12 (1969) 27–37.
Rathery, Francis: La cure de Bouchardat et le traitement du diabète sucré, Paris 1920.
Reboux, C.: Diabète: 300 ans de progrès, in: Bibliographie Annuelle de Madagascar (1976) (350) 400–407.
Reckendorf, Helmut K.: Medizinische Konzeption und Therapie. Die Behandlung des Diabetes mellitus zu Beginn des 19. Jahrhunderts durch John Rollo, in: Therapie des Monats (Boehringer Mannheim) 11 (1961) 17–19.
Reed, John A.: Arataeus, the Cappadocian: History enlightens the present, in: Diabetes 3 (1954) 419–421.
Reinwein, Helmuth: Neuzeitliche Behandlung des Diabetes mellitus, Stuttgart 1946 (= Vorträge aus der praktischen Medizin, H. 19).
Rembert, George William Francis: Diabetes mellitus – old and new, in: New Orleans Medical Journal 85 (1932) 153.
Rentchnick, Pierre: Best, le méconnu, Paulesco, l'oublié, in: Médecine et Hygiène 29 (1971) 956.
Reshef, Abraham: (The history of diabetes, hebrew), in: Dapim Refuiim 16 (1959) 400–412, XVIII–XIX.
Richter, Paul: Ueber Paracelsus und die tatarischen Krankheiten. Ein Beitrag zur Geschichte der Stoffwechselkrankheiten, in: Medizinische Klinik 5 (1909) 1456–1458, 1495–1498.
Ricketts, Henry T.: Robert R. Bensley, in: Diabetes 4 (1955) 334–335.
Ríos, M. S.: Contributo spagnolo alle conoscenze sull'insulina, in: Minerva Medica 60 (1969) 4659–4666.
Risch, Friedrich: Heinrich von Stephan, 1831–1897, in: Männer der deutschen Verwaltung, Köln u. Berlin 1963, S. 151–165.
Robin, Albert: Diabète sucré et son traitement sans régime d'après les auteurs arabes anciens; à propos d'un travail de Dinguizli, in: Revue de Thérapeutique Médico-Chirurgicale 81 (1914) 79–84.
Rolls, Roger: Brewer's yeast and diabetes, in: British Medical Journal (1977) (1) 905.
Ropers, Bruno: Vergleichende Statistik über Todesfälle an Diabetes vor und nach Einführung der Insulintherapie, Diss. med., Hamburg 1933.
Rosemann, Rudolf: Zur Entdeckung des Glykogens vor 75 Jahren. Eine Berichtigung, in: Münchener Medizinische Wochenschrift 34 (1932) 1367–1368.
Rosenfeld, Georg: Wandlungen in der Behandlung des Diabetes, in: Archiv für Verdauungskrankheiten 22 (1915/16) 113–141.
Rosenfeld, L.: Henry Bence Jones (1813–1873): the best „chemical doctor" in London, in: Clinical Chemistry 33 (1987) 1687–1692.
Rosenthal, Helen: Diabetic cure in pictures, Philadelphia 1946, ^{2}1953, ^{3}1960.
Rubner, Max, u. Friedrich Müller: Einfluss der Kriegsverhältnisse auf den Gesundheitszustand im Deutschen Reich, in: Münchener Medizinische Wochenschrift 67 (1920) 229–248.

Sahli, Hermann: Prolegomena zur Einführung der Insulintherapie des Diabetes mellitus, in: Schweizerische Medizinische Wochenschrift 53 (1923) 813–819.

Salomon, Max: Geschichte der Glycosurie von Hippokrates bis zum Anfang des 19. Jahrhunderts, in: Deutsches Archiv für Klinische Medizin 8 (1871) 498–582, auch Leipzig 1871.

Sandison, A. T.: The last illness of Herod the Great, King of Judea, in: Medical History 11 (1967) 381–388.

Sardou, Victorien: Une biographie médicale, in: La Chronique Médicale 15 (1908) 727–730 (Cardano).

Sathe, Ramchandra Viswanath: Diabetes in India – retrospect and prospect, in: Journal of the Association of Physicians of India 17 (1969) 387–398.

Saundby, Robert: Kussmaul's Coma, in: Birmingham Medical Review 17 (1885), auch Birmingham 1885.

Saundby, Robert: Diabetes mellitus in Albutt and Rolleston's system of medicine, London 1908.

Sawyer, Warren A.: Frederick Banting's misinterpretation of the work of Ernest L. Scott as found in secondary sources, in: Perspectives in Biology and Medicine 29 (1986) 611–618.

Schadewaldt, Hans: Die Entdeckung der oralen Antidiabetika, in: Deutsche Medizinische Wochenschrift 101 (1976) 909.

Schadewaldt, Hans: Die Geschichte des Diabetes, in: Adolf Heymer u. Wilhelm Gronemeyer, Hg.: Allergie- und Immunitätsforschung, Verhandlungen der Deutschen Gesellschaft für Allergie- und Immunitätsforschung, Bd. 2, Stuttgart 1968, S. 9–22.

Schadewaldt, Hans: Die Geschichte des Diabetes, Frankfurt a. M. (Farbwerke Hoechst) o. J. (1971) (= Diabetes im Bild, H. 5).

Schadewaldt, Hans: Geschichte des Diabetes mellitus, in: Karl Oberdisse, Hg.: Handbuch der Inneren Medizin, Berlin ^{5}1975, S. 1–44; auch Berlin 1975.

Schadewaldt, Hans: Das Pankreas in der Geschichte der Medizin, in: Norbert Henning, Klaus Heinkel u. Harald Schön, Hg.: Pathogenese, Diagnostik, Klinik und Therapie der Erkrankungen des exokrinen Pankreas, Stuttgart 1964, S. 1–46.

Schadewaldt, Hans: Paracelsus und die Zuckerkrankheit, in: Medizinische Klinik 72 (1977) 875–878.

Schirmer, Alfred Max: Beitrag zur Geschichte und Anatomie des Pankreas, Diss. med., Basel 1893.

Schliack, Volker, Diabetes: Zur Geschichte und modernen Therapie, in: Urania 26 (1963) 407–410.

Schneider, T.: Diabetes through the ages: a salute to insuline, in: South African Medical Journal 46 (1972) 1394–1400.

Schütz, Augustin Jacob: Beyträge zur Geschichte der Heilungskraft des Kalkwassers gegen die Harnruhr, in: Journal der Practischen Arzneikunde und Wundarzneikunst 12 (1801) 129–145.

Schultheisz, Emil: (Trnka Vencel, hung.), in: Orvosi Hetilap 105 (1964) 2293–2294.

Schulz, Caecil: Beiträge zur Geschichte des Glycogen, med. Diss., Berlin 1877.

Schulz, F.: Zeittafel zur Geschichte des Diabetes mellitus, in: Hellmut Mehnert u. Karl Schöffling, Hg.: Diabetologie in Klinik und Praxis, Stuttgart 1974, S. 563–566.

Schumacher, Horst, u. Joseph Schumacher: Einst und jetzt: 100 Jahre Diabetes mellitus, in: Münchener Medizinische Wochenschrift 98 (1956) 517–521, 581–585, 601–604.

Schumacher, Joseph: Index zum Diabetes mellitus. Eine internationale Bibliographie, München 1961 (hist. Einführung S. 1–34).
Schumacher, Joseph: Geschichte des Diabetes mellitus bis zur Insulin-Ära. Daten – Theorien – Forschungen – Fortschritte, in: Deutsches Medizinisches Journal 14 (1963) 707–715.
Schumacher, Rudolf: Die Carl v. Noorden'sche Haferkur. Ihre Weiterentwicklung und ihr Einfluß auf die Diättherapie des Diabetes mellitus. Unter Berücksichtigung ihrer heutigen Bedeutung, med. Diss., Freiburg i. Br. 1966.
Seckendorf, Ernst: Kurze Geschichte des Diabetes mellitus, in: Die Medizinische Welt 40 (1931) 1443–1445.
Seide, Jacob: The early history of diabetes mellitus, in: Acta Medica Orientalia 4 (1945) (4) 126–129.
Seide, Jacob: The first discovery of glycosuria in diabetes, in: Indian Medical Journal 43 (1949) 331 ff.
Seide, Jacob: Diabetes mellitus in the 19. century, in: Hebrew Medical Journal 30 (1957) 93–97, 182–188.
Seide, Jacob: The two diabetics of Amatus Lusitanus, in: Imprensa Médica 19 (1955) 670–674.
Selmi, Giacomo: Gli studi di Claude Bernard sul pancreas, in: Medicina nei Secoli 3 (1966) (3) 29–34.
Sforza, A., R. Lolli, A. Mohamed Hassan, S. E. Gogliandro, u. Attilio Lodi: Il diabete nei tropici. Note tra storia della medicina e attualità anatomocliniche, in: Minerva Endocrinologica 10 (1985) 249–251.
Shaw, Margaret Mason: He conquered death. The story of Frederick Grant Banting, Toronto 1946.
Silva Araújo, Carlos da: L'empereur du Brésil Dom Pedro II à Aix-les-Bains, en 1888, Aix-les-Bains 1953.
Silva Araújo, Carlos da: (Severe disease of the Brazilian Emperor in Milan, in 1888. Italian physicians who assisted him, port.), in: Revista da Associacao Medica Brasileira 14 (1968) 279–284; auch in: 21st International Congress of the History of Medicine, Siena 1968, Atti, Bd. 1, Roma 1970, S. 302–312; auch Rio de Janeiro 1968.
Simowitz, Fredric M.: A short history of diabetes mellitus, in: Journal of the Medical Association of Georgia 51 (1962) 478–481.
Singer, Peter, u. Volker Schliack: Zur Geschichte des Insulins, in: Wissenschaft und Fortschritt 22 (1972) 467–471.
Smyth, J. A.: Diabetes: past, present and future, in: The Ulster Medical Journal 23 (1954) 73–88.
Sönksen, P.H.: The evolution of insulin treatment, in: Clinical Endocrinology and Metabolism 6 (1977) 481–497.
Sós, József: Claude Bernard, Macleod, Banting und Best: Ihr Beitrag zur Diabetesforschung, in: Orvosi Lapja 3 (1947) 1853–1854.
Spiegelhoff, Werner: Die Geschichte der Pankreaserkrankungen, med. Diss., Düsseldorf 1937.
Sprague, Randal George: Diabetes – past, present and future, in: Balance. British Diabetic Association 11 (1965) 124 ff.
Stadie, William C.: Henry Rawle Geyelin 1883–1942, in: Diabetes 6 (1957) 291–293.
Stahl, Jules: La découverte de l'insuline, in: Strasbourg Médical 12 (1961) 871–879.
Stein, Peter: A propos de la découverte de l'insuline. Les travaux de Zuelzer, in: Médecine et Hygiène 29 (1971) 1102.

Stein, Peter: Prioritäten und Prioritätsansprüche ums Insulin, in: Gesnerus 31 (1974) 107–112.

Stepp, Wilhelm: Altes und Neues in der Therapie des Diabetes mellitus, in: Münchener Medizinische Wochenschrift 82 (1935) 1307–1312.

Sternberg, Wilhelm: Die Krankheit der Juden. Die Zuckerkrankheit, eine Folge der rituellen Küche und der orthodoxen Lebensweise der Juden, Mainz 1903.

Stevenson, Lloyd G.: Sir Frederick Banting, London und Toronto 1946, [2]1947.

Steudel, Johannes: John J. R. Mcleod, ein Wegbereiter der Diabetes Forschung, in: Der Diabetiker 1 (1951) 49–51.

Steudel, Johannes: Elliott P. Joslin, der Nestor der Diabetes Forschung, in: Der Diabetiker 1 (1951) 62–64.

Steudel, Johannes: Die Geschichte des Diabetes, in: Diabetiker 3 (1953) 45–46, 61–62, 77–78.

Stockmans, François: Meyer (Jean-Egide-Camille-Philippe-Hubert De), in: Biographie Nationale Belge, Bd. 41, Bruxelles 1979/80, Sp. 523–533.

Stöcker, Wolfgang: Zur Geschichte des Diabetes mellitus, in: Therapiewoche 16 (1966) 1077–1082.

Stöcker, Wolfgang: Der Prioritätsstreit um das Insulin, in: Therapiewoche 21 (1971) 3464–3467; auch in : Pharmazeutische Zeitung 116 (1971) 1764–1765.

Straight, William M.: Notes on the history of diabetes mellitus, in: Jackson Memorial Hospital Bulletin 7 (1953) 5–11.

Strauch, Manfred, u. Norbert Grez: Animal models to induce renal failure: a historical survey, in: Contributions to Nephrology 60 (1988) 1–8.

Striker, Cecil: The song of diabetes, in: Diabetes 1 (1952) 492–493.

Striker, Cecil: Graham Lusk. On his contributions to the science of nutrition, in: Diabetes 2 (1953) 242–243.

Striker, Cecil: Joseph H. Barach, in: Diabetes 3 (1954) 254–255.

Striker, Cecil: The early history of the American Diabetes Association, in: Diabetes 5 (1956) 317–320.

Striker, Cecil: Famous faces in diabetes, Boston 1961.

Striker, Cecil: History of insulin, in: Annals of Internal Medicine 76 (1972) 329–330.

Suzuki, Yoshitami: (Historical survey of visual disturbance due to diabetes mellitus, especially the effect of Li Tong-yuan's prescriptions for diabetic retinopathy, jap.), in: Nihon Ishigaku Zasshi 16 (1970) 49–50.

Suzuki, Yoshitami: (Effects of drugs on diabetic retinopathies and a supplement to the history of the visual disturbance caused by diabetes mellitus, jap.), in: Nippon Ganka Gakkai Zasshi 75 (1971) 1047–1051.

Syllaba, Jiři: (Historical development of czecholovak balneotherapy of diabetes, czech.), in: Fysiatricky a Reumatologicky Vestnik 57 (1979) 65–69.

Tallot, Lutz: Seit wann kennt man Diabetes?, in: Ciba-Zeitschrift 1 (1933/34) 65.

Tee, Garry J.: On Sami Hamarneh's review of „Der Diabetestraktat" ᶜAbd al-Laṭīf al-Baġdādī's, in: Isis 64 (1973) 232.

Teichmann, S. L., u. P. A. Aldea: The other side of the insulin story: Paulescu's contribution, in: New York State Journal of Medicine 84 (1984) 312–316.

Thies, Hans-Jürgen: Der Diabetestraktat, ᶜAbd al-Latif al-Baġdādī's' Untersuchungen zur Geschichte des Krankheitsbildes in der arabischen Medizin, Bonn 1971.

Thompson, Reginald Campbell: Assyrian prescriptions for diseases of the urine (Transliterations and translations of cunei form tablets), Paris 1934 (= Babyloniaca, vol. 14).

Thomsen, Viggo: The history of traumatic diabetes, in: Viggo Thomsen, Ed.: Studies of trauma and carbohydrate metabolism with special reference to the existence of traumatic diabetes, Kopenhagen 1938, p. 9–36.
Todhunter, E. Neigo: Biographical notes from the history of nutrition: Elliott Proctor Joslin – June 6, 1869 – January 28, 1962, in: Journal of the American Dietetic Association 46 (1965) 150.
Torzecka, Wiesawa, u. Ryszard Rogoziński: (Participation of the pancreatic islet system in etiopathogenesis diabetes (an historical survey and present-day views), pol.) in: Wiadomości Lekarskie 29 (1976) 897–901.
Tratner, Eli: A new Talmudic source on the history of Diabetes (late onset), in: Koroth 8 (1982) 197–202, 205–212.
Trowell, Hugh C.: Diabetes mellitus death-rates in England and Wales 1920–70 and food suplies, in: Lancet (1974) (2) 908–1002.
Trowell, Hugh C.: Ants distinguish diabetes mellitus from diabetes insipidus, in: British Medical Journal 285 (1982) 217.
Tuttle, George H.: The changing conception of diabetes as a disease, in: Boston Medical and Surgical Journal 194 (1926) 931–932.
Ullmann, Hans: Die Zunahme der Zuckerkrankheit – eine Ernährungsfrage?, in: Die Medizinische Welt (1928) (3) 87–92.
Umber, Friedrich: Rückblicke und Ausblicke in der Klinik des Diabetes, in: Deutsche Medizinische Wochenschrift 60 (1934) 11–14.
United States National Health Survey, Hg.: Diabetes reported in interviews, Washington 1960.
Vargas, Fernández Luis: (The discovery of insulin and its antagonists and the consequence for the knowledge of diabetes, span.), in: Revista Medica de Chile 92 (1964) 789–794.
Vargas, Fernández Luis: (Historical revision of the contribution of Houssay and collaborators to the role of the anterior hypothesis in diabetes mellitus, span.), in: Revista Medica de Chile 100 (1972) 728–732.
Vasiûkova, E. A., M. G. Margolis u. V. K. Malkovich: (Achievements of Soviet diabetology, russ.), in: Kliničeskaja Medicina 55 (1977) (12) 18–25.
Veith, Ilza: Four thousand years of diabetes, in: Modern Medicine 39 (1971) 118–125.
Vértes, László: (Elliot Proctor Joslin (1869, junius 6. – 1962, januar 28.), hung.), in: Orvosi Hetilap 111 (1979) 750.
Vierordt, Hermann: Todesursachen im ärztlichen Stande. Ein Beitrag zur Ärzte-Biographie, Stuttgart 1926.
Volk, Bruno W., u. Edward R. Arquilla: Historical review, in: Volk u. Wellmann: The diabetic pancreas, New York 1977, ^{2}1985, S. 1–16.
Voss, Franz: Ältere Geschichte des Diabetes, München 1936.
Voss, Hermann: 100 Jahre Langerhanssche Inseln, in: Anatomischer Anzeiger 125 (1969) 333–335.
Wang, Zhipu: (Brief history of consumption-thirst syndrome (diabetes mellitus), chin.), in: Chinese Journal of Medical History 10 (1980) 79–82.
Warburg, Erik: Some cases of diabetic coma complicated with uraemia, with some remarks on the previous history of diabetic coma, in: Hospitalstidende 67 (1924) 809, 825, 856; auch in: Acta Medica Scandinavia 61 (1924/25) 301–334.
Warren, Shields: The pathology of diabetes mellitus. Historical considerations, Philadelphia 1930, ^{4}1966, S. 9–18.
Wendriner, Berthold: Der Diabetes mellitus. Zuckerharnruhr im Lichte der modernen Forschung. Eine Skizze über die Entwicklung der Diabetes-Behandlung bis in

die neueste Zeit. Mit chemischen Beiträgen und Diätvorschriften von Friedrich Kaeppel, Bonn 1905.

West, Kelly M.: Diabetes in American Indians, in: Advances in Metabolic Disorders 9 (1978) 29–48.

Whitehouse, Fred W.: Classification and pathogenesis of the diabetes syndrom: a historical perspective, in: Journal of the American Dietetic Association 81 (1982) 243–246.

Wilder, Russell M.: Introduction to motion picture „The Story of Diabetes" by K. A. Smith, in: Proceedings Staff Meetings of the Mayo Clinic 14 (1939) 15–16.

Wilder, Russell M.: Twenty-five years of insulin era, in: Proceedings American Diabetes Association 6 (1947) 107–116.

Wilder, Russell M.: Karl Petrén. A leader in pre-insulin dietary therapy of diabetes, in: Diabetes 4 (1955) 159–160.

Willms, Jost: Berühmte Diabetiker: König Herodes der Grosse (73–4 v. Chr.). Läusesucht oder Zuckerkrankheit?, in: Diabetiker 16 (1965) 288–289.

Willms, Jost: Berühmte Diabetiker: Jean Paul Marat (1744–1793), Arzt und Revolutionär, in: Diabetiker 16 (1966) 49.

Willms, Jost: Berühmte Diabetiker: Paul Cézanne (1839–1906), der Ahnherr der modernen Malerei, in: Diabetiker 16 (1966) 49.

Willms, Jost: Berühmte Diabetiker: Heinrich von Stephan (1831–1897), vom Postschreiber zum Weltpostmeister, in: Diabetiker 16 (1966) 206.

Willms, Jost: Berühmte Diabetiker, Alexander Girardi (1850–1918), Volksschauspieler, der in Wien den Girardikult entfesselte, in: Diabetiker 16 (1966) 402.

Willms, Jost: Berühmte Diabetiker: Heinrich Zille (1858–1929), Zeichner des Berliner „Milljöh", in: Diabetiker 17 (1967) 176.

Winternitz, Hugo: Über den Anteil J. von Merings an der Entdeckung des Pankreasdiabetes, in: Medizinische Klinik 27 (1931) 1507–1508.

Winternitz, Hugo: Noch einmal der Anteil J. von Merings an der Entdeckung des Pankreasdiabetes (Stellungnahme zu dem Aufsatz von E. Frank, Nr. 44 dieser Wschr.), in: Medizinische Klinik 28 (1932) 138–139.

Wolff, Günther: Kleiner Abriß der Geschichte der Zuckerkrankheit, in: Ärztliche Praxis 6 (1954) 18.

Wolff, Günther: Abriss der Geschichte der Zuckerkrankheit. Zugleich ein Beitrag zur Medizin- und Kulturgeschichte des Zuckers, in: Medizinische Monatsschrift 7 (1953) 253–254, 527–529, 9 (1955) 37–41.

Wolff, Günther: Zucker, Zuckerkrankheit und Insulin. Eine medizin- und kulturhistorische Studie, Remscheid – Lennep 1955.

Wolff, Günther: Die Entdeckung des Insulins vor 35 Jahren durch Banting und Best, in: Medizinische Monatsschrift 10 (1956) 468–475.

Wolff, Günther: Zur Geschichte der Harnzuckeruntersuchung, in: Therapie des Monats, Boehringer (1957) 321–323, 838–846.

Wolff, Günther: Der Zuckerstoffwechsel – eine biographische Studie, in: Medizinische Monatsschrift 12 (1958) 766–774.

Wolff, Günther: Beiträge berühmter Studenten zur Erforschung des Zuckerstoffwechsels, in: Münchener Medizinische Wochenschrift 102 (1960) 1203–1208.

Wolff, Günther: A propos de la découverte de l'insuline, in: Médecine et Hygiène 29 (1971) 1102.

Wolff, Günther: Paul Langerhans – Inseln waren sein Schicksal, in: Der Kassenarzt 18 (1978) (27).

Wolff, Günther: Abriß der Geschichte der Zuckerkrankheit, in: Ernährungs-Umschau 35 (1988) (Sonderheft) 497–501.

Wolff, Günther, u. Hans Schadewaldt: Biographische Adnota zu Paul Langerhans. – Inseln waren sein Schicksal – Teil 1–2, in: Medizinische Welt 28 (1977) 1–7, 91–96.
Woodyatt, Rollin T.: Bernhard Naunyn, in: Diabetes 1 (1952) 240–241.
Wrenshall, Gerald Alfred, Géza Hetényi u. William Richard Feasby: The story of insulin, London 1962, dt. Insulin: Die Geschichte eines Sieges, Oldenburg–Hamburg 1962.
Wybieralski, Andrzej: (Fuller life for diabetics, pol.), in: Polski Tygodnik Lekarskie 26 (1971) 1868–1869.
Young, Blanche (?) A.: The history of the British Diabetic Association, in: Postgraduate Medical Journal 45 (1969) (suppl.) 789–795.
Young, Frank G.: Claude Bernard and the discovery of glycogen, in: British Medical Journal (1957) (1) 1431–1437.
Zander, Karl: Zur Begriffsgeschichte des Diabetes mellitus, med. Diss., Freiburg i. Br. 1973.
Zimmermann, Ole Christian: Die erste Beschreibung von Symptomen des experimentellen Pankreas-Diabetes durch den Schweizer Johann Conrad Brunner (1653-1727), med. Diss., Basel 1944; auch in: Gesnerus 2 (1945) 109–130.
Zimmermann, Ole Christian: Johann Conrad Brunner 1653–1727, in: Diabetes 6 (1957) 537.

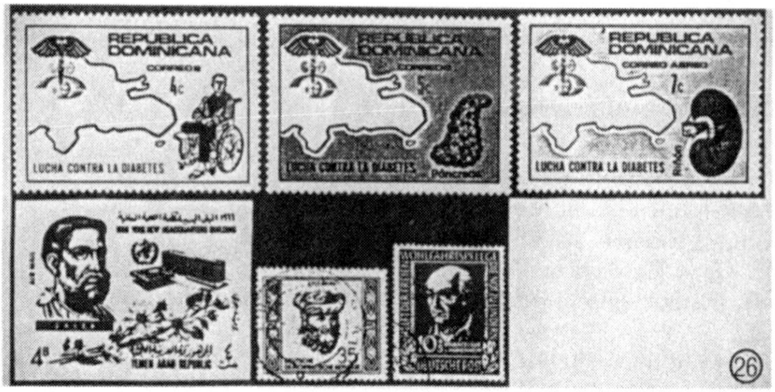

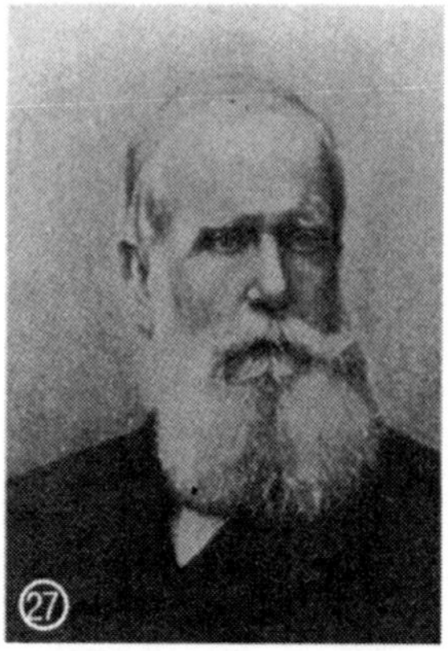

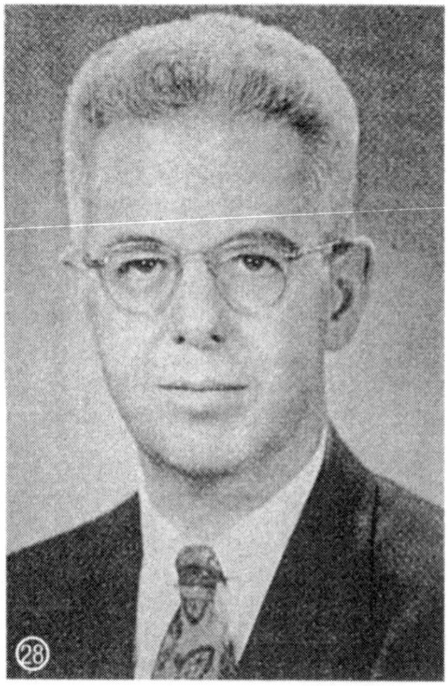

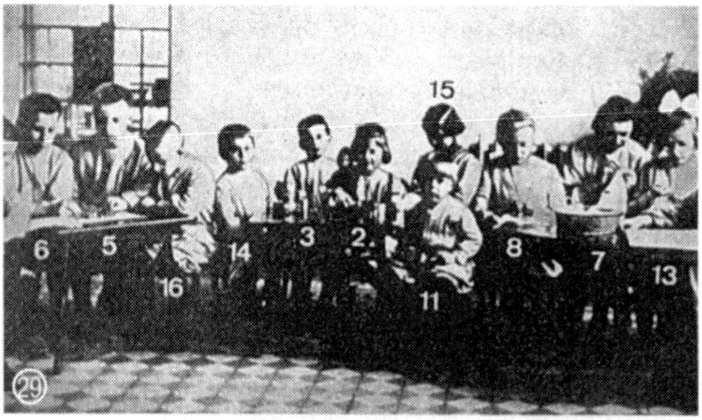

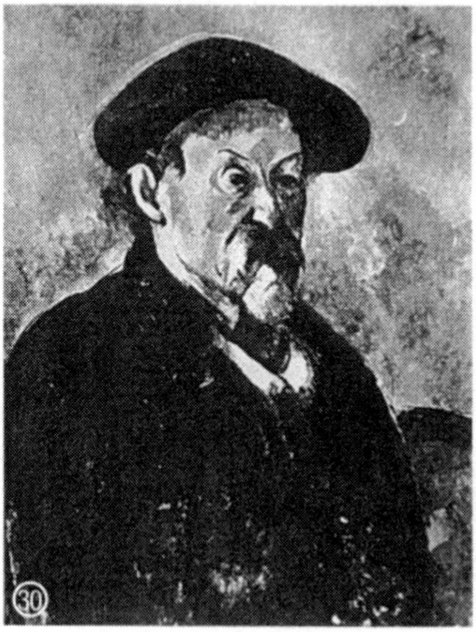

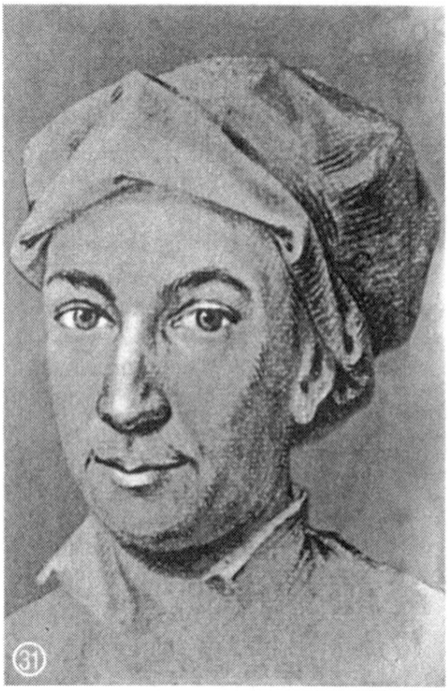

(26) Stamp designs on diabetes and insulin
(27) Pedro II of Brasil (1855–1891), Photograph, 19th century
(28) Randall G. Sprague (born 1906), Photograph
(29) Diabetic children, Vienna University Hospital, 1925. Case 1: the first child treated with insulin
(30) Paul Cézanne (1893–1906), Oil, self-portrait, about 1900
(31) Johann Georg Hamann (1730–1788), Drawing, 18th century

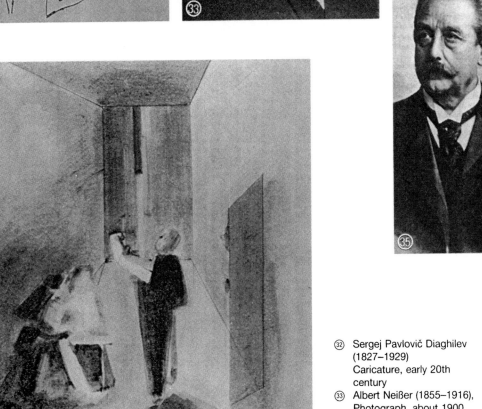

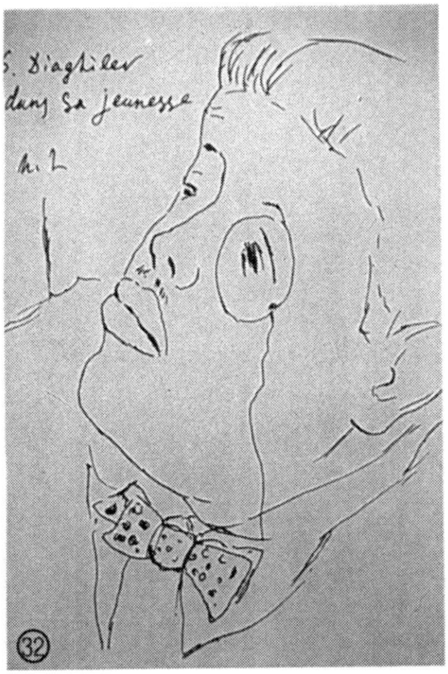

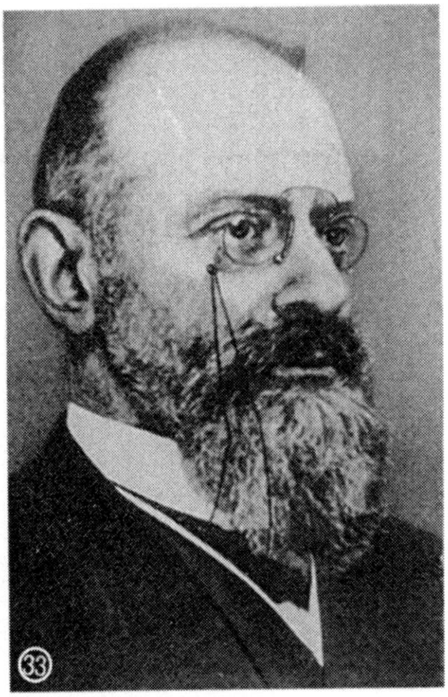

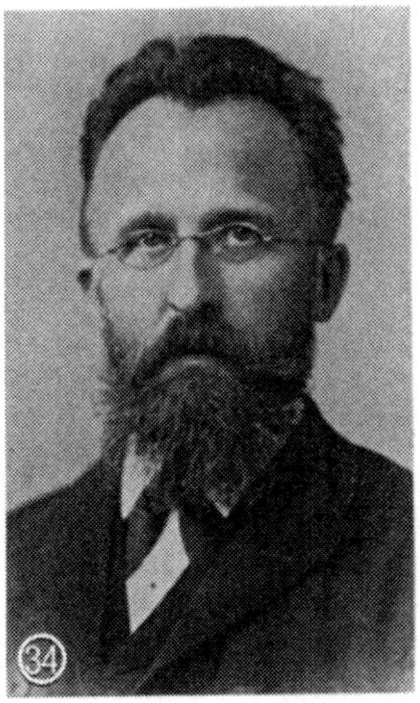

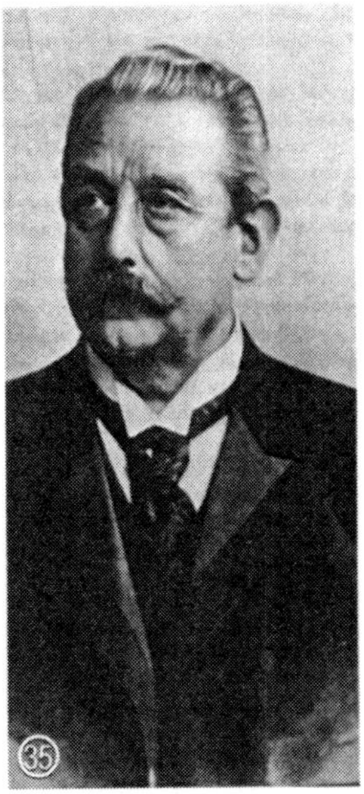

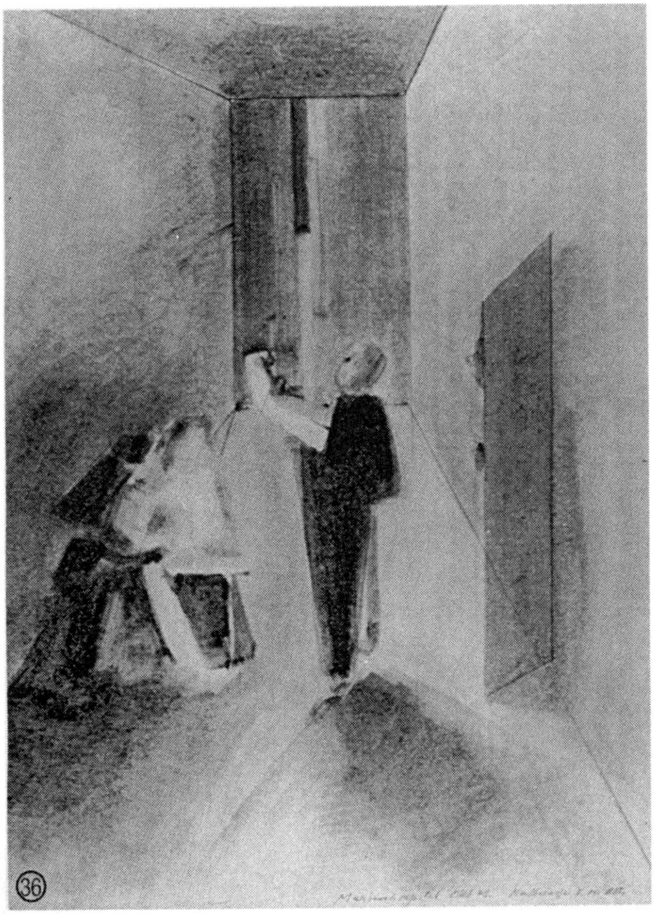

32. Sergej Pavlovič Diaghilev (1827–1929) Caricature, early 20th century
33. Albert Neißer (1855–1916), Photograph, about 1900
34. Max Fürbringer (1846–1920), Photograph
35. Julius von Michel (1843–1911), Photograph, after 1900
36. Oskar Schlemmer (1888–1943), Night-duty and the old man, 1942

Lightning Source UK Ltd.
Milton Keynes UK
UKOW02f0606200913

217523UK00002B/23/P

9 783642 483660